PREFACE

Professional workers with children are becoming more interested in the subject of growth and development because they recognize increasingly the close and important tie between health and development.

It is obvious to all familiar with children that the diseases and other manifestations of ill health from which they most commonly suffer change characteristically with age and, also, that the risks these entail and the problems arising from them change with advancing age. Health obviously is related in various ways to the maturity and growth status of the children concerned. Students from the health disciplines are interested in this subject, not merely to learn how children grow and what developmental events take place, but also to understand what constitutes "healthy development" and how it may best be protected or promoted. The emphasis here is on what is sometimes referred to as "positive health"; not merely the absence of disease or of developmental defects or retardations, but evidences of a full measure of physical fitness, emotional well-being, and developmental progress for age.

This book presents in broad terms a picture of the child and his expected progress at all ages from conception to maturity. It is concerned with him as an individual who is changing or developing according to natural laws and inborn potentialities. It deals with the major aspects of his physical development and the nature of the basic needs which support and promote satisfactory progress. It deals also with psycho-social development and the factors favoring mental health. It attempts to increase the reader's understanding of those features of progress which are characteristics of health or "normality." After an introductory chapter which presents important general principles and meanings of words commonly used, these subjects are developed separately by chapters. Each subject is dealt with as it applies to successive age periods and with consideration of the wide differences between children and the essential individuality of each child's characteristics of progress. Chapter IV is devoted to physical growth and development and Chapters VI and VII to psychological considerations and personality development.

Every child must grow and develop in his particular environment which tends to be continually changing and to which he must constantly make adjustments. One basic characteristic of these changes is the increasing breadth and complexity of the environment, starting with the restrictions of life in the uterus and ending as maturity approaches amid the many forces and contacts of community life. Considerable attention, therefore, is given throughout this book to the environmental factors which may have important effects on the child's health and at times sharply limit his development. Illness experiences are considered in Chapter II as they differ with age periods and stage of development and in this connection the development of immunity to infectious diseases is discussed. However, it is not within the scope of this book to describe individual diseases or their specific effects upon health. The purpose rather is to indicate the ways in which the manifestations of illness appear related to the stage of development and the means by which the ill effects of illnesses may at times be prevented or modified.

Maternal health, particularly during pregnancy and childbirth, is considered in Chapter III and because it is so importantly related to fetal development the latter is also discussed in this chapter. Nutrition is dealt with rather fully in Chapter V because it is a major and constantly operating factor in support of physical health and development. The family and its social components are given separate consideration in Chapter VIII and educational factors in Chapter IX to such extent as they are considered to be related to general health or to physical, emotional, or intellectual development.

It is recognized that all the subjects discussed in these chapters may be conditioned or modified in various ways by cultural differences in populations. The general approach adopted has been in reference to the dominant cultural characteristics in the United States in midtwentieth century. However, many cultures have provided vastly different backgrounds for large sections of American family life and these still influence to varying degrees the cultural components of the lives of many subgroups of this country's population. These differences are referred to from time to time in particular contexts. It is imperative that those who work in the field of maternal and child health be alert to recognize the importance of cultural differences as they influence the habits, ideas, and attitudes of families, and therefore the environment, care, and behavior of their children.

It is becoming widely appreciated that all children can profit from appropriately spaced examinations and reviews of their health histories. Particular attention should be given in these to the progress of each individual's growth and development and to any factors potentially or actually affecting health and progress. To carry out this purpose effectively a broad understanding of growth and development and factors relating to them is required on the part of all those who participate in providing these services. Chapter X considers the relevance of the subjects considered in earlier chapters to maternal and child health services.

A goal of health services for mothers and children is to assure that the care and feeding of children are changed with their advancing age and in accordance with generally recognized requirements, even that these be anticipated through what has come to be referred to as anticipatory guidance. A further goal is that advice be individualized as the need for change becomes apparent after the study of each child. A major problem in making assessments of children is that of variability between them or what is commonly referred to as individual differences. Wide differences are encountered among children in every observable attribute and at every age. Although these to a large extent are intrinsic in character and represent healthy development, some either within or outside the ranges of variations considered appropriate for most children are clearly evidences of interference with good progress. It is often necessary to follow the progress of an unusual child over a considerable period, carefully noting the characteristics of this progress and the features of his environment, care, and health before one can attain a useful although not always a complete understanding of the factors involved and their importance to him as an individual.

The first step required in conducting a health appraisal is usually to compare a child with his peers in respect to age and sex and for this purpose various standards or norms of reference for like groups are useful for identifying the child's prominent features. For example, one may conclude from a single assessment that the child is moderately tall but very light in weight, inactive and somewhat delayed in motor development, lacking in expected appetite or in the consumption of basic foods and subject to excessively frequent and unusual emotional upsets. All these terms are selected on the basis of general expectancies for age. In like manner the types, severities, and frequencies of his illnesses may be judged on the basis of the usual expectancies at his age period. "Norms" are available for rather precise classification of some of these whereas others are based largely on the physician's experience.

The second step, more time-consuming but far more rewarding, is to study the child's progress over time. This permits recognition of the consistency of his progress, the changes in his behavior, and the success of attempted changes in care, diet, and environment.

Both types of appraisal require professional training and experience with children at all ages. The single assessment in which the child is judged only in terms of knowledge of his peers is greatly facilitated by the use of the "norms" referred to, or so-called "standards of reference" such as height and weight tables. These permit rather objective comparisons of the child under study with general expectancies for children of like sex, age, and circumstances. Professional training for this purpose requires extensive study of the knowledge available regarding children at each age in all aspects of health and development. The second type of appraisal under which it is possible to compare the child with his former self rather than with other children is greatly enhanced if the appraiser has had opportunities for continuing experience with the same child over periods of time. For this reason pediatric education is more and more providing such opportunities in connection with internships or residencies. Although these assessments usually are made principally by the physician, the effectiveness of all professional workers participating in such health services is greatly enhanced by a thorough understanding of the chief factors involved in child development and in the protection and promotion of child health. The care of children will be effective and appropriate only to the extent that the understanding and interest of those who contribute to his care are adequate. Although specific instructions for individual care usually come from the physician, much of the guidance and health education provided to the mother or other members of the family comes from other professional workers. In these situations public health workers are contributing to health education. The approach in this book, therefore, is intentionally broad and directed toward providing understanding of general principles rather than details respecting each aspect of growth and development and of child care.

Reference is made in the Foreword which follows to the Longitudinal Studies of Child Health and Development conducted between 1930 and 1956 at the Harvard School of Public Health. Some of the findings in this research are referred to in the chapters to follow. The term "longitudinal" is used in referring to this project to indicate that the children enrolled were studied periodically throughout childhood. Several projects of this general character have been in operation over much the same period in other centers. This type of research is in sharp contrast to the more common and readily conducted studies referred to as "cross-sectional," based on the study of different sample groups of children at selected ages. By using the longitudinal method the progress of each individual enrolled can be recorded so long as he or she can be kept under periodic observations. This permits recognition of differences between individuals and groups in the characteristics or patterns of their growth and development, as well as in their life experiences.

In this research a multidisciplinary approach was adopted, that is, the staff consisted of pediatrician, nutritionist, anthropometrist, psychologist, social worker, public health nurse, and specialists for more limited purposes in other fields. This permitted study of each child's manifestations of growth and development, both physical and psychological as well as his dietary intakes, his illness experiences, his care, and the socioeconomic circumstances of his environment during each age interval.

Data on the characteristic patterns of progress in several of these respects have been published for the maturity series of children, that is those who were followed in this research from birth to their 18th year. A more detailed description of the studies made, a bibliography of past publications, and a series of reports on findings are available in a Supplement to *Pediatrics*, November 1959. Reference is also made to other large projects of longitudinal character. Studies of the interrelations between the various aspects of progress thus far reported are in preparation at the time of this writing.

A word must be said in explanation of the repeated references throughout this book to the role of the mother in child care and the infrequent mention of the father in this connection. Little is said also about the appropriate roles which may be played by grandmothers and other members of the extended family who frequently live in the home and may have important relations with the child. Most discussions of mother-child relationships are simplified by assumption that the mother is available and that the care of the child is primarily her responsibility, because this is the basic framework of family life in our culture. It must be understood, however, that when reference is made to the mother's feeding or management in any other aspect of care, physical or psychological, the provider of this "maternal care" at times is and commonly should be the father, grandmother, or other mother substitute. The father may at times seem neglected in the text, simply to avoid repetitive reference to "mother or father." The growing participation of fathers cooperatively with mothers in all aspects of infant and child care in the modern family is recognized as a source of strength.

Although it is generally accepted that the mother whenever possible should play the dominant role in the nurturance of the child, and that the father's role should be supportive of her in this, the actual degree to which these roles are fulfilled by either or shared by both depends in considerable measure on their personalities. The extent of the father's direct participation in providing "maternal care" depends also upon the occupational status of each parent. The best general approach would seem to be that the father provide continuing support of the mother, physical, emotional, intellectual, spiritual, and material, while recognizing her as the primary nurturant member of the family. This applies especially to the infant and young child with recognition that certain areas of leadership and supervision may properly be taken over by the father in later years. From the child's point of view the more fully that both parents can be identified as united, consistent, and equally contributing, the better. Complete agreement and constant harmony between parents on all occasions cannot be anticipated, but constant sharing of ideas by a loving couple, and of child care from the beginning, can reduce to unimportance these areas of disagreement.

The editors of this volume are indebted to all contributors for cooperation in adapting their sections to the purposes the book is intended to serve. For some this required an unusual approach and deletions of material they would have liked to retain. Several contributors gave valuable advice to the editors regarding sections other than those for which they were individually responsible. In addition to contributors, several persons were helpful in reviewing texts or in planning contents. Miss Christina MacAskill and others who assisted her in the preparation of manuscripts carried out a most complicated task with great care and patience. To all of these the editors express their deep appreciation.

HAROLD C. STUART, M.D.

March 15, 1960
Boston, Massachusetts

CONTENTS

FIGURES

TABLES

FOREWORD

"He who watches a thing grow has the best view of it."
Heraclitus of Ephesus

The publication of this book is the culmination of a number of years' consideration by a group of physicians, psychologists, social workers, educators, and nutritionists of current knowledge and theory of the physical, emotional, intellectual, and social development of children and youth and its presentation in a way that would be useful to all professional persons working with families and children.

The chapters are an extension and rearrangement of the materials used in large part by the authors in a series of Institutes on Child Growth and Development offered by the Department of Maternal and Child Health of the Harvard School of Public Health to workers in state public health programs. The preparation of these materials into book form was conceived by the Department; and its members, past and present, have written a substantial part of the text. They are responsible for its approach and general content. Important contributions, however, have been made by members of several other faculties of Harvard University, as well as by persons connected with other universities, both to the Institutes and to this book.

The list of contributors to this volume shows the multiplicity of disciplines which necessarily have been called upon to cover the wide range of subjects essential to a broad consideration of child development. An attempt has been made to present rather fully important examples of present knowledge which reveal basic principles rather than to discuss all aspects of development. The authors have been selected on the basis of balanced interest and experience in research, teaching, and services to succeeding age groups. A few of them, notably the senior editor, span the decades since the Committee on Child Development of the National Research Council stimulated the initiation of a number of long range studies; others have carried on their work in more recent years. Several contributors were associated for varying periods of time with the Longitudinal Studies of Child Health and Development at the Harvard School of Public Health. This project was directed by the senior editor and has constituted the major research of the Department of Maternal and Child Health since 1930. The experience of these research workers has contributed greatly toward the points of view presented by them in this volume. All of the authors have contributed through their separate disciplines to the great tide of knowledge of child development that has been rising in recent decades with increasing volume and swiftness. Happily the association of a pediatrician and a psychiatrist as co-editors has assured an unusual degree of balance in emphasis and space given to physical, intellectual and psychosocial development.

By giving the book the title of "The Healthy Child: His Physical, Psychological, and Social Development" the editors do not imply that there is a single prototype of healthy development in childhood. On the contrary, long years of research by the editors and their colleagues, and by many others in various child research centers, make clear that there is a considerable range in the patterns of physical and psychosocial growth and development of children that fall within the "normal." Health, too, is a dynamic process varying among individuals, and consisting at any one point in time of a state of physical, mental, social, and emotional well-being. Each individual child has certain general characteristics common to his age and sex, but also others that are unique in his own particular combination of attributes. He must be regarded as an individual in progress toward goals which collectively mean attainment of his full potentialities for health and development at maturity.

Knowledge of child growth and development in its many aspects is a relatively recent acquisition. For this and for other reasons it is an area of knowledge likely to have been covered inadequately in the basic training of many kinds of professional workers who now find themselves involved with children. This applies particularly to an understanding of the interrelationships between the various aspects of child development and the environment in which the child lives. A wide variety of physicians, those in private general practice, in the practice of pediatrics, obstetrics, or any of the specialties caring for handicapped children, and those who work in maternal and child health and school health programs or in academic settings will find in this book subject matter that is pertinent to their interest. The same is true for the multitude of workers in the other health professions, in social work, and in education. Clearly the authors have not had any single profession in mind in planning the content of this book. Rather, they have tried to set forth principles and concepts that should be of common interest to persons in all professions serving children.

MARTHA M. ELIOT, M.D.

THE
HEALTHY
CHILD

His Physical,
Psychological, and Social
Development

I

THE PRINCIPLES OF
GROWTH AND DEVELOPMENT

HAROLD C. STUART

THE ORDERLINESS AND THE INDIVIDUAL VARIABILITY OF GROWTH
AND DEVELOPMENT

There are general patterns of progress in all aspects of human growth and development which are characteristic of each of the age periods of childhood. The changes which occur in each period are for the most part very orderly, one following the other in an easily predictable manner. It is possible, therefore, to describe human growth and development in general terms and thus to anticipate the coming events which create changing needs and different health problems. Since there are marked differences between children, however, in the rates or degrees of change and in the timing of individual events with respect to age much attention must be given to variabilities or individual differences and their possible significance in terms of needs and problems of importance to health. The sequence of events in the infant's progress toward walking is a useful example. It is well recognized that the pattern of progress on the whole is followed with great regularity, however, the ages for attaining each new stage in this progress are subject to wide individual differences among perfectly adequate infants. Appropriate progress toward walking may be delayed by a variety of circumstances. Gain in weight is another example. This is continuous from year to year as a result of continuous growth and the expected rate of gain changes markedly from one age period to another. Although everyone is aware of the marked differences between children in their actual weight at selected birthdays and in their gains by year it is obvious that weight may fail to increase or even be lost under circumstances which require attention. All physiologic processes and their manifestations likewise change normally with the progress of development and for any of them the changes manifest by individuals may be unsatisfactory. The specific applicability of these generalizations differs considerably between the various aspects of development, the orderliness of progress being notably greater in respect to physical than to psychological changes. The principal contrasts of this type will be brought out in the chapters dealing with other than physical development.

The primary purpose shared by all contributors to this book has been to enhance the reader's knowledge of how children grow and develop in the major aspects of their progress during successive age periods, how individuals may be expected to differ one from the other in these respects, and to point out some of the leading indications of the healthfulness or particular significance of various features of difference among children. This applies particularly to some of the environmental circumstances which may contribute to unsatisfactory progress. Another objective has been to describe children's basic needs at each stage of development and some of the ill effects of failures to meet these needs satisfactorily. While attempting to give a broad understanding of child development from the standpoint of health needs and health problems care has been taken to avoid the impression that the reader can acquire therefrom the ability to distinguish between unusual but normal development and pathological development or unfavorable progress. The objective rather has been to make the reader aware of situations which call for health appraisal and to enhance his competence in health education and general guidance to parents.

THE AGE PERIODS OF CHILDHOOD AND THE MEANING OF TERMS COMMONLY USED

The years before maturity may be divided into periods, each of which is characterized by certain features of growth and development. Although these divisions are not sharply delimited and are very artificial they form convenient groupings of children for discussion of the characteristics by age and the differences between ages which are significant aspects of growth and development. These features are of practical value in providing base lines of general expectancies for children of any age and in recognizing the child who is making unusual progress for his age.

Under most circumstances it makes little difference what terms are used to describe the age group to which any individual belongs. However, in a book to which representatives of different disciplines contribute it is imperative that all use the same term or a comparable term in referring to events of a particular period of childhood. In professional parlance there tends to be rather loose use of certain terms, such as adolescence or puberty, and this at times causes confusion in discussion of age-linked problems. There is some evidence that the earliest but hidden changes associated with the adolescent cycle of development properly begin as early as 6 years but one would not be justified in referring to a 6 year old child as an adolescent. By common consent when a term defined below is used in the chapters to follow, the comments made are appropriate under the definition given unless otherwise qualified. Other terms may be used but in such cases the period of childhood being referred to will be made clear in the text.

The criticism is sometimes made that the attempt to divide childhood into precisely defined age periods may lead readers to adopt the notion that a child suddenly becomes a different individual on each of several selected birthdays. There are a few quite rapid transformations in individuals as they "grow up," as when the fetus becomes a neonate (physiologically), or when the preschool child becomes a school child (psychologically), or when the prepubescent child reaches puberty (physically). But in most instances transitions from the characteristics of one period to another are very gradual. Initial descriptions of growth or development, therefore, are made to apply most accurately to the central portion of each period for the average boy or girl. One hesitates to state the obvious but, for the record, two statements should be made here. First, as the defined dividing line between two age periods is reached the characteristics of the first have begun to fade while those of the latter have begun to take their place. Second, the actual ages at which children fit most accurately the descriptions of a period differ considerably among them, there usually being a continuum from the most advanced to the average to the least advanced child. Within the same individuals also differences are manifest in the timing of different attributes.

Acquiring knowledge of the usual characteristics of growth and development by age periods is only the first step in coming to understand these processes as they are revealed by the infinitely varied patterns of children's progress.

Childhood. The span of *childhood* may be variously defined to serve different purposes, but as used in this book it refers broadly to the entire period from conception to adult maturity. Although it is not possible to point to the exact age at which a child becomes an adult, *adulthood* is reached only after a long period of adolescence during which the child has been transformed into a structurally — and functionally — mature man or woman. For administrative purposes the Children's Bureau of the United States Department of Health, Education, and Welfare accepts 21 years as the end of childhood, and since there are wide differences between individuals in respect to the age at which they might be considered fully mature, 21 years would seem to be a practical end point for their purposes. In this book the last period of total childhood is defined as ending on the average for girls at 18 years and for boys at 20 years.

The prenatal period. The period before birth encompasses all the changes following the fertilization of the ovum at conception to the delivery of the fetus at birth. Even in his prenatal life the child changes in different ways during each of the three trimesters of pregnancy. It is therefore convenient to discuss fetal problems separately in relation to them. The *embryonic* period covers the first 8 weeks after conception; the *middle fetal* period covers from the ninth week through the second trimester; and the *late fetal* period covers the final trimester of pregnancy. It should be noted that these time divisions are broadly correct only from the point of view of fetal development, and do not precisely coincide with those indicated when the same terms are applied by an obstetrician with reference to the stages or periods of pregnancy. A final short but very critical period is that of labor and delivery, usually referred to as the parturient stage of the prenatal period.

Infancy. The first 2 years after birth are considered here to cover infancy when unqualified, but for purposes of discussion this must be divided into three phases. The first month after birth is referred to as the *neonatal* period, and constitutes an extremely important time of rapid change, particularly during its early days. This is followed by *infancy proper,* from 1 month to 1 year, and *late infancy,* which covers the second year after birth.

Childhood proper. This is divided for convenience into the *preschool* period, from 2 to 6 years, and the *school* period, which covers the ages 6 to 10 for girls and 6 to 12 for boys. The child of school age or the school child are terms which obviously refer to a different and rather ill defined age, but the school period is a term commonly used and is thus defined for the purposes of this book. It coincides approximately with the elementary school years for boys, or the first 6 grades. It is shorter for girls owing to the earlier onset of adolescent changes in girls, and hence covers approximately the first 4 grades for them.

Adolescence or the adolescent period. These terms refer broadly to the remaining years up to maturity, more precisely 10 to 18 for girls, and 12 to 20 for boys. However, adolescence cannot be described as a whole, but must be considered in three quite distinct subperiods, which are referred to as *prepubescence, pubescence,* and *postpubescence.* The latter term corresponds in general with the age period commonly referred to as *youth.* The approximate ages to which these three subdivisions of adolescence refer are, on the average for girls, 10 to 12, 12 to 14, and 14 to 18. The ages for boys are approximately 2 years later in each instance. *Prepubescence* covers the transitional period from the relative steadiness of the *school age period* to *pubescence* which refers to the central period of most rapid growth and of profound developmental changes. *Post-

pubescence covers a tapering-off period for completing the final steps leading to adult maturity.

Although as stated above it is not possible to draw sharp lines between the periods of fetal life, infancy, childhood, or adolescence or their subdivisions on the basis of chronologic age, the ages given facilitate discussion of the general characteristics of particular periods. The reasons for the arbitrary selection of these particular groupings of months or years into periods will become apparent as the differing characteristics of each period are described. It must be understood that the ages given refer to average children and that during adolescence the differences among children often extend to two or more years earlier or later in respect to the ages at which they change from the characteristics of one to the next age period.

Growth. As used in this text *growth* refers to those increases in the size of the body as a whole, or of any of its dimensions, parts, or tissues which occur as part of the child's progress toward maturity. In this sense excess gain in weight which is due to obesity or edema would not be considered part of growth, although gain in weight is usually a useful measure of overall growth. True growth results essentially from multiplication of cells and increase in intercellular substances.

Development. As here used *development* refers to the many other changes occurring as part of progress toward adult maturity. Some of the changes essentially are part of intrinsic maturing, and occur among all normal children, usually in a similar order. Others are more particularly the results of interplay between the individual and his environment. They depend more largely upon experience and learning, but require developing capacities to adapt or to regulate body functions. These two aspects of development are referred to as *maturation* and *adaptation*. They are both operative to some degree in most if not all aspects of development, and it is well to be aware of both processes, and their differing roles, in specific attainments. Developmental processes include differentiation of cells, tissues, and organs; skeletal maturation, such as calcification and fusion of epiphyses with diaphyses; changes in physiologic and immunologic activities and states, with increased capacities for successful adaptations in body functions; progress in gross and fine motor coordination; intellectual development; and emotional development.

It is common practice to use *growth and development* as a single expression when both kinds of changes are being considered. The purpose is to suggest that although these two words represent quite different aspects of the child's progress, they are actually related closely in one composite pattern of change. In early life it is difficult to find an example of one independent of the other, but after growth ceases in a part, as for example the brain, development progresses in many ways. Commonly, as in the title of this book, the word *development* is used in a very broad sense to cover all of the changes which take place as part of the natural progress of the individual from conception to full maturity and sometimes the word *growth* is used alone in the same sense, in either instance to avoid frequent use of the term *growth and development*. This should only occur when the particular usage is clear from the context.

Health. This term is sometimes thought of as merely the absence of disease. In this book it is considered to encompass physical, emotional, and social well-being in a positive sense. For any one child this means a state of well-being appropriate to him as an individual, taking into account his age, his progress toward maturity, and in the case of the handicapped, his permanent limitations. It implies relative freedom from illnesses but the healthy child is subject to the usual self-limited diseases. Webster defines health as "a state of being hale or sound in the body, mind, or soul." When considering the child soundness must include ability to grow and develop to the full extent of intrinsic endowment without defects or limitations imposed by the environment or chance occurrences. In giving health services to a child the aim is to keep his condition constantly as near as possible to optimum for him. The use of the term health in relation to illness is considered in Chapter II and in relation to physical growth and development in Chapter IV. Its application to mental health and emotional development is considered further in Chapter VII.

"GENETIC" OR "INTRINSIC" FACTORS IN GROWTH AND DEVELOPMENT

Each child grows and develops as he does for a number of reasons. First, he is a human being and must remain within the limits of the "human pattern" which his biological inheritance has evolved through the ages. He also has a racial and familial background of inheritance which will determine some of his attributes and may make him differ in striking ways from other human beings. The inheritance which he receives from his mother will differ from that of his father. His resulting attributes may bear resemblances to one or the other but at times prominent features will appear which are not presented by either parent but are transmitted through one of them from their forebears.

The familial determinants of features of a child's individuality reside as genes in the chromosomes of the fertilized egg cell from which he develops and these genes are transmitted from cell to cell in subsequent divisions. By this means the potentialities for the expression of genetic factors in the course of his growth and development are brought by the multiplying cells to all parts and tissues which must participate in his progress. The actual progress made by a child and the character of the development which he ultimately attains, however, may be modified in a variety of ways by influences acting upon him at any stage of his development. It is customary to divide these factors into two categories referred to as "heredity and environment," "intrinsic and extrinsic," or "nature and nurture." These terms have different shades of meaning but the first in each refers to those forces which in large measure determine his continuing attributes or the basic characteristics of his status, responses, and progress in most aspects of growth and development. The second term in each refers to all the features of environment which may modify the full attainment of intrinsic potentialities in one of many ways and may act at various stages of his development.

The genes inherited by a child account in the main for his continuing individual characteristics such as size, build, rate of developmental progress, and many other aspects of his health and personality. They probably account in large measure for his adaptive capacities and his potentialities, weaknesses, and strengths. The genes determine sex and are responsible for attributes which are basically of racial or familial origins. They account also for occasional characteristic familial diseases and specific defects. However, as will be discussed further when considering congenital malformations in Chapter III, abnormal genes may be present and express themselves fully or only partially or they may remain latent. Apparently, in some instances at least, the result depends upon environmental conditions during the fetal period.

It is not rewarding given the present state of knowledge to attempt to distinguish in all situations among genetic and intrauterine environmental factors which may have operated singly or conjointly to account for conditions found at birth or for the course of early development. However, it is important when possible to recognize those which result from maternal ill health or the conditions of intrauterine environment. It is also important not to neglect the possibilities for contributing toward a child being "well born" by attention to maternal health throughout pregnancy as discussed more fully in Chapter III. The term "intrinsic" has merit as a substitute for "genetic" in that it implies factors which are accountable for many of a child's basic characteristics at birth without implying that they are fully genetic in origin. The term thus includes congenital malformations, certain endocrine disorders, metabolic errors, and other manifestations of abnormality, recognizable at birth or early in life and probably of prenatal origin. In most instances, however, intrinsic factors express themselves as individual variations within normal ranges for human characteristics of status and of progress.

Genetic inheritance can account for innumerable variations in the course and outcome of development. The genes influence the character of a child's growth and development at all ages in a variety of ways. They do so by determining the characteristics of the enzymes which they elaborate and which reside in the developing cells. Presumably variants of normal genes produce variant enzymes and defective genes also account for defective enzymes. These determine in some measure, at least, the ways in which and the extent to which the cells in the different tissues and parts of the body multiply, differentiate, and lay down intercellular substance. They set the pattern, also, for their continuing functioning and responsiveness throughout childhood to circulating hormones, nutrients, and other stimuli. Recent research in enzyme development in early infancy has been reviewed by Driscoll and Hsia[1] in relation to functional differentiation and the maturation of organ systems.

The hormones influence in specific ways the metabolism of the various tissues which they reach through the circulating blood. The character of the growth which takes place in any given period, for example in the tibia, is determined in part by certain genetic characteristics of the cells composing the "growth zones" at the ends of this bone, and in part by the amounts of specific hormones, particularly of the so-called pituitary-growth hormone, carried in the blood to these areas. The amounts of these which are secreted also are determined in part by the genetic characteristics of the cells composing the glands which produce them. The effect of these hormones is either to accelerate or to diminish the intrinsic activities of the local tissues within the ranges of their several potentialities. The usual effect is to promote their metabolic processes in such ways as to accelerate their customary activities.

Embryonic development is determined largely by the components of the individual cells, which are dividing and multiplying with great rapidity and some of which are differentiating into specialized types of cells. These processes continue under locally elaborated enzymes or "organizers" until large groups of like cells are organized to form tissues. The types of cells laid down in these tissues account in large measure for the type of growth and development which will take place in each part of the body, this differing greatly in the different parts. Groups of tissues combine to form organs and other structures which, by the end of the embryonic period, at about 8 weeks of fetal age, simulate the systems and organs of the human body. Their later functional activities result from a grouping of appropriately differentiated cells in proper formation and organization. In order for these growth activities to take place, it is essential that normal cells be laid down, that they be surrounded by intercellular substances of normal composition, and nourished by an adequate circulation in order to permit the maintenance of normal cell metabolism.

The extent to which various maternal or placental hormones influence the course of fetal development has not as yet been satisfactorily established. The rudimentary endocrine glands of the fetus probably have little, if any, influence upon the fetal development during the first trimester but thereafter they may play a part individually in the course of further growth and development. However, the characteristics of these appear to be determined principally by the normality of the fetal cells and the adequacy of the immediate uterine environment, and particularly of the placenta. Maternal and fetal relations and the characteristic problems of the fetal period are considered in Chapter III.

The endocrine glands through the changing amounts of the several hormones which they elaborate and which circulate to all tissues of the body, in large measure, regulate and modify the progress of postnatal growth and development. These hormones affect the functional activities as well as the structures of the organs and tissues upon which they act and accomplish their purpose chiefly through differential stimulation. The central control for this mechanism apparently resides in the hypothalamus, an area of the brain in close proximity to the pituitary gland. The anterior lobe of this gland, in response to hypothalamic stimulation, produces a "growth hormone" which is characterized by uniform general stimulation of growth throughout the body. The response by the cells in the various areas of the body to this stimulation is determined primarily by their constitution, but the magnitude of the response in any area varies with the strength of this hormonal stimulation, which in turn is determined by the degree of pituitary activity.

The pituitary gland produces a hormone which specifically stimulates the thyroid to produce a hormone of its own which is essential for normal growth, for differentiation of tissues and particularly for normal mental and osseous development. During all of life this thyroid component is essential for normal metabolism and for the maintenance of tissue replacement and development generally. The pituitary gland also produces a hormone which stimulates the cortex of the adrenal glands and others which stimulate the primary sex organs. These in turn produce hormones of their own which are importantly related to adolescent development, sex differentiation, and later reproductive functions. The testes produce male sex hormones including androgen, whereas the ovaries produce estrogen and other female sex hormones. Androgen has a particularly stimulating effect on the adolescent spurt of growth, the development of muscle, and other male sex characters. Thus the differences in growth and development between the sexes appear to be in large measure dependent upon the differences in the hormones elaborated by the testes and the ovaries, with pituitary and adrenal cortex hormones playing their respective parts.

The above description is an extreme simplification of a very complicated mechanism of controls established by the body. Knowledge in this field is very incomplete and much further research is required for an adequate understanding of many of its aspects. The few features of the control mechanism presented here are meant solely to point out the varieties of ways in which growth progress may be modified in a given individual. There may, for example, be failure of the development of the brain, particularly of the hypothalamus, with consequent lack of normal stimulation of the pituitary gland, as a result of which it may fail to produce one or several hormones in required amounts. Other pathologic conditions may lead to overactivity of the pituitary in one or more of its functions. Similarly, the thyroid, adrenals, or gonads may fail to respond to the stimulation which comes to them from the pituitary, or they may overrespond because of some pathologic condition. Any one or several of these mechanisms may fail; thus, there are many endocrine-based reasons for abnormal growth.

Throughout late infancy as well as childhood proper the "growth hormone" of the pituitary gland appears to be the principal one in accounting for the magnitude of growth in all parts of the body. A lack of this hormone appears to produce uniform dwarfism, while an excess results in uniform overgrowth. The whole course of adolescence, in contrast to that of earlier childhood, is controlled to a considerable degree by a combination of hormones elaborated by the pituitary gland, the cortex of the adrenal glands, the testes in the male, and the ovaries in the female, and by the interaction among these several glands. These factors which operate chiefly in relation to adolescent development are discussed further in the last section of Chapter IV.

It is not usually possible to assign values to the different factors which are known to play a part in determining the course and outcome of growth and development. Clearly a genetic defect which prevents the functioning of one of the endocrine glands necessary for normal development will be decisive in causing abnormality. Similarly, an injury to an infant in the process of birth may account for a clearly recognizable abnormality in the newborn or young infant. Commonly there appears to be an interplay of factors which account for the health and development of individual children. In specific situations there are clearly recognizable signs of a familial disease or characteristic eccentricities of growth traceable in the family tree which identify the occurrences as genetic. In other situations characteristic manifestations of nutritional deficiencies, infectious diseases or injuries make the resulting abnormalities or retardations of development clearly the result of environmental causes. The present concept is that an individual's basic inherited potentialities for growth and development condition him to a type of response to the various aspects of environment. They certainly account in considerable measure for the success of his adaptations. It is apparent that familial susceptibilities to the development of defects or the acquisition of certain diseases or syndromes such as allergies may be essentially latent, partially expressed, or fully manifest depending upon environmental circumstances.

In some instances inherited characteristics may be so defective that life cannot be supported in an environment which would normally be adequate. In others they may be somewhat defective so that a child's progress is poor only when one or another environmental factor is less than fully satisfactory. In many instances, however, the intrinsic characteristics are so adequate that progress continues surprisingly well despite what appear to be very unfavorable environmental circumstances. This leads to great differences among individual children in their needs and their responses to the same defects in environment or care. The great majority of children who are well fed and well cared for, who live in a suitable environment, and who avoid the chance of destructive effects of serious accidents or illnesses appear to grow and develop largely in accordance with what appear to be intrinsic individual characters.

There are two important reasons for study of the intrinsic causes of differences in children. The first is that much can be done to increase the probabilities that a baby be "wellborn" through preconceptual, prenatal, and natal care as described in Chapter III. The second is that appreciation of the reasons for and the significance of individual differences in status and progress at every age period is important for those who participate in advising on any matters relating to health. It is helpful, for example, to have available the evidence that a very small child has always been a slow maturing individual and that there is familial evidence that this is probably an intrinsic attribute. It is even more important to appreciate that rapid weight gain in later years may represent developing stocky build or accelerated normal growth and not obesity. If either is the case efforts to reduce or restrict gain are contraindicated.

ENVIRONMENTAL FACTORS WHICH MAY AFFECT GROWTH AND DEVELOPMENT

The interest of people who work in the field of public health is understandably oriented primarily toward the control of extrinsic or environmental factors which are more readily subject than intrinsic or genetic factors to correction when unfavorable and promotion when healthful. For this reason much consideration is given in this book to environment and to meeting known needs.

There is obvious need for further research to increase our knowledge of the environmental factors which may affect the child's progress, the means by which or the circumstances under which they do so, and the most effective ways of promoting or protecting growth and development. There is also need for developing means for recognizing exceptional children and their particular problems and for adjusting the environment to meet them.

One of the most common environmental causes for retardation in growth and development is the insufficient provision of the necessary food substances. This may be due to inadequacy of food intake both qualitatively and quantitatively or to defective assimilation or utilization of foods taken.

There is little doubt but that faulty nutrition in one or more of its elements or processes accounts in large measure for the acquired faults in growth progress. All types of deficiency in food intake can lead to poor growth as well as to specific signs of deficiency disease. Inadequate diet apparently can lead to underactivity of the endocrine glands, or to poor responses to the circulating hormones on the part of the organs and tissues.

The effects of undernutrition differ in accordance with the type as well as the degree of dietary deficiency, the stage of development at which it occurs, its duration and the success with which the child is able to adapt to the low intake. A common effect associated with any type of dietary deficiency is a lessening of the rate of over-all growth and development without any signs specifically indicative of undernutrition. Because of the variability among children in the normal or appropriate rate of progress for them, this type of effect is hard to recognize until it has persisted for some time or has become marked. One rather characteristic effect of prolonged undernutrition is recognizably poor progress in muscular development. Even though muscle size and strength for a given age differs greatly among individuals on a genetic basis, as well as on habits of physical activity, it is apparent that the actual development of muscles may be dependent in considerable part upon, or limited by the adequacy of the diet.

When the diet is lacking in a specific nutrient, the signs of pathological growth characteristic of its deficiency may not appear or lead to recognition of the specific inadequacy until general development has been modified to a considerable degree. The principal result of habitually excessive food consumption is the gradual development of obesity. A high protein diet, associated with excessive calories, appears at times to stimulate growth in height as well as in weight. This acceleration of over-all growth may well result from stimulation of the pituitary gland to increased production of its "growth hormone." There is not sufficient evidence, however, to indicate to what extent this is a factor in modifying a child's eventual size. The factors of importance from a nutritional standpoint are discussed in Chapter V.

Physical activity is essential for proper functioning of the body and its various organs and systems, and this proper functioning in turn is essential for normal growth. Regular activities which require use of the large muscles of the body are particularly important for optimum muscular growth. Any interference with nerve or blood supply, or with normal use, may inhibit the growth of the part affected. Thus a paralyzed extremity is unlikely to keep pace with its normal mate. On the other hand, over-activity sufficient to produce recurrent or chronic fatigue appears at times to interfere with satisfactory progress, possibly indirectly by interference with the normal ingestion and utilization of food. A well-balanced program of alternating activity and rest, appropriate for the child's stage of development and his individual capacities, is important in relation to physical growth as well as to optimum nutrition.

Lack of other necessities of life, particularly of adequate sleep, rest, and exercise often account for failure to maintain satisfactory progress in particular ways. Climate may affect the development of children for many reasons. Prevailing temperatures and the amount of exposure to sunlight may affect the child's physiologic processes directly. Seasonal changes tend to affect habits of activity, the availability of essential foods, and, particularly, the presence of various types of pathogenic organisms. For the most part these are basic problems of importance to health officers who are responsible for improving the general healthfulness of the environment. However, they create special problems requiring attention by those who deal directly with mothers and children.

Diseases and injuries may affect growth and development in a variety of ways, directly or indirectly, temporarily or over long periods, or even permanently depending on the parts involved or the nature of the damage brought about. Any disease which interferes over a considerable period of time with physical activity, with nutritional processes or with the functioning of the circulatory, urinary, endocrine, central nervous, or respiratory systems will interfere with normal progress.

The prevention of accidents is a major goal of all groups concerned with the health, education, and welfare of children. Collectively they account for a large portion of deaths, temporary disabilities, and permanent defects among children. Mortality statistics for the United States for the year 1958 showed that for the age period 1 to 14 years inclusive all forms of accidental death collectively nearly equaled in number all deaths in the next four leading categories, namely "malignant neoplasms, including lymphatic and hematopoietic tissues," "influenza and pneumonia," "congenital malformations" and "major cardiovascular-renal diseases." Accidents remain the leading cause of death at all ages from 1 to 34 years.[2]

Accidents differ in the prevailing types and causes and in the incidence of each type by age, because many of the reasons for their occurrence are highly related to the developmental status of the child: mental, emotional, physical, and educational. For these reasons several approaches to their prevention must be adopted, each differing with age and environment, and consistently pursued to keep their incidence to a minimum. "Anticipatory guidance" as part of health services to mothers, particularly in relation to infant and preschool child care and educational programs for older children in schools presently are receiving much attention. Pediatric organizations, public health agencies, and educational institutions are actively studying the nature, causes and methods of control of accidents which are applicable to their groups. Legislatures, law courts, city planners, and the police are all concerned and have important opportunities to promote safety for children. Much will continue to depend, however, upon parents and their awareness of the age-linked hazards and some of the simple steps which can be taken in the home to reduce their incidence. All health workers have opportunities to contribute to the effectiveness of one or more of these preventive programs.

It is distressing to review statistics on the causes of accidents in the home and to realize that deaths of young children commonly result from eating aspirin tablets or other medicines carelessly left about the house or in rural areas from drinking kerosene oil from drums conveniently located in the wood shed.

Children differ among themselves in the types and frequencies of the accidents which they experience, not only by age but within age groups, dependent in part at least upon personality traits, physical characteristics, and major interests. The sharply higher rates among boys than girls, especially during adolescence is one indication of this. Accident rates differ also among cultures and with the basic characteristics of the communities on which the rates are based.

Because of the wide variety of factors related to the causation of accidents and therefore to their control, prevention is not considered further here. Examples of their relations, however, are presented in later chapters, particularly those dealing with physical growth, emotional development, and education. Also, three excellent summaries of the problems of accidents in childhood can be recommended.[3, 4, 5]

Much more needs to be learned as to how most effectively to prevent when he finds various unfavorable circumstances but no positive diagnostic criteria for growth failure is to apply the "therapeutic test." This means simply to correct in as far as possible unfavorable circumstances and to observe the results. The corrections are indicated in any event as part of preventive service and they may be followed by evidences of more satisfactory progress as well.

THE EVALUATION OF HEALTH WITH CONSIDERATION OF INDIVIDUAL DIFFERENCES

Reference has been made in previous connections to individual differences in all attributes of children at any given age and the possible relevance of these differences to health or to individual needs. Most children of the same sex and age have much in common in that, for any measurement, they tend to cluster around the average, derived from study of a large sample of their peers. The further a child is removed from the average in any distribution, the fewer the children usually found like him. In any large group, however, there will be a few who are extreme in their differences from the average. It is important to appreciate that marked difference from the usual is not necessarily abnormal or even undesirable. For a school age girl to be extremely tall or for a boy to be short may create personal problems which deserve attention, but for the individuals concerned their heights are usually appropriate for them and rarely are found to represent developmental abnormality. It is, however, ordinarily though not invariably true that the more extreme the deviation of a child's position, within any range which properly represents his population of peers, the greater the likelihood of its having some health significance.

The characteristics of "norms" for height and weight are shown graphically in Chapter IV, together with examples of striking and consistent individual differences. The use of these norms is intended to supplement general health appraisals and not in themselves to determine a child's normality. Unfortunately, the statistical term "norm" is commonly confused with the clinical term "normality," but the former refers only to findings in studies of populations whereas the latter relates solely to the individual.

The limits of "normality" as contrasted with "abnormality" can never be set and the attempt to do so arbitrarily should be discarded. A question repeatedly asked by a mother or an older child referring to a given weight, height, blood pressure level, or other finding is to the effect: "Is that normal, doctor?" This question is understandable but it should always be explained that the answer given refers to the appropriateness of the value for the individual. Many factors must be taken into account by the different kinds of accidents at different ages. It is probable that so experience with minor accidents is part of development which, as wi infectious diseases, may provide some resistance to them. Overlong cor plete protection certainly delays safe independence but it is difficult t plan safe "immunizing" exposures to accidents.

It is not easy to evaluate the extent to which emotional factors may interfere with a child's development and the ways in which they do interfere. There is no room for doubt but that they do at times have important effects. Emotional factors probably operate by influencing the kinds and amounts of food eaten, the metabolic processes through which normal nutrition is maintained, and habits of rest and activity. In some instances emotional disturbances appear to lead to inadequate or unbalanced food intake but in others they clearly lead to excessive caloric consumption and hence to obesity. They not only may account for abnormal habits of physical over- or underactivity but may affect cardiovascular and respiratory functions and metabolic or endocrine processes. Emotional problems are known to interfere with learning and other aspects of mental development so that neuromuscular development may thus be indirectly delayed.

Part of the process of successful development consists in a child learning to obtain from the environment what he needs and to develop capacities to defend himself from potentially harmful elements or to make successful adaptations to them. Children differ tremendously among themselves in their capacities to make such adaptations but, in general, the younger or more immature the child the greater the need for protection from environmental hazards. However, limited exposures to unfavorable environmental factors probably are the means of promoting successful defenses or mechanisms for adaptations to them. The age and developmental state of the child at the time of their impact undoubtedly are important factors in determining successful adaptations but experience indicates that children differ greatly in these capacities at any age.

In attempting to appraise the effects of unfavorable environment upon a child one cannot recognize with any certainty, except when marked and obviously adverse environmental circumstances exist, just what factors have accounted for any delays which have been recognized in a child's progress, commonly referred to as "growth failure." The most effective procedure in rendering health services to children is to be alert to evidences of growth failure on the one hand and to inquire carefully for specific faults in environment and care on the other. By equating the findings under these two approaches one may obtain important leads as to interrelations. The most common procedure resorted to by the physician

physician before he reaches a judgment as to the normality of any such attribute.

It is important to pay attention to the growth and development of a child when assessing his general state of health and the adequacy of his care. In doing this one tries to distinguish among those characteristics which are appropriate for him as an individual and those which may be inappropriate or which suggest unsatisfactory status or progress. One helpful aid in recognizing the appropriateness of a child's progress is to determine its consistency. Reasonable consistency is a usual manifestation of most intrinsic characteristics, whereas marked inconsistency suggests environmental influences. As an example of consistency, it may be a characteristic of one child to be somewhat delayed in his motor development whereas another may be characteristically well ahead of the average child in this type of progress. If intrinsic constitutional differences account for the former being late in walking, it will usually be found that he was also late in sitting with support and in other steps of progress toward walking. He should certainly not be compared unfavorably with the other child who would always be expected to be ahead of him. However, if a third child failed to make expected progress in motor development to the extent of becoming delayed, after having been advanced for some time, this would be sufficiently unusual to justify further study to make cetain that there was no unfavorable factor operating which had delayed him and needed attention. The first two children described are examples of consistent progress, although in this developmental attribute there appears to be somewhat less consistency in the timing of the steps observed than in some others. The third child, however, exemplifies an unusual degree of inconsistency which may or may not represent abnormality for him.

Consistent differences from average expectancies in the patterns of progress manifest by individual children deserve recognition also when pronounced because they afford leads as to the appropriate timing of changes in care for such children and also, at times, for the understanding of the child's behavior or other characteristics. Pronounced and seemingly sudden changes in rates of progress, particularly marked delays, may characterize a few steps or changes in normal development but in most instances they are unusual. Marked delay or arrest of progress is of far greater significance than being continually late or slow in this regard. Thus, the evaluation of the normality of a child's progress is based more soundly upon comparison with his former self than with his peers in respect to age.

It should be emphasized that the term consistency as used here does not imply identical or even similar patterns of progress throughout childhood for many intrinsic patterns involve gradual changes over the years and at times striking differences. It refers rather to year by year progress which tends to be orderly for the individual. The following are examples of consistency with change which appear to represent varieties in the basic patterns. Some children who are always near average in height from birth to the end of the school period then change to a much more rapid rate of growth in height, which then continues throughout the remaining years. In contrast, other children grow similarly until puberty, after which they grow much more slowly so that by 18 years the two groups may differ markedly. The problems which such changes create are considered further in Chapter IV but this and numerous other differences in progress over time are recognized as normal variants of human patterns of progress and for the individuals concerned they usually represent consistent progress.

Understanding the unique aspects of a child's developmental progress will be facilitated by considering his over-all *developmental age* rather than the conventional chronological age alone. This term may be applied to various aspects of physical progress and refers to the age with which his status at a given time most closely corresponds in terms of average children. Thus, to speak of a child as having a developmental age of 6 years means that on the basis of attributes studied his development corresponds most closely to the average development of a child at 6 years. The child in question may actually be 5, 6, or 7 years of age or even 4 or 8.

"Skeletal development," sometimes referred to as "osseous development," is an aspect of physical development which follows a sequence of changes which occur at different ages in early, average, and late maturing individuals. This is characterized by specific features of change in development of bones, some of which have been extensively studied and are known as maturity indicators. These are recognizable in the living child in appropriately taken X-ray films of the hand. The significance of this and other features of individual differences which can be assessed rather precisely lie in their close association in time with other steps or stages of development. As an example, the infant who is dull and not progressing satisfactorily because of lack of thyroid function will not progress normally in skeletal development and an X-ray of the hand can reveal the age equivalent of this delay. The child who is advanced in one physical attribute tends to be so in most others. It is not surprising, therefore, that the boy who is advanced in his skeletal development is usually found also to be advanced in general growth as reflected in height and in the appearance of his secondary sex characters. The girl of 10 who appears distressingly tall among her schoolmates may be so only temporarily as a result of her advanced pubescent development, one aspect of which is rapid adolescent growth. As shown in more detail in Chapter IV, this advancement leads to early termination of growth and a much more customary adult stature and to menstruation well before the usual age. In short, her developmental age may be that of 12 or 13 years even though she is in fact only 10.

The patterns of physical growth and developmental progress of children have such universal applicability that some coming events for any child may be predicted in broad outline. This applies particularly to the sequences of developmental changes and the events which may be anticipated under ordinary circumstances. Because of the wide variability in the actual expression of these basic human characteristics, however, in magnitudes of change, timing of events, and details of manner of progress, one must be guarded in the prediction of the exact time of occurrence of any given event or the manner of its occurrence. This is important in order not to create anxiety in the minds of parents over perfectly normal individual variations. It applies with special force when applied to an individual event at a particular time, without consideration of the child's former progress. The interpretation of such specific events is most accurate and useful when made in the light of the child's earlier developmental history, which permits a better understanding of his particular potentialities for growth and development.

A most important differentiation which constantly must be undertaken in dealing with children has to do with whether unusual findings are constitutional attributes or the results of unfavorable environment or health problems. This requires careful study by the physician of the child's habits, care, and environment and can be greatly facilitated by periodic studies of his progress. Much of the discussion which follows in subsequent chapters relates to their effects.

II

THE CHARACTERISTICS OF CHILDHOOD ILLNESSES AND IMMUNITY

GENERAL FEATURES OF ILLNESS BY AGE

ISABELLE VALADIAN

Those who work with children are aware that in general childhood diseases change characteristically with age and that a child's health is related to his growth and developmental status. The features of his status which account for these relationships or the mechanisms through which they are brought about are not well understood or perhaps even recognized. Our knowledge and understanding of these relationships, however, is being expanded in a variety of ways. It is the purpose of this section to provide a brief over-all view of the illness experiences of "healthy children" at their successive age periods throughout childhood in the light of present knowledge.

Health means something more than the absence of illness and the presence of illness should not necessarily be taken to mean poor health. There are children who rarely have a definite illness but equally rarely can be said to be in good health in the sense of enjoying physical, emotional, mental, and social well-being. A girl followed in the Harvard Longitudinal Studies of Child Health and Development[1] can be cited as an illustration. She was always small and slender from birth on, growing very slowly throughout childhood and maturing slowly as well. Her skeletal age, based on assessment of radiographs of the hand was constantly delayed, and her adolescent growth spurt occurred late and was small in amount. Her secondary sex characters also appeared late and menstruation first occurred at 14 years. She consistently had poor muscles, poor posture, and her physical activity was strikingly less than average. She was considered slow, lazy, and irritable in school and had a great deal of trouble in all aspects of school life. In adolescence she was constantly tired and irritable. Despite these evidences of poor growth, development and adaptations this girl had no serious or frequent illnesses, in fact she was among those children who experienced the fewest and mildest illnesses throughout their first 18 years.

There are children, on the other hand, who experienced many or serious illnesses without deviating more than briefly from their general status of excellent health. The boy in the Harvard Longitudinal Studies who had the most frequent and most severe illnesses is an illustration. A goodly number of his illnesses were respiratory in type. At the age of $4\frac{1}{2}$ months he was acutely ill with sore throat and high fever and this was followed by a two month period in which he was described as "not well" with chronic respiratory symptoms. At $5\frac{1}{2}$ months he had another acute upper respiratory infection and at 9 months an acute attack of bronchitis. Thereafter he continued to have repeated respiratory illnesses of varying degrees of severity and duration but mostly severe and involving both the upper and lower respiratory areas. These were complicated at times by otitis media and asthma and he acquired most of the acute communicable diseases of childhood. Despite all these illnesses this boy was consistent in his growth pattern, always being tall and of average build with good posture, good muscles, and developing a broad stocky build in later years. His skeletal age was advanced as well as his secondary sex characters. He was also described as well adjusted in school, cooperative, usually active and successful in selected sports. The cases cited, of course, are extreme examples for major illnesses usually affect total health in a variety of ways and may lead to substantial delays in growth and development. The point is that the failure to find a pathologic condition on examination does not justify the conclusion that the child has no health problems deserving attention.

Some of the factors which really constitute health are the resistance the child has when exposed to infectious agents, his ability to make successful adaptations to disease or stresses of other sorts, and in some measure his "learning" or ability to improve his defense mechanisms through illness experience. In appraising a child's total health one must take into account his susceptibilities to illnesses and more particularly how readily he recovers from illness and how satisfactorily he keeps on growing and developing without impairment as a result of them. Any illness may be accompanied by loss of appetite, poor intake and poor utilization of food, while febrile illnesses increase caloric, fluid, and other specific needs. Failure to absorb or actual loss of nitrogen during illness is common. Severe, chronic, or recurrent acute illnesses are likely to have deleterious effects of some type or degree on physical growth or on emotional, mental, or social development. They may initiate or aggravate many health problems. Some illnesses may destroy or seriously damage tissues or organs and impair vital body functions leading at times to permanent defects. As examples, rheumatic fever may cause severe heart damage. Both acquired heart disease and congenital cardiac anomalies may interfere with growth by reducing the oxygen saturation of the blood. Chronic kidney conditions may interfere with the development of that organ and diminish its functions in such ways as to interfere with general growth. Chronic disturbances in metabolic or glandular functions of any type may result from various illnesses and these are likely to have profound effects upon one or more aspects of growth.

Certain pathogenic agents have particular tissue tropism, that is they are drawn to reside in and to cause particular damage to certain tissues. The effects of German measles occurring during the first months of pregnancy on the growing fetus will be mentioned in Chapter III and serves as an example. The virus of poliomyelitis attacks the anterior horn cells of the spinal cord, damaging certain nerves and as a consequence the muscles dependent upon them. The extent of the damage is variable but usually the earlier in the growth period it occurs the greater the total limitation of the growth of the part affected. Physical and chemical agents also may have predilection for some tissues. Lead poisoning may cause encephalitis with resulting brain damage and as a sequel mental retardation.

During serious illness the child is kept in bed or on restricted activity. This means that in addition to the effects on his nutrition and his metabolic processes he does not use his muscles in customary ways and their development may be impaired. He is away from school and from his peers and thus may fall behind in his education and social development. In some conditions anxiety is created by pain or fear; these and other circumstances may be expected to give rise to emotional problems in addition.

Problems often develop insidiously and seemingly as the cumulative result of former illnesses, especially when they have occurred repeatedly. A girl followed in the Harvard Longitudinal Studies is an example. She was the most frequently sick girl in the series. From infancy through adolescence she experienced such major illnesses as recurrent hemichorea, pyelonephritis, and severe episodes of respiratory infections among which there were three attacks of lobar pneumonia requiring six hospitalizations, three of which were of 2 to 3 month duration. Nevertheless, she grew steadily up to 8 years and although small and thin was reasonably active when not sick and manifested good emotional health. These findings indicated quite satisfactory adjustments to her illnesses up to that time. After 8 years, however, her growth and behavior began to deviate from her former pattern. She became increasingly obese and inactive, spending her days in a chair if not in bed, refusing to walk to school and unhappy in school where she had considerable difficulty. At 16 she was a most unresponsive, unhappy, and lonely girl.

The effects of most acute illnesses are usually transitory with few, minor, or no observable effects upon growth and development. Regardless of the nature of the illness there is often disturbed calcification at the epiphyses of one or more long bones, observed on roentgenograms as dense transverse lines. These persist for a variable time but usually fade away. Some infectious diseases may have transitory effects on particular organs, manifested by such signs as palpitations or extra systoles in the heart or the appearance of albuminuria.

There is little evidence in the literature as to the types or incidence of the observed effects of ordinary acute illnesses upon growth. They may be said to vary with the complex conditions which exist at the time such as the severity, frequency, and duration of illness and whether or not it occurs during a period of rapid growth. Some studies have shown no significant differences in the growth of children who had frequent illnesses as compared with those who had been relatively free from illnesses but frequency without consideration of type, severity, or duration is a poor measure of the impact of illness. The degree to which an illness due to infection affects growth undoubtedly is dependent upon the nature of the infecting agent, the individual child, the environment, and many chance factors such as age of onset and portal of entry of the infecting organism. Nevertheless, it is surprising how many illnesses or what severe or prolonged illness a child may have without this interfering much with growth and without any ultimate evidence of failure to obtain full stature and adequate development. Knowledge is still limited as to why some children's growth is manifestly interfered with while others with seemingly equal amount and severity of illness show no recognizable effects. However, our estimates of the severity of an illness may not be based upon its most important aspects as they relate to the physiologic integrity of the child. It appears that the growth of some children is readily interfered with by illness, whereas others fail to manifest interference. Body weight is usually the first measurement to respond to illness and growth in height or other body measurements appears to be much less easily affected. Even with a brief illness weight may drop sharply, possibly from loss of body fluids but also from utilization of body tissues for maintenance purposes. Weight is apt to rise quickly during convalescence, the time necessary to catch up depending in large measure on the impact of the acute episode and the quality of care during convalescence. Some people seem to lose and regain weight or mobilize and store fat much more readily under these circumstances than do others.

The staff conducting the Harvard Longitudinal Studies is attempting to relate each individual child's responses to illnesses in terms of their number, type, severity, and duration as manifest by changes in progress of growth and development, as well as in appetite, activities, and in other ways. Two children, in the early years of the study, a girl at the age of $3\frac{1}{2}$ years and a boy at 2 years had acute respiratory infections with otitis media which required paracentesis. Within a few days both children developed pneumonia and were hospitalized. In the fourth week the girl developed empyema which required incision and drainage, the latter lasting for 4 weeks. The boy developed mastoiditis in the fifth week, which required mastoidectomy and was followed by drainage both from the mastoid and from enlarged cervical nodes. These conditions later were complicated by erysipelas. Both children were acutely ill for about 3 months, the situation at times being critical. Both lost a considerable amount of weight. However, when they came for routine examinations about 3 weeks after discharge from the hospital, they had already regained most of the loss and 3 months later their height and weight curves had risen to accord with their original patterns.

A girl who had enjoyed good health and vigorous growth up to 2 years 5 months, was then severely burned on the left leg and foot, requiring skin grafting and 9 weeks of hospital care. During this time she developed scarlet fever with local pectoral abscesses. As a result of all this she lost 6 pounds in weight but her height remained in its own channel. A few months later she had several acute respiratory infections which succeeded each other at short intervals with recurrent otitis media, catarrhal jaundice, measles, German measles, recurrent boils and styes, and whooping cough. During this period her weight dropped sharply and remained at a low level compared to its former position in the range until 5 years of age but her height progressed steadily at its previous level. After 5 years her weight dropped further and reached the bottom of the usual range for age and by this time her position in the range for height had dropped also. A fracture of the leg at 6 years 2 months required the wearing of a cast for 13 weeks; tonsils and adenoids were taken out at 7 years; and mumps occurred at 7 years 5 months. This crowded history of illness continued until she was about $9\frac{1}{2}$ years, after which her general health began to improve. The girl's skeletal development, which was slightly advanced up to 6 years and average from 6 to 8, fell somewhat behind the average for a time thereafter. Prior to the time of her adolescent growth spurt, when her health had improved, the weight curve started to climb in the range, followed by a similar change in the curve for height and acceleration of skeletal development. As a result her position in respect to the "norms" for all of these returned to the positions which they held at the end of her infancy. This girl illustrates the kinds of effects repeated illnesses commonly have upon the progress of physical growth and maturation. Other cases in the same Longitudinal Studies with similar histories of repeated illness, also show weight, height, and skeletal development falling behind in the same order. This course of events, however, is by no means invariable. In contrast to the girl above, a boy progressed much more in line with expectations, despite a seemingly comparable amount of illness and other children were observed to do the same.

It seems necessary to conclude that repeated illnesses, prolonged or severe, will interfere with normal progress only under certain circumstances depending upon the inherent capacities or adaptabilities of the child concerned or upon aspects of his care and environment, or probably a combination of both. The determining factors, not yet understood, may be largely inherited characters relating to the vigor of the growth potential and the capacity to adapt but health and nutritional status at the time of onset of illness, immunological status, and the care obtained may have equal significance.

All people are exposed to infection and other diseases and at some time experience illnesses. Children are especially subject to illnesses and accidents during their early years. Morbidity studies reported by Collins[2] have shown that morbidity rates from all causes have the highest rates in the youngest and the oldest age groups. The age-specific rates for total illnesses are high in infancy but fall steadily throughout childhood, reaching a low at about 20 years. Total illnesses generally remain low in number during the 14–25 year period after which they gradually rise to higher rates but by 60–65 years at least have not reached the level attained in infancy. Sydenstricker[3] using morbidity survey data calculated the percentages of people who had experienced no sickness, one, two, or over four sicknesses in a year. In childhood 50 per cent had more than four illnesses, while those having none were rare. There have been many limited studies of the incidence of illnesses but there is no general reporting of them and therefore official statistics reveal only evidence as to communicable diseases. The morbidity figures for children are, however, considerably broader than for the general population as a result of numerous studies made in schools, institutions, or well child conferences.

Physicians as well as parents often consider a given child "too frequently sick" or "exceptionally healthy" but if they compare him with his peers they may find that he is either sick just about as often as others or that he is somewhat different in this respect. We are accustomed to comparing a given child with his peers by using standards such as those for height and weight but we have not had any standard for illness experiences. How frequently "healthy" children are "sick" in any given country or community and what types of illnesses prevail have not thus far been sufficiently well studied. It is obviously important to have information as to these frequencies by age periods.

The Harvard Longitudinal Studies[4] showed that each of the 134 children followed comprehensively from birth to maturity experienced from a minimum of 17 to a maximum of 104 total illnesses during the first 18 years; total illnesses as used here include all kinds from all causes with various degrees of severity. The majority of boys experienced from 36 to 70 illnesses while the majority of girls had 20 to 36 illnesses. The median number for boys was 52 whereas for girls it was 42. This greater frequency of illness among the boys than the girls is characteristic of all age periods except from 10 to 14 years but most striking for the age periods 2 to 6 and 6 to 10 and least so during the first 2 years. It was found in this study that the median numbers of illnesses for each age period were as follows: in infancy, boys 6.7, girls 5.8; in the preschool period, boys 16.6, girls 12.7; in the school period, boys 12.2, girls 9.4; in early adolescence, boys 6.1, girls 6.2; and in late adolescence, boys 5.6, girls 4.0. The illnesses experienced by the group tended to be mild to moderate on the average throughout total childhood. In both infancy and in the preschool period the great majority of boys and girls had about equally mild and moderate illnesses. In the school period there were considerably more girls in the mild category than in the moderate but boys were still more nearly equal in each. The highest values for both the numbers and severities of illnesses were in the preschool period with relatively high values in infancy and the school period and a definite decrease after 10 years. They reached their lowest levels in late adolescence.

Children can experience the same amount of illness during the 18 years in different ways. Some have illnesses spread throughout these 18 years but the great majority experience illness more predominantly in a given period. The greatest number of individuals showed this predominance in the preschool years, with fewer illnesses in infancy or the school years and only rare illnesses in adolescence. Regardless of the amount of illness experienced in infancy, the preschool or school age periods, adolescence was always freer from illness.

In considering individuals we have observed changes with time in their illness experiences and have found marked differences for each child by age periods and also between individuals at the same age. These differences are based upon differences in type, severity, and frequency of illness. Although stressing the individuality of each child we have found a number of children alike or closely similar in their patterns of illness experiences. In fact 14 different patterns were recognized based on similarities within the group forming the pattern, in number and severity of total illness throughout childhood, on similarity of the age period at which illness predominated and on similarity of number and severity of illnesses within that given period.

The patterns including the greatest number of individuals were found to be the following:

(1) Mild total illnesses in moderate frequency for total childhood; illness predominating during preschool years.
(2) Mild total illnesses in moderate frequency for total childhood; illness predominating during school age period.
(3) Mild total illnesses in moderate frequency for total childhood; illness predominating during infancy.
(4) Mild and infrequent total illnesses, spread throughout childhood.
(5) Mild and infrequent total illnesses, predominating in the preschool age period.

Not only are there differences in the total incidence of illnesses but there is considerable difference from age to age in the relative importance of categories of diseases. Some will occur at any age, others occur chiefly at certain age periods and are the exception at others. Again the Harvard Longitudinal Studies brought new light on our knowledge.[5] The greatest proportion (over 75 per cent) of all illnesses experienced by 134 individuals were of the respiratory tract. This applies to all age periods as well as when the total 18 year span is considered. This proportion varies with age periods. It is lowest during the preschool period and highest in adolescence when other illnesses are relatively rare. Respiratory illnesses were predominantly infections but allergies constitute a sizeable proportion. The infections were mostly mild to moderate and of the "common cold" category. For example, during the age period 2 to 6 years, 67 boys accumulated a total of 1216 illnesses of all types, of which 997 were respiratory ones. Of the latter, 418 were mild and of short duration (less than a week), 320 were moderate while 134 were severe involving both upper and lower parts of the respiratory tract, the remainder having specific area involvements or complications. Respiratory illnesses predominated to such an extent that not a single child escaped them during their 18 years.

Gastrointestinal infections were at their highest levels in infancy, after which they declined steadily in frequency. Other illnesses occurred with a wide range of diagnosis but most of them were single events with no one that can be cited as occurring with particular frequency.

Accidents occurred relatively infrequently among these children as compared with total illnesses. This is of interest because although total deaths from all causes of illness exceed total deaths from all causes of accidents, accidents appear as the leading cause of death for most periods. This has been explained more fully in Chapter I. In the Harvard Longitudinal Studies accidents occurred more frequently in boys. They occurred least frequently in infancy for both sexes, most frequently among girls during the preschool period and among boys during the school period.

Compared with respiratory illnesses, the "communicable" diseases are relatively low in frequency but constitute the majority of all "other," nonrespiratory illnesses. These diseases occurred infrequently in infancy except whooping cough which occurred more frequently from 0 to 6 years; they increased rapidly between 2 and 6 years, remained high during the school age period, then rapidly declined; 93 of a total of 139 children had at least one of these specific illnesses between 6 and 10 years in contrast to only 10 having one or more in late adolescence. The most frequent communicable disease was measles. This occurred most commonly in the 2 to 6 year period while in contrast mumps occurred most commonly between 5 and 10 years for girls and 6 to 12 years for boys.

Many aspects of each of the three variables which account by their interactions for the course of disease, that is the pathogenic agent, the environment, and the individual child must be taken into account in attempting to understand the features of illness in any child. A very important one, however, is the age or stage of development of the child who is sick. Certain diseases may be expected to occur only during certain developmental periods or at least only rarely at others. The same disease may be expected to manifest itself very differently depending on the age at which it occurs. Examples of age-linked characteristics of illnesses are presented here but it will be seen that some are due essentially to the child while others are importantly influenced by the environment provided at this age.

An example of a factor within the child is the presence of the umbilical wound in the newborn, which may be the site of entry of local infection varying from the mild through the gangrenous and sometimes leading to septicemia. The newborn is poorly equipped to defend himself against invading microorganisms, and the premature infant even more so. He is particularly susceptible to pyogenic microorganisms such as the staphylococcus, or the gonococcus.

Again the neonatal period may provide an example of factors related to special environment. Thus obstetrical trauma occurring during delivery may cause conditions of various sorts which manifest themselves at birth or during the first days. Another example is the use of excessive oxygen with premature babies which may occasionally lead to retrolental fibroplasia.

Some anatomic attributes characteristic of given ages have an important influence not only on the pathology of the region involved, but also on that of the body as a whole. The influence of developmental anatomic changes in the respiratory tract on respiratory infections is an example of the relations between development and the susceptibility to disease. At birth nasal passages, particularly at the level of the posterior orifices, are narrow and easily obstructed which gives rise to difficult and noisy respiration and sometimes difficulty in eating. The eustachian tubes are short, wide, and almost horizontal; infections progress easily through them to the middle ear so that otitis media is relatively common in infants. The changes in the lymphoid tissues of the respiratory tract with age are responsible for some of the manifestation of respiratory infection in children. In general lymphoid tissue is relatively slight at birth, increases progressively, reaching a maximum at 6 to 10 years and regresses thereafter; after the age of 3 years the tonsils become relatively large and tonsillitis becomes a major problem for some years thereafter.

Different parts of the body develop functionally at unequal rates and this leads to different susceptibilities to involvement with disease at different ages, particularly age-specific responses to infections. The digestive tract is particularly vulnerable to infection by many pathogenic agents, regardless of the part or system originally involved. Gastro-intestinal disturbances are frequently the principal if not the only symptoms of infection in infancy with diarrhea and vomiting commonly being part of the symptoms of any illness at this age. The accompanying dehydration is also related to the physiologic characteristics of that age. In infancy water content in proportion to body weight is much higher than in later years; but although richer in water, the tissues lose it more easily and infants suffer from lack or loss of water much more quickly and severely than adults. Dehydration is one of the factors which causes infections in infancy to be more severe. Again, in infancy, pneumonia, whether pneumococcal or not has a lobular dissemination, while in the older child and the adult it is lobar.

A characteristic way in which an infectious disease tends to manifest differences with age is its decreasing tendency to spread from the initial location. Impetigo in the newborn, for example, tends to spread over much of the body, whereas in the older child it tends to be localized. Tuberculous infection in the infant when untreated is apt to spread from the lymph nodes to the meninges, or by miliary distribution throughout the body, whereas in the child during the preschool and school periods it is more likely to remain relatively quiescent in the tracheobronchial or cervical nodes, or possibly spread to the bones. These represent primary types of tuberculosis. During adolescence, on the other hand, quiescent lesions tend to become active, and the adult or secondary type with pulmonary involvement becomes more common. This is a destructive process, usually localized but spreading gradually within the lung tissue.

Here again tuberculosis demonstrates how the local response may vary according to the development of the host.

Change with development in immune responses to infection is another characteristic of age difference which is considered in the next section.

Within any particular age group similar clinical manifestations may be due to a variety of causes. This is particularly true in infancy. Regardless of the site of infection and of the causative agent, the clinical features may be much alike. Symptoms tend to be generalized and often the onset of illness is abrupt. A happy, active infant becomes languid, refuses food, is listless, cries or is apathetic with a sad expression; stools may be loose and temperature misleading. Physical findings are vague and difficult to relate to the cause. It is difficult, for example, to localize the abdominal pain of appendicitis in the young child. In the preschool and school years general reactions, such as high fever and convulsions may occur but gradually illness tends more and more to be accompanied by symptoms which are identifiable. As the child grows into adolescence clinical entities become more defined and more similar to the adult type.

THE DEVELOPMENT OF IMMUNITY
JOHANNES IPSEN, JR. AND HAROLD C. STUART

Natural Immunity

Man is constantly surrounded by a great variety of living organisms ranging from entirely harmless saprophytes on the one hand to dangerously pathogenic viruses, bacteria, or parasites on the other. Some of these live and multiply on his skin or respiratory mucous membranes, or in his gastrointestinal tract. To avoid infectious illnesses he must keep those capable of producing disease from invading and living within his body tissues where they may multiply and cause their specific kinds of infectious processes and pathological states. Some organisms such as influenza viruses appear in epidemic form periodically, each causing a characteristic disease in great numbers of susceptible individuals. Others (e.g. measles, mumps) are constantly within population groups and account for a continuing recurrence of epidemics of communicable diseases depending upon the frequency of susceptible individuals. These pathogens constitute a continuing threat to those who have not developed specific immunity to them or who have lost previous immunity due to the passage of time without sufficient exposure to maintain it.

Pathogenic organisms differ enormously between themselves in their communicability, method of spread and of entering the human body, likelihood of causing serious illness or death or of leaving specific permanent disabilities. Under natural circumstances a balance is established between man and these infectious organisms which permits survival of both with some continuing sacrifice of life on both sides and a high total incidence of infectious diseases in man.

The ideal method for man to prevent a serious infectious disease is to eradicate the specific organism involved from areas inhabited by human populations and to set up procedures for preventing their return. Much has been accomplished along these lines in many areas of the world, particularly in regard to the organisms causing yellow fever, malaria, typhoid fever, and parasitic diseases but constant vigilance is necessary to prevent their recurrence.

The development of the processes which lead to defensive reactions against infections in general and may provide specific and effective prevention against certain diseases is a most important aspect of development in childhood. At the time of birth the infant is protected to some degree against certain types of infection by immune substances transmitted to his blood from the mother's blood via the placenta. This protection, referred to as passive immunity is effective only against those diseases for which the mother herself has developed immune bodies in sufficient amount to be passed this way. These include measles, mumps, diphtheria, tetanus, smallpox, and poliomyelitis. The immune substances are gradually lost from the blood and for continuing effectiveness they must be replaced by substances produced by the infant's own immune mechanisms. The duration of passive protection varies considerably among diseases and individuals but it is usually lost by six months, and before this the infant if infected can develop some natural immunity without disease. Artificial immunizing procedures are usually more effective the less maternal antibody that remains. The young infant also has much lymphoid tissue which probably plays an important part in modifying or localizing infections for which he has as yet no well developed immunities. The newborn and particularly the premature infant appears to be especially susceptible to staphylococcus organisms and the colon bacillus (E. Coli). He does not acquire measurable passive immunity to whooping cough.

The natural development of immunity and immune responses to infectious diseases is for the most part on a specific basis, that is specific immune bodies or antibodies are formed to cope with a given organism. This specific defense is stimulated by contact with that organism so that the individual has a heightened resistance following such contact. In addition, there are numerous physiologic and cellular changes with development which add greatly to the competence of the individual to deal not only with infections but with other disease processes and thus to reduce the seriousness of these diseases when they occur. The specific antibodies which are developed to cope with single or closely allied infections come from the tissue cells, the lymphoid tissue being the principal source of them and they mainly appear in the gamma globulin fraction of the blood plasma. These substances begin to appear in the blood stream a few days after infection and last for a long but variable time. Even after the substances disappear from the circulating blood the cells which have been adapted by previous exposure to produce specific antibodies, will maintain for a long time the capacity of rapid production as a response to renewed exposure. These aspects of naturally acquired immunity have been mentioned principally because they provide the basis for many of the procedures adopted in connection with artificial immunizations to be described below.

The reason why certain infections persist in our society as "childhood diseases" is largely because of the natural increase in immunity toward adulthood. However, the peak incidence of these diseases usually occurs around the age of entry into school. This is not due to a change in immune status in respect to these infections between infancy and school age but rather to an increasing frequency of exposure to these diseases which comes with the development of the child's social contacts. Because of fewer social contacts, a single child is apt to contract childhood infections several years later in life than children in large families, as evidenced by studies of age incidence of measles[6] as well as of age prevalence of naturally acquired antibodies against poliomyelitis and streptococcus infections.[7]

The severity of infectious diseases has been shown to vary with age. In infancy they are likely to be relatively severe, due in large measure to the immaturity of physiologic processes. The changes due to physiologic development tend to localize infections, that is to prevent their becoming disseminated throughout the body. Tuberculosis is an example because changes in immunity have nothing to do with the striking changes in the pattern of its expression, as described in the preceding section. Their dependence upon physiologic changes is specifically indicated by the increased tendency for tuberculosis to become acute, and particularly for the adult type of tuberculosis of the lungs to occur about the time of the rapid physiologic and endocrine changes which occur during the pubescent period.

There are certain complications of infectious diseases in adolescence or early adult life which can be prevented by acquiring the diseases earlier in life and these infections tend to be more severe when older people have them. Examples are the common occurrence of acute involvement of the gonads as part of mumps in adolescence and more importantly the production of congenital defects in the fetus when the mother has German measles during the early weeks of pregnancy. These preventive possibilities make it advisable to permit children in good health to have contact during the preschool and school age periods with the usual communicable diseases of childhood which cannot fully be prevented by artificial immunization.

Allergies and Allergic Reactions

The responses of some individuals to the materials which provide immunity as well as to various complex large molecule substances, usually foreign proteins, may be grossly exaggerated. The resulting reactions are referred to as allergic and the hypersensitive state of the individual who thus reacts as an allergy. The substances which commonly cause such reactions are sera of various types, antitoxins, pollens, animal hairs or danders, whole proteins from food, and some drugs or other chemicals. The exaggerated responses occur when one or more to which an individual is allergic or hypersensitive comes in contact with skin or mucous membranes, is inhaled or ingested or is injected into the tissues. The responses tend to be more severe in the young and usually to occur after previous contacts which have initiated the abnormal immune response. The resulting symptoms may be urticaria (hives), angioneurotic oedema or certain rashes, vasomotor rhinitis, asthma, acute digestive upsets, or more severe generalized reactions. In infants and young children who inherit a trait which predisposes to this excessive response of immune mechanisms, there is a tendency to acquire specific allergies readily and to outgrow them. Hence a child tends to change the substances to which he is allergic and gradually to outgrow all or most of them as immunologic processes become stabilized.

Thus one child may start by being sensitive to egg white, then to several other foods, then to cat or dog hair and finally to pollens, losing one after another in the process. Allergies cause or complicate respiratory illnesses very commonly in infancy and the preschool years, at times being difficult to differentiate from respiratory infections. They account for a considerable amount of recurrent or chronic rhinitis, bronchitis, and asthma in childhood.

Artificially Induced Immunities

There are various means of stimulating immunity to certain specific infectious diseases, in some producing almost lifelong immunity, while in others obtaining varying degrees or durations of immunity. In the latter prevention can be improved with occasional small repeat immunizations or booster inoculations.

So-called passive immunization is similar to the temporary passive transfer from mother to fetus through the placenta. It may be accomplished for the infant artificially by taking blood from the mother or other immune individual and injecting it into the susceptible infant.

A further extension of this method involves use of pooled and concentrated hyper-immune serum from the blood of highly immune groups, now mostly in the form of gamma globulin prepared from these pools. The limitations of this method of protection as in the case of natural passive immunity are due chiefly to the short span of its effectiveness. It may be used appropriately with the intent to prevent the disease in question when exposure is known to have occurred and when the child is very young or sick. It is used more commonly to modify the course of a disease while permitting it to occur in mild form in order to secure truly acquired and usually lifelong immunity for the child. With the first purpose in mind a relatively large dose of immune serum is given as soon as possible after exposure, whereas with the second a small dose is given nearer the end of the incubation period of the disease in question. Injections of gamma globulin are used for measles to modify but usually not to prevent the disease, with this purpose in view. Current research with measles living-virus vaccine has produced a modified disease, with much the same immunity effect as with gamma globulin in modifying dosage combined with the natural disease. The usefulness of such a vaccine would be to produce mild disease at an appropriate time rather than to completely prevent it.

Vaccines are prepared from cultures of the bacteria or viruses causing the diseases which they are designed to prevent. There are two general types, killed vaccines and living but attenuated vaccines. Killed viruses require two or usually three injections to stimulate the organism for antibody production. Living vaccines may be used if they have been sufficiently altered or attenuated so that they can no longer produce the typical disease but still can induce immunity to it. A killed vaccine is easier to prepare, standardize, and safeguard than an altered living one, but usually it is less effective, that is it must be given in several consecutive doses as a "basic course." Periodic reinjections commonly referred to as "booster injections" are required to maintain adequate immunity in later life. A vaccine of this type provides fairly effective immunity to whooping cough (pertussis). Living cultures which have been attenuated to the point of safety but without loss of immunizing power have the advantage of a single dose for basic immunity, because they multiply in the human body for increased stimulus. One dose may even provide lifelong immunity. However, smallpox vaccine is an example of one which does not do so. Although a live smallpox virus is used which leads to multiplication of virus in the body and thus adds to the stimulation of immunity, revaccination from time to time is required. In contrast, yellow fever virus vaccine is the best example of one that produces long lasting immunity without disease. Still, experience with yellow fever vaccine is only 15 years old. The present BCG vaccine is an example of an altered but living bacterial vaccine used under special circumstances to induce immunity against tuberculosis. The vaccine currently used for the prevention of anterior poliomyelitis is a killed one and requires periodic revaccination to maintain an adequate level of immunity. However, there appears to be good promise of developing a safe preparation of an attenuated living virus vaccine. One type of immunizing procedure is the use of toxoids either individually, or in combinations with bacterial vaccines for pertussis, typhoid, or poliomyelitis. This is the effective method for prevention of diphtheria and tetanus.

Toxoids are prepared from toxins, which are specific protein substances excreted by the diphtheria and tetanus organisms. The toxins can be separated from the bacilli and purified, almost to chemical purity. Formalin treatment transforms toxins into toxoids with the effect that their disease producing power is erased while the antibody stimulating capacity is preserved.

Toxoid immunizations follow the rules of immunization with killed vaccines, that is, several doses are necessary for basic stimulation, and booster doses are needed at not too frequent intervals (4–10 years). Readiness to respond quickly to booster stimulus is maintained for at least ten years and possibly for considerably more.

This form of immunization has the remarkable feature that it exceeds the natural disease in its capacity to produce immunity. An efficient toxoid program can eradicate diphtheria from a community. However, it must be kept in mind that eradication of natural disease deprives the population of natural means of maintaining its immune status by incipient infections. In a modern society, the adult population is often found more susceptible to diphtheria than the children.

Active immunization with tetanus toxoid makes it possible, over the years to come, to replace the prophylactic dose of horse serum (passive immunization) with a booster dose of toxoid in case of injuries. Horse serum can cause severe allergic reaction (serum sickness), particularly in individuals that have had such previous injection. The immunity afforded by booster toxoid is more solid than that of antitoxic horse serum, but toxoid should only be used as emergency prevention if it is ascertained that the individual has previously had tetanus toxoid.

It is not intended here to discuss the presently recommended procedures for the routine administration of sera, toxoid preparations or vaccines, or the combinations of them in the care of infants and children. The products to be used are constantly being improved or extended and recommendations as to dosages, frequency of administration, number and combinations of substances to be used are constantly changing. Hence in planning programs or in advising mothers the latest recommended schedules should be referred to. The American Academy of Pediatrics issues a report on the control of infectious diseases which is revised from time to time by the committee assigned to keep abreast with the new knowledge relating to these procedures.[8] Another reason for not including more specific information about routines for clinical procedures is that these routines should be drawn up with consideration of the community in which they are to be applied. A report to the World Health Organization by a group of consultants convened by the Director-General agreed "that epidemiological conditions often vary greatly from country to country, from town to town and from time to time rendering it difficult to lay down any universal recommendations on immunization . . . , the morbidity and mortality of a disease will be determined by such factors as the number of infected persons, both cases and carriers, the number of susceptible persons, and the amount of opportunity for effective contact between them. Such considerations should govern the choice of the immunizing agents, the methods to be used, and the age groups and specially exposed groups of population in which these should be applied." [9]

It is important that professional members of any clinical staff providing health services for children should understand the principles and purposes of their immunization programs. Mothers who bring infants or children for immunizations should be informed what has been done and what further steps are to be taken; in fact, it is desirable that they be given a record of all tests or inoculations applied on specified dates. The habit of telling a mother that her child has now "completed his shots" is to be condemned. Usually she has no clear idea as to what diseases he has been protected against and this causes uncertainty as to what steps should be taken subsequently when the child is exposed to a communicable disease, in particular tetanus infection at injury, for which there is an available immunizing agent.

The current immunization programs carried out almost routinely in most of the United States include vaccination against smallpox, immunization against diphtheria, tetanus and pertussis (whooping cough), usually carried out together, and against poliomyelitis. All of these require one or more "booster" reinoculations but at varying intervals of time. It should be pointed out that there are three varieties of virus which cause poliomyelitis and that persons who have had one form of this disease require the protection of the vaccine which contains all three strains.

The Control of Tuberculosis

The BCG tubercle bacillus vaccine (Bacillus of Calmette and Guérin) is used in massive immunization programs in some countries where tuberculosis is rampant and control of spread by other means quite impossible. In the United States BCG vaccine should probably be used when there are special hazards as for example when infants are born into homes with open tuberculosis cases or with young doctors and nurses about to enter upon the care of patients. A disadvantage in the widespread use of BCG vaccine in a country with limited exposure is that this vaccine produces a positive tuberculin test and therefore destroys its diagnostic value as discussed below.

The control of tuberculosis in infancy and early childhood deserves special discussion here because of its own importance and the general principles which it exemplifies. It requires prompt recognition of active cases particularly within the family because at these ages infection is readily acquired and the disease tends to spread actively to various parts of the body. The mother with pulmonary tuberculosis and positive sputum must be separated from her newborn infant and young children until her sputum becomes negative under therapy. Finding positive cases in the population before they have caused infection in children is an important problem for public health departments. All efforts in the United States currently are focused on case finding, prevention of exposure, and early treatment of the diminishing numbers who acquire this infection. There are many ways in which the presence of tuberculosis may be suspected in a family by any alert visitor to the home and follow-up by clinical examination and chest X ray in such cases may prevent a series of childhood cases. A most effective method of case finding is the use of the tuberculin test routinely at selected ages, depending on circumstances, as part of health services to infants and children.

A positive tuberculin test indicates that the child has been infected with tubercle bacillus in sufficient extent to incite a natural immune response. It does not mean that the child did have more than microscopic or short lived infection or that he has active disease at the time of the test. For this reason an X ray of the chest is called for with all children found positive and close clinical follow-up should be provided. The fact that a young child is found on routine testing to have a positive tuberculin test provides an important lead to an active, but previously unrecognized case, usually an adult in his immediate environment. Such a finding should alert the health department to search for and bring under suitable treatment and temporary isolation the case in question. In view of the great risk of spread of tuberculosis when infection occurs in infants, positive tuberculin tests discovered during that period at least are customarily viewed as evidence of active and potentially serious infections which call for therapy with safe drugs like isoniazid without waiting for symptoms or positive signs of active disease. Diagnosis of the latter usually requires the taking of chest X rays of all suspect close contacts. With these useful tools available, tuberculosis in early life has been tremendously reduced in recent years and with further effort both in prevention and early treatment it can be reduced to an infrequently encountered problem. Today positive tuberculin tests are found in very small percentages among adolescents whereas a generation ago almost all had acquired infection by this age. This reduces the magnitude of the problem of eradication and the newer therapeutic agents enhance the possibilities for control of this disease among young adults as well as children. However, success depends upon intensive effort and prompt use of the measures at hand. This infrequency of positive reactions among young people enhances the usefulness of the test in high schools and colleges, again because it identifies those with probable active disease or recent infection.[10]

III

THE PREGNANT WOMAN, THE FETUS, AND PREPARATION FOR MATERNAL CARE OF THE INFANT

INTRODUCTION

Modern pregnancy care takes a full view of the family and sees its needs in a broad concept of the physical, emotional, and social environment in which its members live. The physical requirements of the mother-to-be, as a pregnant woman, are met with the best care that present day medical and surgical obstetrics can offer, and rightly so, for the first goal of pregnancy care is the safety of the mother and her baby in this great event. But "safe delivery" implies more. For the mother this is a chance to play her part in the development of her family unhampered by any injuries of childbirth and emotionally able to meet her increased problems. For the baby it is the right to be born well, uninjured, and with his potential for developing a useful life enhanced by an understanding family and community.

In a practical way, this concept of total care places responsibility upon many people, each with his own contribution: the mother, the father, the grandparents, in-laws, other relatives, friends, neighbors, doctors, nurses and other professional workers, the school, the church and the government. In spite of the variety of these influences, it is possible to maintain a coordinated program when there is wide understanding of the principles upon which this broad-spectrum care rests. They may be stated as follows:

(1) Physically, pregnancy produces changes in the entire body, which may be both normal and pathological, and require the service of the entire range of medical and surgical obstetrics.

(2) Pregnancy is part of a series of events which collectively affect the entire life span of the woman (and much of that of her husband), and is not an isolated 9 month incident.

(3) Each phase of pregnancy has its own particular problems, and each person his own reactions to them, which can be anticipated, prevented, or met with appropriately directed measures.

(4) The family is the unit around which all pregnancy care centers, but

it must be recognized that the family group is composed of individuals and that it must exist in a community larger than itself.

In this chapter the physical, emotional, and sociological bases for a broad concept of pregnancy care are examined, and the essentials of such a program outlined.

THE PHYSIOLOGY OF PREGNANCY AND CHILDBIRTH
SAMUEL B. KIRKWOOD

When any woman becomes pregnant she is no longer the same person, physically or emotionally. Pregnancy is not something that involves the uterus alone, but it causes profound changes in the structure and functioning of a woman's entire body and psyche.

An Understanding of the Menstruation

The physiology of pregnancy starts with the study of menstruation. Menstruation is, most simply, a periodic preparation for pregnancy. It is a mistake, however, to look upon menstruation as confined to a few days out of every month. There is no day during which a part of this process does not occur.

The average menstrual cycle — that is, the time from the beginning of one periodic flow until the next — is most commonly 28 days in length, and can be divided into two phases, each lasting approximately 14 days. The first phase starts with the actual flow and ends with ovulation. The second phase starts with ovulation and ends with the onset of the next flowing. In general, the first half of the cycle is concerned with building up the lining of the uterus, and is, therefore, often called the proliferative phase, while in the second half the structures of this built-up uterine lining are prepared as the bed for the fertilized egg. This second half of the cycle is called the secretory phase. Both the proliferative and the secretory processes are continuous and progressive.

Ovulation, which marks the change from one phase to the other, consists of the discharge of the egg, or ovum, from the ovary. This is the result of a steady development which has produced daily changes, culminating in the mature ovum, ready for fertilization.

All of these processes are under the control of the endocrine glands, especially the pituitary, ovaries, thyroid, and adrenals. The process is a complicated one, involving chemical substances, the hormones, which are secreted by these glands into the blood stream and are carried to other organs, where their action takes place. The pituitary gland seems to take the lead in this mechanism, although the control of the cyclic changes more properly lies in the interaction of these several endocrine glands.

Not only is the uterus affected by these hormone changes, but many other parts of the body as well. The character of the skin alters in the different phases of the cycle. The appetite varies. Weight changes, through a shift in the amount of body water excreted. Bowel and kidney function are not the same throughout. Wide swings in mood and temperament occur.

If the egg is not fertilized, further shifts in hormones take place, rather suddenly, and the lining of the uterus breaks down and is discharged as the menstrual flow. All other bodily changes that have occurred also are reversed. The whole process then starts over again.

On the other hand if the egg is fertilized in its passage through the Fallopian tube, it embeds itself in the soft, well-prepared, uterine lining and begins its 9 month development into the full term baby.

Pregnancy

When pregnancy occurs, more profound changes result. These go far beyond delivery of the child. Only when every organ and structure of the body has reverted to its normal, nonpregnant condition can the pregnancy be considered over. It is essential, therefore, to recognize these changes.

Psyche and Nervous System. Both the central nervous system and the autonomic nervous system become more labile during pregnancy. These are entirely normal changes, but they may cause symptoms which are disturbing unless understood. The psychological changes that occur are discussed in full in a later section. Here it is sufficient to make note of the wide swings in mood that are an entirely normal part of pregnancy, if seen in their proper perspective.

The autonomic nervous system loses its usual stability of control throughout pregnancy and indulges in a new lability of action. This is particularly noticeable in the control of the cardiovascular system. Flutterings of the heart — extra systoles — are common. Blushing occurs much more readily than before and, paradoxically, many women experience a sort of hot flash, otherwise usually associated with the menopause. Often a feeling of faintness comes on without warning. All these are disturbing but not serious. Other vagaries of the sympathetic nervous system lie behind many of the symptoms of other organ systems to be described below.

Blood and Circulatory System. The total volume of the blood increases during pregnancy by approximately one-third. Because the plasma volume increases relatively more than the red cells, a "pseudo-anemia" results, a physiological fact of great importance. From the point of view of treatment, the necessity for accurate differentiation between this and the true anemias is obvious. This additional blood volume supplies the needs of the enlarged uterus, and offers a margin of safety for the blood loss at delivery. Other changes in the blood enhance its ability to clot at the termination of pregnancy.

This added blood volume inevitably throws more work on the heart, estimated by Eastman to be at least 25 per cent. From the clinical viewpoint it is important to note that this increased load reaches at 28 weeks of gestation a peak from which it decreases as term approaches. Mostly because of the changing position of the heart as the uterus enlarges murmurs appear. While these are almost always functional, the possibility of organic disease must be kept in mind.

Varicose veins of the lower legs appear to some degree in almost every pregnancy, due in part at least to the increased intra-abdominal pressure of the enlarged uterus. Fortunately much can be done to alleviate this condition, even during the course of pregnancy.

Partly because of the changes in circulation in the legs, and partly because of an alteration in water retention, some edema of the ankles may occur. It can usually be controlled without difficulty.

Respiratory System. Pregnancy causes a congestion in the mucous membranes lining the entire respiratory tract. A majority of pregnant women suffer from a stuffiness of the nose and many are bothered by hoarseness and symptoms of a sinusitis. X rays of the lungs taken during pregnancy show increased markings that can be misinterpreted unless understood.

In spite of the encroachment of the enlarged uterus upon the excursion of the diaphram, the vital capacity is not reduced. The expansion of the thoracic cavity in width compensates for this encroachment.

Digestive System. Whether through changes in nerve control or hormone action, or both, the mobility of the entire gastrointestinal tract is reduced in pregnancy.

At the same time and perhaps for the same reasons, the amount of free hydrochloric acid and total acid in the stomach is reduced. Finally, the stomach, as pregnancy advances, finds itself pushed out of its normal position to a considerable degree. All these factors contribute to the heartburn, flatulence, nausea, and vomiting that plague almost all pregnant women. There is no doubt, however, that a large psychological element enters into the severity of these symptoms.

Constipation is the rule during pregnancy, but can usually be controlled through proper diet and exercise. Routine use of cathartics is to be avoided.

The decreased intestinal mobility, the resulting constipation, and the increased venous congestion of the pelvis all conspire to produce hemorrhoids. They occur in almost every pregnancy that approaches term. Fortunately, relief, if not cure, is always possible.

There seems to be a slightly increased tendency to attacks of gallbladder disease in pregnancy, but no significant alteration in liver function takes place.

Urinary System. That the urinary system is affected by pregnancy is apparent to every pregnant woman. Frequency of urination often accompanies early pregnancy, while the same condition recurs consistently in the late weeks. Infection attacks the urinary tract in pregnancy much more often than otherwise. Back of these changes is a profound alteration of the structure and action of the kidneys, ureters, and bladder.

Most prominent of these pregnancy changes are dilation of the kidney pelvis and dilation and tortuosity of the ureters. The cause of this probably lies in the same altered hormone-nerve reaction that affects the gastrointestinal tract. In any event, the result is a change in the usual pressure gradients, with ensuing slowing of the urine excretion. This amounts to a relative stasis which, as always, predisposes to infection.

The bladder suffers more acutely from mechanical displacement and pressure, both of which lead to congestion of mucosa and alteration of the outlet mechanism.

At times lactose may be excreted in the urine, but glycosuria must raise the question of diabetes.

Endocrine System. The best indication that pregnancy is a total bodily change lies in the changes occurring in the endocrine glands. To some degree all apparently take part, and it is through the proper interplay of their secretions that the normal progress of pregnancy is assured.

The pituitary gland shows unusual shifts in its cells, both the lobes taking part. The posterior lobe seems associated with the control of the contractions in labor, while the anterior contributes the ovarian stimulating hormones so necessary to maintenance of early pregnancy.

The thyroid, parathyroid, and adrenal cortex all show increase in size, indicative of added activity.

Most remarkable of all the organs producing hormones, however, is the placenta itself. This structure not only provides for the nourishment of the developing fetus as well as its excretory necessities, but manufactures the quantities of hormones necessary to carry the pregnancy to term. There is every reason, therefore, to watch the function of the placenta throughout pregnancy. Many of the routine questions and examinations that form a part of good pregnancy care are directed toward checking the condition of the placenta.

Skeletal System, Supportive Structures, and Skin. Pregnancy imposes a particular load upon the skeleton ligaments, muscles, and connective tissues of the woman's body. In the male the problem of weight-bearing and motion — the prime functions of these structures — is uncomplicated, and can be met by a single-purpose design. In the female, on the other hand, all of the pelvic structures must be formed for a dual purpose — weight-bearing and child-bearing. Periodically, with each pregnancy, even further modifications occur to meet the physiological needs of parturition.

The pelvic bones, joined by the three pelvic joints, normally are united firmly and therefore function as a single structure. In pregnancy, again under hormone influence, these three joints separate slightly. The two sacroiliacs absorb water into their tissues, relax and the synoviae increase. The pelvis becomes a mobile, plastic structure, well able to ease the stresses and strains of delivery, but far less capable of supporting the woman's body and the transmission of motion. As term approaches these changes grow steadily more marked.

With this loosening of the base through which weight is borne and motion transmitted from the spine to the lower legs, it is only natural that the body mechanics of posture and walking should be considerably altered. Particularly, as the uterus enlarges, the center of gravity of the body shifts forward. A compensatory increase in the curve of the low back permits the shoulders to be held farther back and balance maintained; but in so doing the typical, somewhat waddling gait of pregnancy is acquired. Unfortunately the strains thus produced often cause discomfort if not actual pain. With proper care much of this can be alleviated.

It is quite wrong to think of the pelvis in terms of its bones alone. Much more important in respect to possible injury to the mother are the soft parts which line the bony canal. These are the muscles, the connective tissues, blood vessels, and mucous membranes which support the uterus, line the vagina, and form the pelvic floor. During pregnancy all these structures take up fluid and become much more vascular. Elastic tissue increases. All these changes are purposeful, directed toward reducing resistance during delivery but the obstetrician must be alert to the symptoms which may result from this increase in the vascular bed.

Other joints in the body are affected. Most commonly a thickening of the tissues surrounding the finger joints leads to stiffening of their action, a situation most distressing to typists and musicians. The toes are occasionally affected in the same way. The feet tend to spread as pregnancy advances, due certainly in part to the increased weight of the body, but also in part to a change in the supporting tissues of the foot. Rarely, the knees, elbows, and shoulders may be involved.

Increased pigmentation forms the most common change of the skin in pregnancy. Characteristically, the skin darkens about the nipples, the genitals, in a vertical midline of the abdomen, and on the face. The last may become so prominent as to resemble a mask. Abdominal scars often enlarge. Tiny, spidery blood vessel formations appear in the skin over different parts of the body. The palms of the hands show reddening, though whether from hormone or dietary influences is not certain. The skin elsewhere in the body, but particularly in the face, may become more or less turgid so that the features grow blunted. All of these skin changes gradually disappear after delivery.

Reproductive System. The uterus during pregnancy grows from an organ weighing barely 2 oz to one weighing more than 24 oz. Paradoxically, its wall grows thinner but vastly increases its muscular power to produce some of the strongest contractions of any organ in the body. Its blood vessels enlarge so that they may meet the greatly increased oxygen demand of the uterus itself, the placenta, and the fetus.

As pregnancy advances the consistency of the outlet of the uterus, the cervix, changes to permit it to dilate during labor.

Through an increase in elastic tissue and an uptake of fluid in its walls the vagina becomes both more distendable and elongated. The reason for these changes is obvious.

The external genital organs likewise become turgid with fluid and increase in vascularity. The breasts grow somewhat softer and larger throughout pregnancy and the pigmentation of the nipples and areolae is markedly increased. The full effect of pregnancy on the breasts, however, is not accomplished until lactation becomes established after delivery. The breasts need good support during pregnancy and especially during lactation.

General Metabolism. In most studies the average weight gain of the mother during pregnancy is 24 lb. The ideal gain during pregnancy, however, must be adjusted for each individual, since proper gain is related both to the nonpregnant weight and a "desirable" weight. Several elements compose this figure in approximately the following amounts: fetus $7\frac{1}{2}$ lb; placenta 1 lb; amniotic fluid $1\frac{1}{2}$ lb; breast enlargement 3 lb; uterine enlargement 2 lb; maternal protein storage 4 lb; maternal water retention $4\frac{1}{2}$ lb.

From the beginning of the fourth month of gestation onward there is a steady rise in the basal metabolic rate. It is likely that the metabolism of the fetus and the placenta accounts for most of this increase.

Pregnancy alters the metabolism of all the essential nutritional elements. Water is retained in the body, partly in the increased blood volume and partly in the tissues themselves. This accounts for almost 5 lb in the total weight gain, and it is lost rapidly after delivery. Sugar metabolism is not well understood. It appears that there is a lowered tolerance for sugar; certainly a considerable number of pregnant women show glycosuria. What the significance of these two observations is, especially in reference to later development of diabetes, remains to be settled by future research. The storage of nitrogen by the mother varies, but it approximates 300 gm, equivalent to 1875 gm of protein. The fetus and its adnexa utilize, in addition, approximately 140 gm of nitrogen, equivalent to 875 gm of protein. An increase in the fat content of the blood occurs. The purposes for which this maternal storage takes place and its ultimate utilization are discussed later in this chapter.

Labor

Although there is considerable variation, the average normal pregnancy reaches term about 266 days after fertilization of the ovum. This corresponds approximately to the traditional 280 days after the first day of the last menstrual period. This latter method of estimating date of confinement is valid only for those women who flow regularly on a 28 day cycle.

At a given time a chain reaction is set off which leads to the birth of the baby. Throughout pregnancy the uterus has been contracting, though slightly, with fair regularity. In the last three months these contractions grow more definite and can be felt as a rhythmic hardening of the uterus. These so-called Braxton-Hicks contractions often come in bouts, and are usually painless. During this period the cervix has softened and flattened. What actually stimulates the onset of labor remains unknown. Certainly hormone secretion shifts are operative to a considerable degree, and changes in the blood vessels supplying the placenta are particularly apparent. Both of these factors, however, occur relatively gradually. Reynolds feels that the determining factor is the distensibility of the uterus. Probably the trigger mechanism is the interaction of all these elements, labor starting when a critical point is reached in the changing of controls, with stimulation being increased while inhibition is lowered.

In any event the contractions acquire new characteristics. They become definite, establish a true rhythmic pattern, and become painful. As labor progresses the pains increase in severity, in frequency, and in duration. A blood-tinged mucous is discharged from the vagina — the "show" of labor — evidence that the cervix is further thinning and stretching to provide the opening through which the baby can emerge from the uterus. Sometimes at the beginning of labor, more often during its course, the membranes which surround the baby and confine the amniotic fluid ("the waters") rupture. Labor usually intensifies thereafter. When the cervix has become fully dilated the "opening" of the uterus is complete and the first stage of labor has been concluded.

There still remains the obstruction of the birth canal to be overcome. Because the pelvis is no simple bony ring, the baby must follow a tortuous course from the inlet to the outlet of the canal. This it does by a series of automatic maneuvers, directed by the uterus, abdominal wall, and diaphragm, accompanied by the "bearing-down" pains, the contractions forcing the fetal head and body against the varying planes formed by the ligaments, muscles, and bones of the pelvis. As the vagina and vulva stretch, the baby is born. This ends the second stage of labor.

Contractions continue, for the placenta and membranes must still be discharged. As they are delivered, one of the most critical periods of the entire labor is reached. At this moment the huge blood vessels which have supplied the placenta throughout pregnancy are wide open. Unless the uterus contracts properly at this point, squeezing shut those open vessels, the mother is in imminent danger from hemorrhage. Here the reserve she has built during pregnancy, the skill of her attendants, and the facilities available come to her aid. With the continuation of good uterine contractions bleeding is controlled, the third stage of labor is over, and the puerperium begins.

Puerperium

The postnatal period physiologically brings return to a healthy, uninjured nonpregnant state. Involution marks all these processes save one, lactation.

With the observation of the lochia — the normal postnatal vaginal flow — and the reduction in size of the uterus, the process of uterine involution can be closely followed. Particular attention should be paid to the involution of the cervix. Only when its vaginal portion is properly and completely covered with intact squamous epithelium can the cervix be said to have returned to normal, and then only if there is no abnormal discharge from the mucous glands of the canal. During this time the excess fluid in the pelvic tissues is absorbed, and the local vascular bed is reduced gradually to normal. Pelvic joints, ligaments, and muscles tighten up, and the pelvis again becomes a firm foundation for the woman's body. Severe edema disappears and the skin loses its marks of pregnancy. With exercise and time even the abdominal wall regains its former firmness.

The other organ systems gradually resume their nonpregnant state. The blood elements revert to normal ratios, and the dilated blood vessels shrink to usual size. Congestion of the respiratory tract disappears. The customary mobility of the bowel is resumed. Urinary function is stimulated in the early puerperium as the body loses its stored water. The bladder resumes its normal position as the uterus involutes, and the ureters become narrow tubes once again. In spite of this, infection acquired during pregnancy may persist well into the puerperium.

Following delivery, excess hormones are excreted, but the change back to normal is not completed for the entire endocrine system until lactation is concluded and the menstrual periods have been reestablished. Usually the monthly cycle is not resumed during lactation, although it occurs sometimes and without affecting nursing. Nursing is, therefore, no sure protection against conception. If the mother does not nurse, the periods on the average return within 3 or 4 months, although they may be delayed as long as 8 or 9. Sometimes a definite change in menstruation follows even an entirely normal pregnancy — periods previously irregular become regular, while a regular cycle may return entirely out of rhythm. Unless other symptoms are apparent, such menstrual alteration need not cause concern. Fortunately, painful menstruation many times is cured by pregnancy.

The breasts, under hormone influence and the mechanical stimulation of nursing, enlarge postpartum, reaching a point of maximum congestion by the third or fourth day postpartum. Following the early secretion of thick colostrum, the milk becomes more liquid and flows freely. Gradually the supply adjusts to the baby's demands. Soreness of the nipples may be present at first, but usually disappears as the milk flow increases. Following weaning the breasts gradually soften, and milk secretion ceases. The breasts are usually left somewhat less firm and slightly more pendulous than before pregnancy.

Although changes in her figure are accepted during pregnancy, following delivery the mother looks hopefully to a return to her former self. This is not a vain hope, for the "pregnant waddle" disappears with a refirmed pelvis, and posture returns as back and abdominal muscles gain strength. Breasts may need slightly more support than before, but this is readily available, and is further enhanced by improved carriage.

Sexual desire reappears gradually, though subject to considerable variation. Local physical soreness, fatigue, and the diversion of baby-caring all tend to reduce the urge to resume sexual relations. A considerate husband recognizes this, but a loving wife steps back into her role without unnecessary delay.

Postpartum there are usually two periods of depression. Both tend to be acute and occur apparently without reason, least of all to the mother herself. The third and seventh days are most usually affected. It is likely that hormone shifts contribute largely to this situation. Reassurance is all that is needed. It should be noted, however, that the present necessity of early hospital discharge may be poorly timed in relation to these emotional lows.

COMPLICATIONS IN PREGNANCY AND CHILDBIRTH
SAMUEL B. KIRKWOOD

Most gestations are entirely normal, but many have minor upsets, and a few develop serious abnormalities.

The minor complications for the most part rise from slight deviations of the normal physiological changes that have been described in the preceding sections. Their worst effect is usually annoyance, and their relief is relatively simple.

The major abnormalities, however, can be serious to the extreme. They tend to group themselves by type into the natural divisions of pregnancy.

By far the most common abnormality of the first 3 or 4 months of pregnancy is vaginal bleeding. Many women have some slight vaginal bleeding during early pregnancy, but it must always be considered a danger signal. There is no way of telling for sure at the outset whether or not a miscarriage is threatening. Abdominal pain is another symptom that should be reported to the doctor. The combination of the two may mean real difficulty, miscarriage or tubal pregnancy.

The middle 3 months of pregnancy are usually quite clear of complications.

In the last third of gestation, although premature labor sometimes complicates the picture, there are two main concerns. Bleeding is the first and is ominous. At this time it indicates the possibility of a separation of the placenta before delivery, or finding later an abnormal position of the afterbirth, in either of which cases expert care is needed. The second is toxemia; high blood pressure, albuminuria, and weight gain being its "great 3" symptoms. This disease is peculiar to pregnancy, and still rather poorly understood. It can lead to the most serious complications of pregnancy. But it can be controlled with continual watchfulness by doctor, nurse, and patient. The management and control of toxemia is considered at some length below to demonstrate the manner in which representatives of different health disciplines may work together for best results in maternal health services.

During labor itself the dangers to both mother and infant are primarily from abnormalities of the birth process such as poor contractions, obstructed passageway, malpositions of the baby, and lacerations, ruptures, and bleeding. All of these dangers can be avoided or lessened by well trained accoucheurs and good facilities. Any of them can lead to abnormalities in the infant at birth, especially as a result of damage to his nervous system. These effects may threaten his survival immediately after birth or limit his capacity to develop normally. Smith[1] has listed the principal natal causes of difficulties encountered in the infant shortly after birth as anoxia, analgesia resulting from drugs administered to the mother, anesthesia given to the mother during delivery, as well as the birth trauma and premature delivery resulting from maternal conditions discussed above.

The major problems after delivery is over usually fall into one of three groups: infection, bleeding, and toxemia again. Even in these days of the antibiotics infection still plays a major role in postpartum complications. Uterus, urinary tract, and breasts are the most common locations. Bleeding in this period usually occurs because of retained bits of the placenta or an improper resolution of the placental site. It can be serious. Much less common than before delivery, toxemia nevertheless can cause difficulty at this time.

While the dramatic abnormalities do not appear in the interval between pregnancies, this is an important time to watch for chronic difficulties that may have arisen during pregnancy and have persisted. Heart disease, hypertension, pyelonephritis, vascular nephritis, and anemias would fall into this class.

The Team Management of Toxemia

The control and treatment of toxemia of pregnancy is a practical example of team work in care during pregnancy.

In his early instruction in connection with prenatal care the physician has discussed the symptoms and signs of toxemia: headache, unusual or untimely nausea, swelling of the extremities or face, blurring of vision, abdominal pain. He has explained the significance of increase in blood pressure, weight gain, and of albuminuria. The first line of defense, a preventive one, is an informed patient.

Because all forms of health education require repetition, the nurse reiterates this teaching in her informal discussions with the pregnant mother in the doctor's office or in the clinic. Frequently, the nurse is responsible for more formal classes in which these matters are considered. Even more important is the observation by a visiting nurse in the patient's own home. Instruction in the office is inevitably abstract to some degree, but teaching in the home assumes an intimacy and ease of application that greatly increase its value.

The initial history may have raised warning signals of old nephritis, pyelitis, or previous hypertension. The physical examination would have shown any lability of blood pressure or preconceptual overweight. An estimate of the mother's nutritional status and usual diet as well as the general emotional and social climate of the family are useful guides to underlying environmental conditions that may spell later trouble. At this stage this information should be easily obtainable by the physician and his nurse.

The routine prenatal visit offers a continuing check on all these premonitory signs. It is here that first evidences of an increasing blood pressure should be noted. Although an arbitrary 140/90 is taken as a guide line between normal and abnormal, a significant rise in either diastolic or systolic even though below these limits is a warning. Only with blood pressure recorded regularly, often best by the nurse, can any such important change be noted. The same may be said of the test for urinary albumin. Rapid weight gain is a cause for concern. Weight change is a highly sensitive indicator of hidden edema, part of the early picture of toxemia. But it requires a careful evaluation taking into consideration usual weight, individual family history and body weight, a desirable pre-pregnancy weight, and a desirable total weight gain and rate of gain. It is obvious that successive weights throughout pregnancy must be taken as nearly as possible under standard conditions.

This type of preventive care depends upon an adequate minimum number of visits. The usually accepted routine calls for visits every four weeks for the first 28 weeks, every two weeks for the next 8 weeks, and weekly thereafter until delivery.

If any symptom or sign of toxemia appears, closer supervision is mandatory. The frequency of visits is increased. A most valuable contribution to the control at this time is a home visit by the nurse between office or clinic visits. This gives an additional series of observations of particular value since they record the patient in her own environment free of the tensions of a visit in the physician's office.

Control of the disease at this stage is accomplished through additional rest and diet regulation. Two additional members of the team contribute to this phase of treatment, the nutritionist and the social worker.

The nutritionist by her training has developed special skills in appraising dietary histories and evaluating nutritional status and needs. In general, the diets used are high in protein and low in salt to varying degrees. Calories are adjusted to individual needs. In fact, the entire diet must be tailored to each patient, for the more severe the symptoms the greater is the stringency of the diet. Unfortunately, diet control is not always simple. The patient's will to cooperate in most instances is the deciding factor. In some way the mother must be motivated to follow the prescribed diet, either for her own sake or her baby's or both. Particularly in clinic work the obstetrician and the nutritionist work in close coordination. It is unfortunate that very little of the same type of consultation service in nutrition is available to the obstetrician in his private practice.

The prescription of additional amounts of rest for the mother at home is not always easily followed. The difficulties lie largely in the social and economic interactions of the family. In recent years particularly the social worker has been more and more involved, and her contribution is very considerable. When possible, home visits by the social worker have added much to the comprehension of underlying problems. Solutions may not be found at all in traditional medical therapy.

In a disease so intimately connected with alterations of the vascular system and its neuropsychic control some answer to emotional difficulties must be sought from the beginning. A mental health worker helps greatly either in working directly with the patient, or, more often, through consultation with the obstetrician and his other co-workers.

The use of mild sedative drugs, vascular dilators, diuretics, or hormones in this ambulatory phase of treatment comes strictly within the direction of the physician. The nurse may act in the role of assistant, and through her home visits is in the best position to observe critically and at first hand their effects.

It is axiomatic that toxemia is never "cured" without ultimate termination of pregnancy and postpartum involution. Hence, once a patient enters toxemia control she remains under it. If the measures thus far described prove to be inadequate, the patient must be hospitalized. The actual treatment in the hospital does not vary much from the outpatient period. Some measures can be pursued more vigorously, but in general the advantage lies in the complete control of the environment and the opportunity for continuous close observation. The physician and nurse of the team are most fully involved, but the other members still may assist in the over-all therapy of the family.

Hospitalization does permit use of the most effective method for attacking toxemia, induction of labor. Naturally, induction of labor before term carries varying risks of prematurity. This is a hazard that must be judged against increasing danger to the mother and her baby of continuing and increasing toxemia. Great professional ability is needed to balance these opposing factors and to choose the optimum time for induction. Quite apart from the toxemia, the final determining factor, of course, is the condition of the cervix, that is, its "inductability."

If control measures fail to stop the progress of the disease in its pre-eclamptic or preconvulsive phase, eclampsia results, one of the most dread complications of pregnancy. In the sense that eclampsia is always preceded by pre-eclampsia, the occurrence of convulsions in a patient marks a failure of treatment. For the most part, this means that control measures were begun too late, were poorly chosen, or were applied with insufficient vigor. Although the mortality for both mother and fetus is high, eclampsia is not a hopeless condition. But prompt, skillful, and continuous treatment is necessary. The patient must be admitted to a hospital. The convulsions are controlled by judicious sedation, temporary anesthesia, quiet, and the usual protective measures for patients having seizures. Neurosedatives and vasodilators are used, often intravenously. Intravenous fluid is given under careful balance control, and meticulous watch is kept over the electrolytes of the body fluids. Cardiac action and pulmonary ventilation are guarded. Edema is treated vigorously; pulmonary edema is a particularly ominous development. In most clinics, once the convulsions have been controlled and the patient's condition somewhat stabilized, labor is induced, usually from below, though at times delivery is by Caesarean section. The successful treatment of eclampsia is a triumph for the hospital staff.

The full team comes back into the picture after this period of treatment. Because of the tendency of toxemia to repeat in subsequent pregnancies, all efforts are directed in the time between conceptions to measures which will prevent its return. Much the same methods apply here as were used in treating the ambulatory phase in pregnancy, reliance again being placed upon rest, diet, and weight control. Hormone treatment has been helpful, but long term therapy with vasodilators less so. Often most effective is rearrangement of family habits to reduce tensions and stress of work for the mother. Obviously, this is broad spectrum management.

In this discussion of the team approach in the treatment of toxemia, each member of the team has been represented as an individual person. Once again it must be stated that the broad concept of the team approach is not necessarily dependent upon the presence of each worker. The treatment outlined above includes fields of service which are properly represented in the most effective attack upon this disease. Whether all these areas are supplied by one professional worker, or with the aid of others, is secondary to the fact of their recognition.

FETAL DEVELOPMENT AND CONGENITAL MALFORMATIONS
HAROLD C. STUART AND THEODORE H. INGALLS

Nature has provided in the uterus of the normal, healthy woman the only safe place for the fetus during most of the 9 months of its development. During the first 2 months after conception, known as the embryonic period, the basic tissues, organs, and systems of the human body are formed through a series of complex and rapid developmental changes, brought about principally through cell multiplication and cellular differentiation and organization. This is a crucial and hazardous stage of fetal life for two reasons. The first is that during the few days after conception the fertilized egg must become successfully implanted in the uterine lining, and soon thereafter the placental circulation must be developed so that the fetus may receive nourishment from the maternal circulation. Chance errors in development may occur during these days and lead to the death and expulsion of the embryo. Being microscopic in size at this time, such loss is not observed. The second reason is that during the succeeding weeks, development is extremely rapid and complex, although quantitatively growth is still very small in an absolute sense. It is in connection with these rapid developmental changes that many gross malformations have their origin.

By the end of the first trimester the fetus has taken on a form with general human resemblances but with striking differences in segmental proportions; all of the body systems, tissues, and organs have been laid down in a basic way. The fetus then is less than 10 cm in length and weighs less than 15 gm. If there are no faults of implantation and if no teratogenic infections or stresses have occurred during early pregnancy, development of the embryo proceeds normally.

The second trimester of fetal life is a relatively safe one, characterized by the most rapid linear growth of any period of development, but with only moderate increase in body weight. Further development of all the systems of the body continues during this middle period of fetal life up to the point of rudimentary functioning of most organs and tissues. At the end of this period survival may be possible outside of the uterus if premature birth should take place but the risks are very great because of the extreme immaturity of most vital parts.

The third trimester is characterized by continuing rapid growth and increased development of muscles. There is also an increase of fat in the subcutaneous tissues, providing an important insulating covering as protection against the lower temperature of the external environment after birth. Increase in body weight during this period on the average is more rapid than in any period in childhood. There is also further maturing of all body organs and tissues toward more adequate functional capacities in anticipation of the needs of existence after separation from the mother. This development attains its highest stage in respect to the structure of the central nervous system and head area and particularly the mouth, the respiratory mechanism, and the heart and blood vessels. When full term is reached these organs are usually prepared to make promptly the necessary adjustments to extrauterine life. The major hazard during the third trimester is that labor will be initiated prematurely and that as a result the normal risks of the early neonatal period will be increased by the immaturity of the mechanisms essential for survival. The second hazard is that labor may be delayed, introducing different risks, an important one being difficulty during delivery due to overgrowth of the fetus.

The events of the short period of labor and delivery have an important bearing on the health and survival of the infant, both at the time and during his later development. Some of the complications which may lead to injury of the fetus in his passage through the birth canal have been mentioned in the preceding section. The developmental changes which must occur in the infant during the neonatal period for successful adaptation to extrauterine existence may be interfered with by injury during delivery and thus prevent his survival, or affect in a variety of ways his immediate or subsequent health or development.

The gross malformations which are found in infants at birth, or shortly thereafter, for the most part result from errors in embryonic development during the first 3 months of gestation. Abnormalities of growth or development may occur during the second or third trimesters of pregnancy and occasionally fetal parts may be so damaged by disease or injury at these times as to lead to defects. For general purposes, however, the term congenital malformation refers to anomalies or defects resulting from errors in embryonic development. If the initial malformations are such as to make fetal existence impossible, death and expulsion of the fetus occurs early in pregnancy. If the malformations are not incompatible with fetal existence, however, the infant will probably be born alive but may be unable to adjust to extrauterine existence. Many neonatal deaths are, in fact, the result of congenital malformations, these usually being secondary only to the complications of premature birth as a cause of death during early infancy.

All parts and organs of the body are subject to errors in development and the defects in individual cases frequently are multiple and may involve several different systems. There are also many stages or degrees of the expression of a particular type of defect, as for example the extent of the defect in an infant with a cleft palate. If the combination of defects is not sufficiently disabling to cause the death of the infant during the early days or weeks of postnatal life, the child may survive to adult life, but with continuing physical or mental handicaps. These may differ enormously in type and degree, and differ in the extent to which they may diminish life expectancy or the possibilities for satisfactory life adjustments.

Malformations of the skeleton are the leading cause of crippling in childhood. Fortunately many malformations, including intestinal and other atresias, are now subject to surgical correction. Unless immediately corrected, many malformations would be incompatible with life. Certain cardiac defects can now be corrected which otherwise would greatly shorten life expectancy or lead to chronic invalidism. Many disfiguring defects, which may not be important to physical health but are handicaps to personality development and life adjustment, also can be improved.

The causes of congenital malformations are many and complex, and often cannot be identified. The primary objectives are their prevention when the causes can be identified, early recognition and correction when they cannot be prevented, and, for the remainder, long continuing care,, education, and training to minimize lifelong disabilities. The last approach requires special consideration of the growth and development of the individual so handicapped, with the objective of utilizing to the full his normal assets and protecting and promoting his total development to the fullest extent possible.

It must be appreciated that there rarely is only one cause which can account for one type of defect, but rather that several different causes can do so. Also, most known causes of congenital defects can produce different types of defects or combinations of several. A single agent, such as infection with German measles virus in pregnancy, to be described further below, often may lead to more than one defect in the unborn baby. The kinds produced usually depend as much on the fetal age at which the injurious cause operated as on the nature of the cause itself.

Much is still to be learned about the interaction of prenatal environment and heredity. The part which the genes play in leading to malformations cannot be ascertained with accuracy except in lower forms of life. Some defects appear to be predominantly inherited characters that are encountered repeatedly in some families, whereas others, such as mongolism are of unpatterned occurrence. Genetic traits which are familial in their occurrence lead repeatedly to characteristic syndromes but even in such cases the degree of expression of the characteristic defects varies considerably among the afflicted young, depending apparently in part upon the environmental circumstances which are operating during the embryonic period. The concept presently favored is that the degree to which the defects become manifest depends significantly upon environmental circumstances, particularly during the critical initial eight week period of embryonic life. Environmental circumstances at this time can produce a variety of gross defects operating indirectly through their effects upon the mother. The particular environment involved is the immediate one of the uterus which is dependent upon the condition of the mother's entire body.

The environmental conditions which it is known may damage the embryo and lead to various defects are numerous and there are probably many others which have not yet been recognized. The administration of quinine medication to the mother may result in the congenital deafness of her child. This is a chemical cause of embryonic injury. Maternal anoxia will result in the oxygen deprivation of the fetus and when the mother experiences very high body temperatures injury to the embryo has a thermal cause. Excessive radiation as a result of overexposure either during roentgen therapy or atomic explosion can affect the fetus. An endocrine disorder of the mother such as hypothyroidism may lead to cretinism in the infant. Mechanical trauma to the mother can occasionally cause lifelong crippling of the unborn child though far less often than usually supposed. Finally, nutritional deficiencies in the mother may be responsible for congenital malformations in the baby, although the extent and character of this relationship in human beings has not as yet been established. In animal experiments it has been shown clearly that marked deficiencies of specific nutrients or of oxygen do register their effects on the offspring.

Maternal syphilis can be transmitted to the fetus during pregnancy, causing defects in the tooth buds and damage to the ears or eyes, and causing anomalies which lead to deafness or blindness. These are consequences of fetal infection, however, and differ from developmental defects resulting from metabolic disorders of the mother. Other than syphilis, the most striking example of a specific maternal disease that may cause embryologic defects is that of rubella, or German measles. If this virus infection is acquired by the mother during the first 8 or 10 weeks of embryonic life, there is a strong possibility that the fetus will be so damaged that it may present at birth such defects as deafness, cataract, or heart abnormality, or combinations of such defects. Similar defects have rarely been reported following other viral infections in early pregnancy.

Congenital malformations may be classified structurally according to the nature of the disturbance in development. Some are simple arrests as, for example, when the palate fails to close or the lips fail to unite at the midline, or when the chambers of the heart do not fully close or differentiate. Other malformations are duplications of normal structures, such as a double ureter. Identical twins basically belong in this category. Some defects represent persistence of rudimentary fetal structures which normally disappear or change with late development, but in these cases fail to do so.

Mongolism appears to be a form of arrested development of the whole organism, including the brain that has its onset at about the eighth week of gestation. No single cause is believed to operate, but a significant feature is that most infants manifesting this defect are born to mothers late in their reproductive lives. The average age of mothers of mongoloid infants is over 40 years, whereas that of most mothers is under 25. This fact suggests the probability that chronic disturbances of mothers, such as endocrine upsets and diseases of the uterus, may register their impact at selected vulnerable stages of growth rather than evenly throughout pregnancy.

MATERNAL NUTRITION DURING PREGNANCY

BERTHA S. BURKE

As a preventive factor nutrition can offer its greatest benefits in the field of maternal and child health. During pregnancy the physiological processes of the body are greatly altered and additional demands are imposed on the maternal organism. Digestion and absorption are often impaired in the early months. Nutritional requirements are considerably increased as pregnancy advances.[2] Considerable evidence from both animal and human research has accumulated in the last quarter of a century which indicates that faulty nutrition during pregnancy may affect the pregnant woman and/or her fetus in ways not usually considered as signs of malnutrition. Much has been learned from studies of the natural course of pregnancy, particularly from repeated observations of pregnant women and of the physical condition of their infants at birth. Several such studies have pointed to faulty diet as a factor associated with unfavorable course and outcome of pregnancy.

The principal relations which have been found to exist between the nutrition of the mother and the events and outcome of pregnancy concern: (a) the incidence of premature births, neonatal deaths, stillbirths, congenital malformations, and other unsatisfactory physical findings among infants born alive and surviving; (b) the size of the infant at birth, as reflected in length and weight; (c) the over-all course of pregnancy including the incidence of toxemia. Evidence[3, 4, 5] as to these relations will be discussed briefly.

In a study of 216 pregnancies conducted by the Department of Maternal and Child Health, Harvard School of Public Health in cooperation with the Boston Lying-in Hospital research dietary histories were obtained from each woman at successive stages of pregnancy; these histories included a careful "cross check" to validate the mother's statements.[6, 7] Independent clinical studies by obstetricians and pediatricians were made of the course and outcome of pregnancy and the condition of the infant at birth. The mothers and infants were each divided into four categories, the infants according to their physical condition at birth and their mothers according to the ratings of their dietary intakes. These maternal dietary ratings probably reflect not only the diets eaten during pregnancy but also longtime food habits of the majority of these women. Figure 1 reproduced from a report of this study[8] shows that in the "very poor" maternal dietary group there was a high incidence of infants in "poorest" physical condition at birth (stillbirths, neonatal deaths, premature infants, major congenital malformations, and infants called "functionally immature"). In contrast, there was an extremely low incidence of these "poorest" infants in any of the three upper dietary groups. This indicates that at a very low level of maternal dietary intake a nutritional threshold exists below which a high incidence of these so-called "poorest" infants may occur. The findings in the upper three dietary groups also are highly significant: a consistent shift in physical condition of the infants is demonstrated with each change in maternal dietary rating. The average birth weights and lengths of the infants are also shown in Figure 1; a consistent decrease of the average weights and lengths was apparent as the maternal dietary ratings became poorer. In the same study a significant, although less-pronounced relationship was found between the maternal diet and the course of pregnancy.[9] Furthermore, there was a high incidence of toxemia in the lowest maternal dietary group, none in the top dietary group and almost none in the two middle groups.

A more recent study of stillbirths, neonatal deaths, premature infants, and major congenital malformations occurring over a five year period has

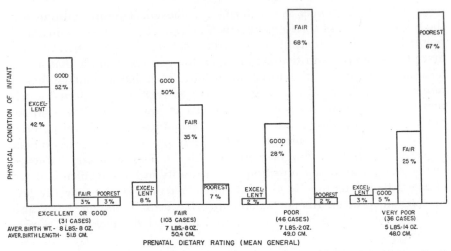

Figure 1. Relation of prenatal dietary rating to physical condition of infant at birth
Source: *Reproduced from Fig. 2, B. S. Burke, et al.,* J. Nutrition 38 (1949), 458.

been conducted in the Boston Lying-in Hospital. Smith, Worcester, and Burke[10] published a report on the autopsied cases of this series. The weight and composition of the fetal liver was shown to be significantly related to maternal dietary intake, and especially adversely affected when the maternal diet was very low in protein. Other relationships of statistical significance were demonstrated between the fetal liver content of certain of the vitamins and the maternal dietary intake of these nutrients. The approach utilized here was suggested by Wallace's studies on sheep. He demonstrated that in sheep the weight of the fetal liver is particularly responsive to maternal diet. Grossly deficient diets fed to the ewes during the gestational period produced lambs whose birth weights were as much as 50 per cent lower than those attained in the same animals on good maternal diets. Their liver weights were even more drastically affected. These relationships were sufficiently striking to suggest that they might be repeated under the less well-controlled conditions of human research. In the human study reported above it appeared from the nutrition histories that the majority of the women had not changed their dietary habits measurably during their pregnancies. Many of these women disliked or for other reasons did not consume much milk, eggs, and meat either before or during pregnancy. Their diets, therefore, furnished extremely low intakes of animal protein, total protein, and many other essential nutrients.

Research data on both animals and humans indicate clearly that if the mother becomes sufficiently depleted nutritionally the fetus may suffer to spare the mother. In other words the fetus appears *not* to be a total parasite upon the mother as was formerly believed. Barcroft in discussing the relative claims of the fetus and mother to available nutritive material pointed to the limitations of the doctrine that the fetus as a parasite has first priority on the nutritive material, on the general grounds that it is a necessary condition of the development of a fetus that its mother should remain alive. The incidence of prematurity in relation to maternal nutrition in a study carried out on 404 women of low income has been reported by Jeans, Smith, and Stearns.[11] Prematurity rose sharply as the maternal diet became poorer; the incidence of prematurity was more than twice as high in the group of mothers with the poorest dietary habits as in the group with better nutrition. The majority of these women had not changed their long-time food habits and their diets were especially low in calcium, protein, riboflavin, and ascorbic acid. Woodhill [12] has also shown a relationship between maternal diet and the incidence of prematurity.

An indication of the national importance of present fetal, neonatal, and maternal losses is that collectively they ranked fourth among the main causes of death at all ages in 1955 in the United States. About 350,000 infants are born prematurely each year. Dr. Eliot has said that "since most of the babies who die soon after birth are born prematurely our best chance to reduce deaths in these first few days lies in finding effective ways of insuring that the mother can carry her baby to term." [13] Unpublished data by Burke et al. indicate that the improvement of the nutritional status and diet of mothers both before and during pregnancy are important environmental factors in reducing prematurity.

Animal experimentation dealing with manifestations of antenatal nutritional deficiency has shown that good nutrition in pregnancy is effective as an environmental factor in the prevention of some types of congenital anomalies. If the work on animals[3] is even in part applicable to man a good nutritional foundation should be laid even before pregnancy begins for the prevention of nutritional deficiencies in the early months of pregnancy.

The evidence available indicates clearly that attention to the dietary habits and nutritional status of all women of childbearing age is an important aspect of health services for them in connection with preconceptional, prenatal, and postpartum care.

The nutritional allowances as recommended for pregnancy by the Food and Nutrition Board are given in Chapter V, Table 3 along with allowances for the nonpregnant and for the lactating woman so that changes from one period to another may be easily compared. Although the entire period of pregnancy is one of increasing physiological stress the greatest demands for additional nutrients are during the latter part. For this reason increased allowances are recommended for the "second half" of pregnancy. The assumption is that a woman enters pregnancy with a background of long-time good food habits and continues in the early months to consume a diet meeting her daily needs. However, such is far from true in a large percentage of pregnant women. If long-time food habits have been poor, evidence already discussed suggests the need for nutrient increases earlier. The nutritional status and diet of many pregnant women still receive insufficient attention as a part of routine prenatal care. In addition, many women still do not seek prenatal care early enough, and in many areas of the United States health services for pregnant women are insufficient in kind, quality, and quantity. As far as nutrition is concerned the fetal period, while vitally important to the entire life cycle, is still one of the most neglected.

In a practical and intelligent nutritional approach to the pregnant patient much can be accomplished from a preventive standpoint, if the physician at the first visit discusses with the patient a desirable weight considering her height and build, and her expected weight gain during pregnancy. The aim is usually to permit a gradual total weight gain of 20 to 25 pounds above a desirable nonpregnant weight. This implies that the underweight woman should be allowed to gain more, while the overweight woman's diet should be controlled carefully by restricting her calories *only*, in order that protein, mineral, and vitamin needs are fully provided. The physician, nurse, nutritionist, or other clinic personnel who are to help her will have to spend sufficient time with the patient to motivate her to want to improve her food habits, when indicated, by explaining the suggested changes in terms of possible benefits to both herself and her unborn child.

The diet needed during pregnancy is a much more special one than is generally appreciated, because as pregnancy advances the needs for proteins, minerals, and vitamins are increased proportionally more than is the caloric requirement. The caloric requirement is never more than approximately 20 per cent above nonpregnant needs even in the latter part of pregnancy, and since many women decrease their activity during pregnancy this may partially or almost wholly offset the increased energy costs of pregnancy. *It takes approximately 1800 to 2000 calories of carefully selected foods daily to meet the increased needs for nutrients other than calories.* This means that a woman's free choice of food is considerably narrowed during pregnancy, if the important structural and regulatory foods are to be eaten in optimum amounts daily. The nonpregnant woman can obtain her normal needs for protein, minerals, and vitamins in about 1200 calories to which must be added almost another 1000 calories in food to meet her daily energy requirement. The recommended adult caloric allowances are for a "reference" woman and adjustments should always be made on an individual basis.[2]

The amount of protein recommended for pregnancy provides 20 gm daily for the second half of pregnancy in addition to the usual allowance of 1 gm/kg of body weight assuming a diet adequate in calories and otherwise well-balanced. The pregnant woman's intake of protein is very important to both mother and fetus. Nitrogen balance studies have shown that women during pregnancy store relatively large amounts of protein over and above the amounts needed by the fetus and its adnexa.[3, 5] Protein is stored from about the eighth week of gestation until close to term, the amount determined to a degree by the woman's own nutritional status. The maternal storage of nitrogen during pregnancy may be regarded in part as a natural mechanism to provide for the relatively larger needs of the fetus toward the end of pregnancy, the large losses of nitrogen occurring just before and during delivery and in the puerperium, and in part in preparation for the high requirement of lactation.

The importance of a liberal protein intake is borne out by several studies. Burke et al.[14] have shown a statistically significant relationship between maternal intake of protein and birth length, birth weight, and physical well-being of the infant.

Although the cause of toxemia of pregnancy is still a controversial subject, it is generally accepted that a high protein diet may act as a preventive agent. Three independent groups[15, 16, 17] have demonstrated convincingly the importance of a high protein well-balanced nutritional regime in the control of toxemia. They call attention to the fact that a normal, gradual gain in weight during the first two trimesters is important; otherwise borderline symptoms of toxemia if watched for and recognized are likely to appear in the second trimester. When this occurs strict dietary control becomes a necessity, as the patient is then recognized as a potential toxemic and so treated by her physician. It is perhaps significant that the second trimester is also the period when the fetus makes its most rapid growth in length; in fact there is no other period in the entire growth cycle of man when rate of growth in length is so rapid.

If 75 to 80 gm of protein daily represent the protein goal during the last five lunar months of pregnancy, few women attain this target by their own volition. Burke et al.[14] in studies at the Boston Lying-in Hospital found that only 32 per cent of their group were consuming 70 gm or more of protein daily, 38 per cent consumed less than 55 gm and 14 per cent less than 45 gm during this important period of fetal growth and development. Similar findings have been published from other areas in this country. While our socioeconomic conditions have so improved that these conditions probably do not exist now to the extent they did, a large number of women today still do not eat a diet well-supplied with protein even for normal needs, and they do not change their food habits appreciably during pregnancy unless motivated to do so.

The demands of pregnancy also require increased intakes of minerals and vitamins over nonpregnant levels. For specific information regarding the recommended allowances for these, the studies upon which they are based and how these needs may be met by diet, the reader is referred to the review references[3, 4, 5] and to the text of the 1958 revision of the National Research Council's recommended dietary allowances.

From a practical standpoint, when the pregnant woman's daily protein needs are met by a proper choice of food, all other nutrients except ascorbic acid and vitamins A and D will be provided in reasonably good amounts because of their natural association with protein in food. When protein is deficient in the diet because milk is in short supply, calcium and possibly phosphorus will also be deficient. Iron, riboflavin, and other B-vitamins are also likely to be deficient in a low protein diet. If protein is not adequately supplied by the diet there is no other practical and palatable way of obtaining it. Table 1 is a summary of foods or their

Table 1. Daily food nucleus to insure optimum nutrition throughout pregnancy

Food	Amount	Protein (gm)
Milk, whole	4 8-oz glasses (1 quart). Patient should label her milk and see that entire quart is taken each day	32
Meat (lean), poultry, fish, cheese. Liver is desirable at least once each week	2 servings daily, in all at least 4 oz or equivalent in grams of protein	26
Egg	1	6
Fruit, citrus	At least 2 servings (1 serving = 4 oz orange juice, 1 medium orange, 8 oz tomato juice, or ½ grapefruit)	2
Potato	1 medium (150 gm)	3
Other vegetables, cooked or raw	2 or more servings (1 serving = ½ cup). Dark green leafy or deep yellow vegetables often	3
Bread and cereal	3 or 4 servings (1 serving = 1 slice bread or ½ cup cereal), whole grain or enriched	6–8
Butter or fortified margarine	1 tablespoon	
Vitamin D	An amount to supply 400 I.U.	
		78–80

nutritional equivalents which would insure optimum nutrition during pregnancy. The approximate protein values are given to indicate the contributory values of different foods or food groups to the protein in the diet.

The foods listed in the table in the amounts suggested or their equivalents supply less than 2000 calories. The ascorbic acid allowance is met by citrus fruit or equivalents. The amount of vitamin A recommended will be furnished by the whole milk, butter, egg, and dark green leafy or deep yellow vegetables as suggested. This assumes that the foods are processed and prepared so as to conserve their nutritive values. Additional food, either more of these foods or others of the woman's own choice will be required to furnish sufficient calories to produce the desired weight gain.[18] The doctor may find it necessary to vary the amounts and kinds of foods suggested to meet individual needs.

For the normal pregnant woman fluid intake should be adequate, approximately two quarts of total liquid daily including milk, fruit juices, tea, coffee, etc. Under normal conditions salt may be eaten in moderate amounts but excessive use should be avoided. Further restrictions should be under the doctor's direction. Iodized salt should be recommended, especially in regions where goiter is endemic.

The pregnant woman, whatever her cultural, social, or economic status, needs a physician with not only obstetrical skill, but also one with an appreciation of the nutritional needs of mother and fetus and of all other factors that make for excellent prenatal care.

THE SOCIAL IMPLICATIONS OF PREGNANCY
ELIZABETH P. RICE

For persons concerned with maintaining the stability of family life and the development of sound mother-child and family-child relations, the period of pregnancy has come to be recognized as an important time to consider the social situation into which the child is to be born, and to take whatever preventive measures may be necessary.

Since it is important for the child to have the love and affection which is necessary for his proper development socially as well as emotionally, the attitude of the mother towards her pregnancy and the responsibilities of motherhood is a first consideration. This will depend in large part on her past experiences, and the goals which she has set for marriage and motherhood. Where the closely linked emotional and social needs of the mother have not been met adequately, she finds it difficult to accept the role of motherhood and to meet the child's need for social development. The mother's ability, also, for easy social relations, as well as to be relaxed and secure in her handling of the child, will affect her role as a mother not only in caring for the infant but for the family as a whole.

The degree to which the mother's own family situation meets some of her basic needs will determine also the extent to which she is able to contribute support and strength to the growing child. It is important, therefore, in understanding a mother during pregnancy, to evaluate her experiences over a period of time and to see how her experiences contribute to her role as a wife and mother.

In considering the family into which a child is to be born, it is helpful to understand the relations of one member of the family to another, since this relation will affect the family as a whole. Tensions between any two will contribute to over-all strains within the family. The part played by other persons in the mother's environment, including the wider circle of relatives and friends, will also affect the mother's attitude and will contribute to the atmosphere of the family as a unit.

It is helpful also to know the role which the cultural background plays during the pregnancy. In all cultures, at the time of births, marriages, and deaths, there are more fears and superstitions, as well as traditional customs, than at other periods of life. These contribute at once both to the mother's feeling of security and comfort, and of anxiety and fear. Thus, to know the mother's cultural attitudes and points of view towards the experiences of pregnancy and birth, will help to give a clearer picture of her tensions and strains. Mothers who have had a broad educational background have a tendency to intellectualize their experiences as a result of reading the conflicting points of view in the literature concerning the period of pregnancy and the care of children. Because of this they ask innumerable questions in regard to the various aspects of pregnancy and delivery. Women who habitually intellectualize most experiences may find it hard to experience pregnancy emotionally. Mixed marriages will often provide additional sources of conflict for the couple in their differences of nationality, race, or religion. At the time of pregnancy and anticipated confinement, any social differences tend to cause extra strains and anxieties, and sometimes insecurities, in the marriage relationship itself. Similarly, the tendency of parents and friends to encourage the mother during pregnancy to carry out methods used by them or within their culture, as against what is recommended by the doctor, may confuse the mother. For the young, immature mother who has not yet worked through her dependence upon her own family, this pressure of parental culture will have a strong influence.

Another factor of consequence is that the mother's attitude toward her unborn child will be influenced by the specific motivations and reasons which created the marriage. Since in all cultures marriages are made for various reasons, and often without reference to positive emotional factors, the purposes and motivations for marriage and the attitude of the woman towards her pregnancy and the new baby will be related. An understanding of this aspect of the marriage background can illuminate some otherwise obscure problems of a woman's pregnancy adjustment.

In reviewing the various reasons for marriage one can readily see marked differences in the ways in which these reasons for marriage contribute to the stability of the marriage at the outset. Most marriages, hopefully, are made because of mutual interest of the mates. In this type of marriage both husband and wife find a real companionship, a pleasure in being together and in sharing common interests and thinking. Marriage made on this basis tends to be more lasting, providing a sound foundation ready to withstand the strains of marital life. Another reason for marriage is that of romance. In this type of marriage the couple have in their minds an ideal pattern of the mate they would like to choose. Unfortunately, the perception gained later through experience with the real person frequently does not fit the mate's ideal, and so the illusion is destroyed and no other basis for permanency of the marriage exists. This newly objective perception of the mate leads inevitably to marital insecurities and maladjustments, and often to separation and divorce.

In most cultures today there is still the expectation that young adults should be married in order to fulfill not only their own expectations and desires but also to meet the requirements of society. Most young people have the desire to meet these personal and cultural expectations as well as to choose a mate with the furtherance of mutual happiness and interests in view. For others, who have had some emotional deprivation in their lives, the driving force towards marriage may be the need for acceptance and attention, for the love and affection which they did not receive from their mothers and family in earlier life. Several studies have been made indicating that adolescent girls, deprived of the love and affection needed for emotional and social development, often seek attention from men who can fulfill some of their unmet needs. Some men and women who have not made a satisfactory adjustment to adult life and the assumption of responsibilities need the comfort and security of someone to care for them. Such dependency needs exist among both women and men. Others, alone in the community without a home or without relatives on whom to depend, seek the security of family life and a home. Still others, bored by the occupations in which they are engaged, find marriage an interesting escape from an occupation that no longer holds their attention. Some women may choose marriage, and therefore pregnancy, because of their interest in children. If, however, one of the mates desires to have children and the other does not, difficulties may be created in the marital relations and for the child when he is born. Many mature men and women, of course, also desire the responsibility of family life and are ready to undertake this broadening experience. Others see marriage as a means of achieving economic security, and this is true of both men and women when the spouse brings to the marriage certain economic assets on which the other may rely. With our increase in aging, some see children as their security in old age. For those more religiously inclined, marriage and children indicate the fulfillment of God's will and a culmination of the purposes for which people are created.

It is clear from these varied reasons for marriage, therefore, that some marriages are laid on the foundations of success while others from the start indicate problems in marital relations, in the security of the marriage, and for the children who will be born to the union.

Pregnancy may be utilized to meet various needs of the husband or wife. Marriages which are somewhat insecure may be held together through the presence of a child, and thus pregnancy is used as a means of cementing the marriage. In such cases, unfortunately, the child tends to be the buffer between the mates, or worse, a tool used by one parent against the other. Thus serious complications may arise for the child, and the marital difficulties are rarely solved by such a step.

Pregnancies may be unwanted for various reasons. At the time the mother becomes pregnant, the family may not be in a desired economic situation. The parents may have planned to delay pregnancy in order that the wife or husband could complete further education, or in order that the wife could help support her husband's education, or until the couple were able to maintain a higher standard of living. Due to the increasingly younger age of marriage, many young couples still have financial responsibilities which were acquired in order to pay for education, or for household equipment, and pregnancy interferes with the budgeting for these previous obligations. Furthermore, many women who marry early are not yet ready to give up their occupations, or their opportunities for a career, in order to settle down to the role of motherhood. For them, especially in the first pregnancy, it is hard to discontinue their associations with friends and colleagues in the community, and they feel lonely and isolated. They miss their social and recreational outlets. For many such mothers a part-time occupation or community interest may help to relieve a difficult transition from full-time employment to waiting for the baby.

Some mothers hesitate to be tied down to the responsibilities of a child, seeing pregnancy as a threat to their freedom and their independence. They see the care of the home and the baby as a rather routine, monotonous, and even menial job. Many of them dislike giving up their own income, over which they have had complete control. Thus, the occupationally oriented society in which young women live and are trained today creates for them several challenges in accepting the role of housewife and mother. However, among young couples today, this point of view seems to be rapidly changing, and one senses that new values are now being placed on homemaking and motherhood.

Some women hesitate to accept pregnancy because of their inability to relate to children. Having never been interested in children and not being comfortable in their presence, they feel themselves inadequate for motherhood and are hesitant to assume its responsibilities. Others feel that their age is against them, that they are either too young or too old for these responsibilities. This is likely to be only a rationalization for a deeper resistance. Some mothers are still immature, and some fathers still want to be treated more like a child and to be the center of attention, looked after and protected. Such parents find it difficult to share their mate with a baby because they themselves still need the undivided affection and attention of their spouse. Immature women, too, uncertain of the affection and constancy of their husbands, are concerned about their figures. Pregnancy, they feel, may make them less attractive to their husbands. Others feel that pregnancy is inadvisable for them because of poor health, either real or imagined. Many mothers, too, are anxious lest they deliver a deformed or abnormal child, and this anxiety may become severe if such a familial history exists in either branch of the family.

There are, in addition, realistic problems, such as the pregnancy coming too close to a previous one, creating an obvious problem in regard to the care of two young children; beyond this, however, there may be a feeling of guilt and shame. Some mothers may believe they already have as many children as they can support, and thus an additional pregnancy means a burden not only to the mother herself but also to the whole family, who thus will be further handicapped by the family's limited assets. For many of the young women with their first babies, housing problems create difficulties. Young couples who are not yet satisfactorily established in permanent housing may likely find their temporary quarters inadequate for a child. Financial problems may be created by the mother's giving up work when the father has not yet become well established occupationally, at a time when additional expenses must be met for medical and hospital care of mother and baby. Additional living space for the new baby may require a larger apartment, and extra costs for the baby's food and equipment will place additional strain on the family's budget. These costs often come at a time when the family with the first baby is still in debt for education or for household expenses incurred in establishing a home.

Husbands share these social problems of pregnancy. Some may show anxieties during the period of pregnancy and delivery, not only in regard to the wife's experiences, but also in facing the responsibilities of father-

hood. Some fathers attempt to escape their new responsibilities by turning to alcohol, temporary desertion, or to other women for satisfaction.
A few fathers may desert permanently. Others may feel jealous of the
new child, who deprives them of their wives' interest and attention. In
a group of thirty-one fathers interviewed in a special family health
clinic,[19] the fathers raised questions for discussion which fell into the
following four major categories: (1) general information about pregnancy, the function of the clinic and hospital procedures; (2) environmental subjects such as finances, housing, study and work schedules, and
postpartum care for the mother and baby; (3) feelings related to parenthood, to themselves, and their wives as persons, to their capacity for
fatherhood and motherhood, and to the stability of the marriage; (4)
past personal history and family relationships of the husband.

Children already born into the family will react to the expected birth
according to their age, the nature of their preparation for the birth, and
the extent to which they have had their emotional and social needs
satisfied in the past by members of the family. For many siblings some
plan of care by a substitute for the mother during her hospitalization
will be necessary when relatives or friends are not available. In many
communities homemaker or housekeeper services have been established
to help a father provide the care and supervision of his children and
the home during the mother's absence and for a period after her return
home with the new baby. This program is established with the belief
that the sibling will be less upset by the mother's absence and the new
baby's arrival into the family if he does not have to leave his familiar
setting and his father at the same time as he misses his mother. In
families where such an arrangement cannot be worked out either because there is no such service available or because the home is unsuitable or the parents unwilling, children may need care in a foster
home under the skilled supervision of a child care agency. Whatever the
plan, siblings need consideration and loving care from the father and a
substitute mother at such a time of crisis in their lives.

To a large degree, the situation in the family into which the child
is born will be determined by the reason for the marriage, which will
have affected the relationships of the parents to each other throughout
the marriage, and which will affect the relationships of the parents to
the child. Thus an understanding of why any two people came together
in marriage will give a clear indication of what strengths and limitations
there will be in their roles as mates and parents in establishing a new
family.

Some of the most serious social problems of pregnancy arise when the
mother is unmarried or the father is not her husband. Such mothers show
variable reactions during pregnancy, depending on their experiences in

the past and, basically, on the relationships behind these experiences.

Most young couples, fortunately, will look forward to having children as a rounding out of their mutual interests and satisfactions, and will provide these children with warmth, interest, and affection. During the period of adjustment to the pregnancy and birth of the new baby parents and siblings may be able to provide the reassurance and mutual support to each other which will keep equilibrium within the family and within the various members of the family. The physician and nurse can give valuable support to the mother during this period. Through anticipatory guidance they can help her and her husband to look ahead to usual experiences which occur at such a time, thus lessening the strains which would result if these were unexpected or not understood. For other parents or children who have greater difficulty in meeting the stresses which occur in pregnancy, other community services may be needed. Depending on the difficulty, guidance may be available from physicians, public health nurses, social workers in the prenatal clinic, or from community agencies such as family counselling services, child care programs, or, for financial assistance, from public welfare.

EMOTIONAL IMPLICATIONS OF PREGNANCY AND INFLUENCES ON FAMILY RELATIONSHIPS
GERALD CAPLAN

Knowing something about the usual emotional changes during pregnancy allows us to relieve some of the discomforts of this period by reassurance and anticipatory guidance. Anxiety and guilt feelings can thus be kept to a minimum. This will also contribute to helping the woman make most effective use of medical care during this period. More importantly, this knowledge allows us to deal more effectively with many of the influences of these changes on family relationships. The idea is that a knowledge of the patterns of unfolding of the emotional life of the pregnant woman may help us in directing her toward paths which lead to the development of a healthy mother-child relationship with the newborn infant. We may also safeguard the emotional life of the family by paying attention to the way the changes of pregnancy complicate the equilibrium of relationships.

Pregnancy is to be regarded as a biologically determined period of psychological stress. Both the intra- and the interpersonal forces in the pregnant woman and her family are in a state of disequilibrium during this period. The future mental health of both may be dependent to a considerable extent upon whether the balance weighs down on the positive or negative side as a result of her experiences in relation to the key figures in her environment during pregnancy.

The emotional changes during pregnancy involve a dynamic unfolding process. Clinical experience with pregnant women shows that at the different stages of pregnancy there are fairly characteristic emotional pictures which mirror to some extent the developing physiological process, although individual women show differences in the rate and rhythm of emotional change. Comparison of the emotional picture in different women is useful if the appropriate stage of pregnancy at which the emotional manifestations occur is indicated. Certain emotional manifestations appear early in pregnancy and then disappear. Others do not make their appearance until the end of the first trimester. Still others appear only toward the end of pregnancy. There is considerable individual variation, but it is possible to indicate general patterns which commonly occur.

Although little is known about the causes of the emotional manifestations of pregnancy it is suspected that there are two main systems of factors.

Somatopsychic factors based upon hormonal and general metabolic changes. Therese Benedek[20, 21] has proposed the hypothesis that the secretion of progestin has a profound effect upon the psychology of the pregnant woman, increasing the emotional investment of her body and herself, while producing also a general introversion and increase in passivity. The changes in emotional irritability and sensitivity, as well as the generalized mood swings, may possibly be based upon complicated metabolic changes.

Psychogenic factors. These are linked on the one hand with the reactions of the woman to the sexual aspects of the reproductive process, which are associated with the details of her personality structure and the vicissitudes of her sexual development, and on the other hand to the process whereby during the course of pregnancy she develops psychologically into the role of mother, a process influenced especially by the details of her relation with her own mother and the mother figures who will serve for her as role models. The controlling factor most likely will be her imagined and subjective recollection of her mother, and not necessarily a realistic and objective view. Since a child is often in conflict with the mother, the question here is how the conflict was resolved.

Common emotional manifestations are:

Alterations in dominant mood, and mood swings. It is usual for the prevailing mood of the woman to change during pregnancy, and this does not seem to be related to easily ascertainable causes. Some women feel better during pregnancy than at any other time. Others feel generally depressed throughout pregnancy even though they may have very actively wished for a child. Sudden unexplainable mood swings are not uncommon, perhaps associated with hormonal and metabolic changes of pregnancy. These may be quite unlike the emotional picture of the woman when she is not pregnant. Short phases of fairly deep depression are not unusual, and unless they have been warned about them, some women become fearful that more serious psychological disturbances will arise. Most of the depressions of pregnancy are benign and do not appear to be correlated with subsequent puerperal psychosis.

Emotional lability, irritability, and sensitivity. Common changes during pregnancy include a tendency to become angry at slight provocation, to laugh and cry easily, and in general to have rapid fluctuations in mood as a result of minor external stimulation. There is also commonly an increased sensitivity of the special senses of taste and smell, with an increased tendency to disgust in response to stimulation of these senses.

Introversion and passivity. This is one of the most characteristic emotional changes of pregnancy. It often begins around the end of the first trimester, and gradually increases in intensity, reaching a peak around the seventh or eighth month. The woman who may previously have been an outgoing person and whose role as wife and mother has been one of nurturance and giving, gradually or suddenly becomes preoccupied with herself, feels lazy and "cowlike," and develops the need to be cared for instead of caring for others. She has increased needs for love and affection. The adequate fulfillment of these needs is of primary importance in preparing her for the role of mother. This is another area where anticipatory guidance is important, not only to ensure the comfort of the pregnant woman but also to prepare her adequately for motherhood. In our culture, husbands often get upset by this change in role of their wives; they fear that they are demanding to be "spoiled." If they refuse the demonstrations of affection which their wives demand, this lack of satisfaction, together with the increased irritability, may provoke hostile patterns of disharmony in the family. A joint interview with the marital partners will be valuable here. The husband can be told in front of his wife what changes to expect in her, and that she will probably have increased needs for demonstrations of affection, which he can satisfy by helping with household chores as well as by manifesting love in other ways. In this manner he will be helping to prepare an emotional nest for the coming baby. He should be reassured that this attitude is likely to change after the baby comes, and his acceptance of his wife's needs now is not likely to set a precedent for their future role pattern.

Changes in sexual desire and performance. Such changes occur in many women at varying phases of pregnancy. Some diminution of sexual desire is common towards the middle of pregnancy, and may be accompanied by frigidity, but some women have increased desire. These changes in the wife's sexual interest and performance, if not anticipated, may lead to marital difficulties, especially when associated with increased irritability. This is one of the areas where anticipatory guidance also can add very much to the comfort of the marital couple and to the stability of the marriage. This guidance may best be given in a joint interview with husband and wife by the physician or other professional worker as early in pregnancy as possible.

Shift in intrapsychic equilibrium. Special mention should be made of this characteristic psychological manifestation of pregnancy, which has not been widely recognized in the past. Experience in clinical situations with normal pregnant women is corroborated by projective psychological test findings, and shows a significant alteration in the relationship between ego and id forces, that is, between the rational controlling aspects of the personality and the unconscious and basic inner emotional drives. This begins towards the end of the first trimester, reaches a peak about the seventh month, and reverts to the usual prenatal state about three or four weeks after delivery. Unconscious conflicts, which were formerly repressed, gradually come up to the surface of consciousness as pregnancy progresses, with the arousal of relatively minor anxiety. Established defenses against the pressures of unconscious conflicts appear to lessen. In some instances this picture can be confused with an incipient psychosis, but there is no associated break with reality or distortion in the perceptions of the outer world. Old problems are revived, and this means that new solutions to them become possible. Especially significant is the emergence of unsolved or partially solved problems in the relationship with mother and siblings from early childhood, as well as problems in adolescence, with particular reference to sex life and masturbation.

The possibility of more mature solutions to these old problems at this time explains the frequent observation that during pregnancy a woman may either spontaneously, or through the help she receives from her medical and nursing advisors, develop greater maturity of personality. There is also, however, the possibility that unhealthy solutions to the problems may be linked with the developing relationship to the coming baby. This frequently takes the form of identification of the baby with some significant figure from an early childhood traumatic experience, or with some element such as "sexuality," "aggression," etc., from the woman's own intrapersonal conflicts. This is an outstanding source of disturbance of mother-child relationship. It can be observed during pregnancy and it can be dealt with very effectively at that time by simple psychological techniques.

Although usually suppressed irrational fantasies and impulses emerge surprisingly freely into consciousness during pregnancy, this process does not take place without the arousal of some anxiety. This characteristically is "free floating," but it attaches itself to many varying phobic symbols during the course of pregnancy. This is the source of the characteristic anxiety and fears which mainly focus on the possibility of danger to the woman herself or to the health or life of her baby. Many of these fears show clearly that they are linked with the idea of punishment because of guilt aroused by old, forbidden wishes. The numerous superstitions associated with pregnancy are connected with cultural methods of handling these anxieties.

The development of the relationship to the baby can be seen in three separate areas:

Attitudes to conception and pregnancy. The writer has observed that approximately 85 per cent of primiparae of the lower middle and upper lower socioeconomic classes show some initial rejection of the conception and are upset by feelings of grief and anger when they become pregnant. Reasons include economic hardship, thwarted ambitions for self or husband, housing difficulties, as well as intrapersonal difficulties of wives which focus upon the change to the maternal role, etc.

There is apparently no correlation between such attitudes of initial rejection of the pregnancy and disturbances of the future mother-child relationship. It is the pregnancy which is rejected and not the baby, which rarely becomes an emotional reality to the woman until after quickening.

Most husbands and wives very quickly adapt to the initial rejection of the pregnancy. By the end of the first trimester 85 to 90 per cent of women who initially rejected the pregnancy have accepted it. Most of those with delay in adaptation change their attitude at the time of quickening. Very few mothers go right through pregnancy with stable attitudes of rejection, although a certain degree of ambivalence is common. During the last few weeks of pregnancy earlier negative attitudes are often revived in connection with the increased physical burdens of this period, which lead to some increase in the "free floating" anxiety and its focus upon the impending birth.

There is no valid evidence that the nausea and vomiting, so common early in pregnancy, are linked to the attitudes of rejection of conception, beyond the fact that both patterns are very common and may overlap. The fact that the nausea and vomiting can often be controlled by psychological techniques, such as suggestion or hypnosis, is no evidence that the etiology is psychosomatic.

Pernicious vomiting, on the other hand, is very often an hysterical symptom, and occurs in women with gross personality disorders who have reacted to traumatic events repeatedly in the past by gastrointestinal symptoms.

Attitude to fetus. The fetus rarely becomes a reality to the pregnant woman until quickening. Women vary in their feelings and attitudes towards the fetus. To some women it never becomes a reality as a living organism even though intellectually they are able to appreciate this fact.

Reactions to the fetus, in any sample of normal pregnant women, vary on a scale. At one pole are women who very rapidly after quickening begin to conceive of the fetus as a real, live person inside them. They endow it in their imaginations with a special personality. They think of it as a boy or girl and they often give it a name. They are very conscious of its movements, and ascribe feelings to it. They "play" with it and often involve the husband in these games. Such women usually have quite intense feelings towards the fetus, and many will say that they have a real maternal love for it in utero. They get a pleasurable thrill when they feel its movements. Such women are often somewhat narcissistic in their general personality makeup and show an intense interest in other aspects of their own body and personality.

At the other pole are women who never conceive of the fetus as a human being. They may think of it as a depersonalized "foreign body." They usually have no feelings towards it, or else they have negative feelings which are stimulated by its movements. Sometimes they will complain about it as a burden; e.g., its movements keep them awake or distract them from their daily activities.

Knowledge of these attitudes during pregnancy allows us to predict something about the initial reaction of a woman to her newborn baby. Attitudes towards the fetus have an influence upon the length of the time-lag after birth before the development of full maternal feeling. Women who are close to the narcissistic pole mentioned above have the shortest time-lag. They describe their relationship to the newborn baby as being a continuation of their relationship to the fetus, which was interrupted only by the birth process. Type and duration of anesthesia are of importance in this interruption. Such women show a remarkable sensitivity in their relationship with their baby immediately after birth, and show a picture of the happy "nursing couple."

The maternal time-lag after birth is longer in the case of those women who have had no active emotional relationship with their fetus. They have to build up a new relationship with a separate person who is a stranger to them. Broadly, then, it can be said that if the fetus seems a nuisance to the mother, the child will often be a nuisance; if the mother is too attached to her fetus, she may be unable to separate herself psychologically from her infant.

In trying to predict the length of the maternal time-lag and the type of early mother-child relationship we are guided not only by these findings but also by:

Fantasies about "baby-to-be." Starting early in pregnancy, and possibly increasing after quickening, many mothers develop an increasingly rich fantasy life in regard to the image of their baby as they imagine it will be after it is born. These daydreams, nightdreams, and imaginings are usually quite separate from whatever feelings there may be in regard to the fetus. However, we can learn a great deal about the woman's psychological preparation for her baby by paying attention to the details of these fantasies. Especially significant are details about the age and sex of the baby in the fantasies, details about the activities in which the woman imagines herself to be involved with the baby, and the emotional tone which colors her thinking.

These fantasies can also be used in predicting the length of the maternal time-lag and the initial reaction to the newborn baby. Women who fantasy tiny babies and imagine themselves breast-feeding or taking care of them in a nurturing way are likely to have a shorter maternal lag and less difficulty in dealing with the newborn than those women who cannot fantasy babies under about 3 to 4 months of age, who even may have daydreams only about grown-up children and make plans about their college education, etc., and who may have anxiety-ridden fantasies about mishandling the details of child care.

After birth, the mother may try to fuse her perception of the real baby with her previous fantasy images of it. This may result in gross misperception, with the danger of subsequent disillusionment in the mother-child relationship. Women who may be preparing to use the baby vicariously to suit their own purposes as a solution to problems of their own may sometimes be recognized from the content of their fantasies during pregnancy, which are characterized by seeing the child in roles which fit more closely into the mother's own ambitions than into any expectation of the child as a separate person with his own needs and individuality.

The emotional changes of the woman during pregnancy have a marked effect upon her husband and her other children, and on her own emotional well-being, just as her preparation for motherhood is in turn affected by the attitudes and behavior of her family. It is well to think in terms of "a pregnant family" rather than just in terms of a pregnant woman.

The most important emotional change during pregnancy which affects the family is the increased introversion and dependency of the woman. In our culture the wife and the mother role are associated with giving and activity. During pregnancy the sudden change towards passivity and receiving may upset the husband and the other children greatly.

The children, especially if they are young, are likely to be quite sensitive in their perception of the mother's withdrawal of interest in them, and she herself may not realize it is happening. If they are older, they may also be upset by observations of external signs of pregnancy or by overhearing talk about the new baby. Behavior disorders which may occur as a reaction to these threats to their security are not dealt with as effectively as previously by the mother because of the pregnant woman's irritability and emotional lability and because of her general passivity and lowering of ego strength. Vicious circles can easily be set up.

The increased demands for nurturance which are a characteristic of pregnancy, especially in its later stages, have to be adequately met for successful preparation for motherhood. The pregnant woman can be regarded as a battery which has to be adequately charged up so as to render her capable of giving nurturance to the newborn baby. She needs to be "spoiled." Her family may not welcome this, and may need help from nurses and obstetricians in adapting to this temporary phenomenon.

In the same way that her general behavior has some degree of consistency linked to her personality type, the reactions of a woman during pregnancy cannot adequately be understood without having some knowledge of her enduring features of character. Women who have experienced earlier emotional deprivation may have a particularly difficult time during pregnancy because of the increase of their dependent needs. As a result they may react negatively to attitudes of obstetricians and nurses interested in achieving a good result for the coming baby. The attitude of these women can be understood along the lines of "I, who have never received enough, am now expected to provide such a lot for someone else." Management of such cases can be effective if this point is recognized, and if the nurses and doctors pay particular attention to "giving" to the woman herself, and to mobilizing as effectively as possible external sources of love and affection in her family.

Hysterical personalities commonly have excessive phobias and other manifestations during pregnancy, but paradoxically there may be a lessening of hysterical symptoms during the last two trimesters. The reason for this seems to be that the normal somatic manifestations of pregnancy may replace hysterical conversion symptoms. These women characteristically show a special disgust at the biological manifestations of pregnancy, birth and child care which they see as signs of "animal" sexuality. They have, for example, special problems in regard to breast feeding, commonly expressing fears that people will make suggestive remarks about their suckling their babies, or that someone will come into the room and "catch them in the act." Appropriate management consists of discussing pregnancy and delivery with them in a sentimentalized way, stressing "the wonders of nature," and playing down the carnal aspects. In these and other ways their defenses can be strengthened and some of their fears relieved, so that the psychological distance between mother and child may be increased sufficiently for them to have a chance of perceiving the baby as a separate, individual person and not as a part of their own sexuality.

Obsessive-compulsive personalities characteristically have a more comfortable time during pregnancy than is their habit of life outside such periods, but obsessive symptoms usually return shortly after labor. Such women are greatly helped during pregnancy if nurses and doctors pay special attention to providing them with a good deal of intellectual knowledge about the process of pregnancy, birth, and delivery.

The increased introversion and passivity of pregnancy is often associated with an increased need to use food as a source of emotional gratification. This sometimes leads to trouble, since it occurs at a stage in pregnancy where overeating may involve danger of toxemia. Metabolic changes earlier in pregnancy may also increase appetite; and food cravings, the origin of which are not clear, may also complicate the issue.

Professional workers, such as the nutritionist, who deal with the pregnant woman's dietary intake frequently encounter difficulties which are complicated by the unconscious transference to the nutritionist of old feelings towards mothers and mother figures. Problems from the pregnant woman's childhood involving conflict with her mother, which may have been manifested by feeding battles, may be revived and played out in the relationship with the nutritionist. In particular, the pregnant woman may have difficulties in drinking milk, difficulties which are directly related to her early experiences with her mother.

Management consists in attempting to break the link between the person giving nutritional advice and the image of the woman's mother. This may sometimes be accomplished by arranging for the obstetrician to recommend the diet. Another method which has been found useful in difficult cases is for the person giving advice about diet to sidestep the emotional aura of foodgiver or mother by giving "prescriptions" in terms of proteins, vitamins, etc., emphasizing the role of physician or scientist.

Emotionally deprived women usually have especial difficulty when advised to cut down their food intake. This can be dealt with by taking care to phrase formulations as a "giving" process and not a "taking away," and by making it quite explicit that the nutritionist is interested primarily in the health of the woman herself, and by not making too much mention of the baby.

Stress situations during pregnancy may not be adequately dealt with by the mother as a result of the general lowering of her ego capacity, an effect of the increased physical and emotional burdens of this period. The danger is that unsolved problems during this time may become linked with disturbances in the relationship with the future baby. Particularly significant are illness or death of near relatives, especially another child or the husband.

There is some evidence that women who are aware that they have Rh negative blood may be overanxious during pregnancy. Such women may develop anxious forebodings regarding the baby which may lead to disturbances of the mother-child relationship.

There is clear evidence that attempts by the mother to terminate her pregnancy, and which fail to lead to abortion, are particularly likely to lead to characteristic disorders of mother-child relations. This is particularly likely in cultures where abortion is regarded as a crime and a sin. The woman often hides her act as a guilty secret, which she does not share even with her husband. When the baby arrives she is characteristically overanxious, and continually searches for illnesses or defects which she imagines must be due to her having injured the fetus. This whole pathological process can frequently be interrupted if, during pregnancy or immediately afterwards, the mother is encouraged by the nurse or obstetrician to discuss what she has done, in such a way as to reduce her pathological guilt to normal proportions.

There is some evidence that difficulties during labor may be associated with emotional difficulties during pregnancy.[22] Women who are able to adapt adequately to the emotional changes of pregnancy tend to have easier and more trouble-free labor. Certainly, anticipatory guidance and education about the details of labor and delivery help women adapt to this experience.

Unless they have been especially trained beforehand, most women do not think very much about the baby during the process of labor itself. During this period they normally are preoccupied with their own condition, and only begin to think of the baby after delivery. Anesthesia during labor, and consequent delay of contact with the child after birth, is likely to increase maternal time-lag without leading necessarily to serious problems.

When a baby is born with a congenital anomaly the mother is presented with an important emotional problem, upon the healthy solution of which will depend how realistically she will subsequently be able to collaborate with physicians and nurses in providing the necessary special care.

She needs special help from her obstetric and nursing attendants particularly in the first six weeks after the birth. Except under extraordinary circumstances she should always be allowed to see the baby, and if possible to handle it, soon after birth. This allows her to get a reality-based perception of the problem, which is usually milder than her fantasies.

She will usually link the baby's defect with the punishing predictive fantasies of pregnancy, and will often ascribe the baby's condition to something bad done by her or her husband, such as having had sexual intercourse after the doctor told them to stop, or lifting another child, or playing too much golf during pregnancy, etc. These guilt feelings should be explored and relieved as soon as possible by matter-of-fact discussions. The woman and her husband should then be emotionally supported by the nurse and pediatrician during the period of weeks or months which may be required for them to work through their problem of accepting the reality of the baby's condition. This is likely to be more difficult and more prolonged if the baby has to stay in the hospital in the first few weeks for surgical operations, in which case the parents' adjustment may take several months.

COMPREHENSIVE MATERNITY CARE
SAMUEL B. KIRKWOOD

The concept of total pregnancy care places a considerable demand upon those responsible for providing maternity services. Fortunately, it is a demand of understanding and attitude more than a requirement for numbers.

Safety and Physical Care. First and foremost, this point of view means strict adherence to the best quality of medical and surgical procedures. Safety takes precedence over all else in pregnancy. This cannot be emphasized too strongly. Furthermore, this attention to good medicine in a physical sense begins long before pregnancy and continues well beyond the childbearing period. It is far better to prevent rickets in the child than to do a Caesarean in the adult for a deformed pelvis. Premarital and preconceptual examinations, including a careful history, give warning of abnormalities that may exist, and permit corrective measures. The interval between pregnancies offers another opportunity for repair of physical deficiencies that may have arisen during the previous confinement. Finally, the menopause and postmenopausal periods require expert medical care to prevent long-run sequelae.

The prenatal period brings two demands upon the physician. He must watch for the physical signs and symptoms of complications and he must assure himself that normal fetal and maternal development is taking place. Since pregnant women are subject to the general ills of all women as well as the special disorders of gestation, the physician must be prepared by his own efforts or through consultation services to meet the gamut of physical abnormalities.

During the confinement and delivery the technical abilities and judgment of the accoucheur are most acutely taxed; so are the physical facilities of the hospital. Several sets of standards have been developed as detailed guides for maternity services. They all provide for meeting surgical emergencies, treating hemorrhage, and isolating infection as minimum essentials.

The purely physical problems of the puerperium are again a combination of possible abnormalities and normal physiological change. Protection against infection is the greatest responsibility in this period. However, care to aid in the return of the mother's body to its normal nonpregnant state cannot be overlooked. The care of the breasts and lactation is a particular problem at this time.

Care of the Newborn. Too often care of the newborn baby is considered as not a part of the puerperium, due in part to the widespread custom of handing this responsibility to the pediatrician. Whether the pediatrician is called in or the baby is cared for by the general practitioner who has done the delivery, the mother and the baby, each reacting to the other, must be treated in a fully integrated manner.

The recommendations of the American Academy of Pediatrics[23] serve as a guide for detailed standards for the care of the newborn. Basic safety measures require constant attention and strict regulation and relate to hospital sanitation and techniques to assure against transmission of infection. Unnecessary procedures, such as bathing the infant, are avoided. Though constant observance for evidence of abnormalities is routine, actual handling of the baby is kept to a minimum. Facilities must be readily available to deal promptly and adequately with each unsatisfactory development. Beyond this, simple routines are followed in respect to feeding and other care, subject to prompt modification in accordance with the responses of the individual child, and the mother is brought into the aspect of care as rapidly as her condition permits and conditions justify, in preparation for an easy shift to home care on discharge from the hospital.

There are always a few babies who require very special care because of problems such as premature birth, congenital defects, or difficulties in making neonatal adaptations successfully. These usually require much closer observation, special and at times constant individual care, and occasionally frequent and complicated treatments. It is customary and advisable to separate these from the normal newborns and to have a special nursery for them, under particularly highly qualified nursing supervision and with special facilities.

Certain Special Features of Maternity Care. Much interest has been centered around the practice of "natural childbirth" in recent years. In general, this has been associated with the concept of "childbirth without fear" as proposed by Grantly Dick-Read.[24] It emphasizes consciousness throughout labor and delivery so that the advent of actual birth may be experienced and the baby's first cry heard. In preparation for this, full explanation of the birth process is given in the prenatal period along with exercises designed to promote voluntary relaxation during labor. The husband is brought intimately into the labor and delivery rooms to share the birth experience. There is no doubt that this approach is highly satisfying to many couples. Furthermore, as a reaction to the custom of overmedication during labor it has been of great value. Unfortunately, many young women and some physicians too have looked upon experiencing the baby's birth as the end in itself, with an almost fanatical concentration, which has robbed it of what could be a truer lasting meaning. Viewed in the terms of the concept of total care here previously presented, the baby's birth is a part of the life experience of the mother, the father, and the family. As such it is always a "natural" childbirth.

Whether birth is accomplished with or without medication and anesthesia is not important except on the basis of personal choice and proper medical indications. If no pain-relieving drugs are used there is actual pain for the mother, and a kind of "pain" for the father. But for both it is a "normal" type of pain, one that brings happy results. If this is recognized and the actual birth viewed as one major event in the total pregnancy and the new life of the baby, the desire of the mother to be awake and fully aware of the birth, and to hear the baby's first cry, is a great deal more than mere curiosity. It is the satisfaction of a deep feeling that unites her to the baby, to her husband, and to her family.

Some mothers start with all good intentions of experiencing their entire labor, but tire before delivery and require medication. Others are emotionally so constituted as to be unable to endure the very real pain of childbirth, and should be given effective relief. For both these groups childbirth without analgesic or anesthesia becomes a nightmare, the most "unnatural" childbirth conceivable. But they can still be given an insight into pregnancy and the baby's birth as a family event, even though they may not take conscious part in the delivery.

The real "natural childbirth" then is the way husband and wife, doctor, and nurse look on the whole event of pregnancy. It is not a method but a broad concept.

Rooming-in is in somewhat the same situation. To have the baby kept in the mother's own hospital room after delivery permits a closer early rapport between the two. Usually, though not always, it is the mother who wishes to nurse who also wants rooming-in, and it is often combined with "natural childbirth." Rooming-in at its best reproduces the advantages of home delivery in the close association of mother and baby, and to some extent the father. First-time mothers, while perhaps more fearful of rooming-in at the beginning, more often obtain greater benefit than multiparae. It is a valid attempt to adapt hospital routine to the more "normal" situation of home delivery. The shift from the hospital environment to the home is eased, for the mother has from the first day had responsibility for the baby and has learned its care as an individual. She has had the advantage of expert supervision at all times in this. The advantages of rooming-in are negated if the hospital staff accepts the request for rooming-in as a desire to be left alone with the baby. Rooming-in calls for patient and prolonged supervision. If given in this spirit the period is one of the most fruitful of all the teaching opportunities in pregnancy care. Perhaps one of the most valuable, if somewhat subtle, effects is physically bringing the family together from the beginning.

However, some mothers do not respond to this immediate full responsibility. These mothers, who none the less can develop full maternal feeling, benefit from a more gradual introduction. The physician and nurse must always be watchful for symptoms of undue fatigue and tension as a result of overzealous attention to the infant. In these instances periodic removal of the baby, even to temporary return to the usual nursery routine, is appropriate. Once again the emphasis should be upon fostering a natural and easy adjustment to the new situation as part of total family living.

The advantages of consultation have been stressed throughout this chapter. However, it is of no value unless consultants are qualified and readily available. Because much of the need for assistance is in emergency situations, obstetrical consultation is often difficult to provide. Yet there should be a constant effort to secure this aid. Consultation can be utilized successfully in anticipating problems and in leading to their prevention.

Separate note must be made of the opportunities throughout the maternity period for teaching the positive side of pregnancy hygiene. If this is consonant with the broad concept of maternity care, the obstetrician and his associates may build with the wife and husband not only a physically healthful pregnancy, but a philosophy of family living. This requires counselling of the family at all of its stages as a group and at all ages of its separate members. The impressionable stage of childhood responds readily to teaching by example. Adolescence brings an almost desperate seeking for new factual knowledge on the one hand, and, to adults a confusing, conflicting disregard of advice on the other. Premarital and preconceptual counselling offer opportunities for sound instruction in physiology as well as help in the great emotional and social changes that accompany these events. Pregnancy, in its rapid physical transformations and strong feelings toward the fetus and baby, is a time that demands and tries the capabilities of the physician-as-teacher to the utmost. Finally, the period of the menopause and the age of the grandmother call for patient and tactful guidance in the physical stress of endocrine changes and in the emotional and social conflicts of the old and the young generations.

The question of hospital or home delivery is, in the light of this broad approach, more or less an academic one. There are advantages and disadvantages to each. Wherever the delivery takes place, safety is the first priority. While in this country the hospital usually offers the least risk, this may not be so in other countries. Furthermore, the generally beneficial emotional and social climate of the home can to some degree be simulated in the hospital.

I V

PHYSICAL GROWTH
AND DEVELOPMENT

CHANGING CHARACTERISTICS OF GROWTH
AT SUCCESSIVE AGE PERIODS THROUGHOUT CHILDHOOD

HAROLD C. STUART

The physical aspects of the child's total growth and development are isolated in this chapter for convenience in discussion. His actual growth and development progress is an interrelated whole, involving concurrent progress in psychological and social development. Time needs to be viewed also in arbitrarily selected units or periods whereas a child's progress presents a continuum of changes appropriate to his stage of growth and development.

Great progress has been made in physical growth and development before birth. During the first two years changes continue at a rapid pace and the child accomplishes many important developmental tasks. The most rapid and critical of these changes are the physiological adaptations of the newborn period when he must quickly initiate respiration and make necessary postnatal adjustments in circulation and other functions. The rest of the year is characterized by particularly rapid growth and maturation of organs and tissues which permit increased functional capacities in most body parts but especially of the nervous system. During his second year growth decelerates but many developmental tasks are accomplished, the most conspicuous being co-ordinated reflex and voluntary motor activities, including walking and increasing control of excretory functions. During the preschool period growth proceeds at a slower, more even year to year rate while physical activities increase in scope and vigor. There is further mastery and co-ordination of many functions and motor mechanisms and rapid learning. During the school years a faster pace of growth gradually becomes established, particularly in broadening out of the trunk, increase in size, strength and tone of muscles, and usually in body weight. Following this, the rapid and striking changes of the adolescent period set in.

The customary changes in over-all growth by age periods are best revealed by considering the gains in weight and height separately. During the embryonic period there is very little growth quantitatively, although as described in Chapter III the organism is going through most rapid developmental changes by cell multiplication and differentiation, with organization of rudimentary organs, tissues, and body systems. During the middle fetal period, however, growth in length is very rapid, the increment for this trimester being greater than for any subsequent three month period in life. However, body weight does not increase proportionately because there is little increase in muscle or fat and relatively little mineral deposit in the bones. The head and chest are growing rapidly to accommodate the organs which must be functioning by birth. During the third trimester, or the late fetal period, the body begins to fill out, the skeleton becomes heavier with more fat being deposited in the subcutaneous tissue to provide the fetus with better insulation after birth. Hence, although growth in length slows down appreciably, gain in weight becomes much more rapid. Because of this, it is understandable why a baby born prematurely will be relatively much thinner and lighter in weight than short in length and generally more scrawny in appearance than when born at full term.

From birth to maturity growth in height and increase in weight continue at different rates in the different age periods and for the two measurements. The changes with age in the rate of progress in height reflect somewhat similar changes in other body measurements. Figure 2 shows the average gain in weight, length or height, chest circumference, and pelvic breadth by year of age from birth through 18 years. It also shows average gains in head circumference to 4 years and in circumference of calf from 5 years. The gains for boys and girls are plotted separately because of important differences in the ages at which the adolescent changes in rates of gain take place and in the magnitudes of these increases. It will be seen from this figure that gain in weight is greater in the first than in any subsequent year, declining abruptly in the second and being very small in the third, fourth, and fifth years. During the school age period there is slightly more rapid gain but with little year by year change. Weight gain then increases moderately in early adolescence, then rapidly to a peak in the fourteenth year for boys and thirteenth for girls, after which it declines sharply for three or four years. Gain in length or height is far greater in the first than in any subsequent year, being on the average at least double that in the second year. During the later years of childhood proper the gains in height tend to diminish slightly, then increase yearly during the early part of adolescence to reach a maximum

---

[a] Measurements for the first five years were obtained from white children in Boston in connection with the Longitudinal Studies of Child Health and Development, Harvard School of public Health. Measurements for the years 5 to 18 were obtained from children studied in Iowa and are available through the courtesy of Howard V. Meredith, Iowa Child Welfare Research Station, the State University of Iowa.

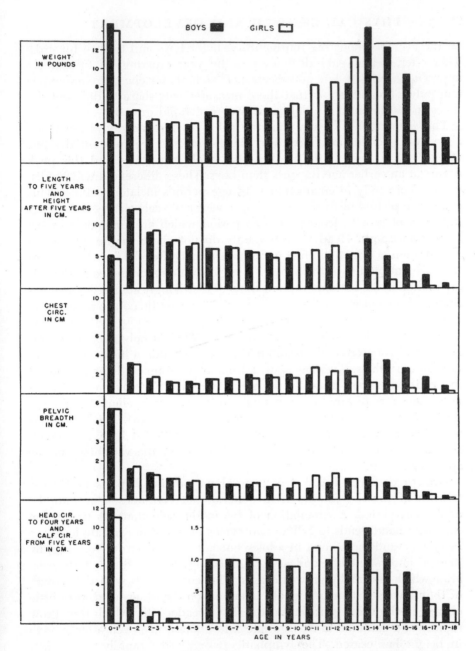

Figure 2. Average gains in selected body measurements for boys and for girls by year of age[a]

Source: *Reproduced from H. C. Stuart and S. S. Stevenson, "Physical growth and development," in* Nelson's textbook of pediatrics (*Saunders, Philadelphia, 7 ed., 1959*), *p. 14.*

on the average about the fourteenth year for boys and twelfth for girls. Thereafter, height gain declines year by year tapering off to scarcely appreciable gains in late adolescence. The charts for chest circumference and pelvic breadth show that these measurements share to different degrees in the infant and adolescent cycles of rapid growth.

This figure shows clearly that the gains for girls and boys are much alike during childhood. However, the increments are substantially less for girls than boys at the peak of the adolescent gains and this peak occurs at an earlier age for girls than boys. These differences will be discussed more fully in connection with age periods in later sections. This composite picture of total childhood, however, reveals clearly the changing rates of growth from period to period which are common to most body dimensions. Head measurements do not share in the adolescent acceleration of growth, in fact gains are so small after the fourth year that they are not plotted in this figure. The gains in circumference of the calf are plotted in the bottom graph to show how strikingly adolescent changes in growth of muscle and increase of subcutaneous tissue are reflected in this measurement.

It must be remembered that this figure presents only average occurrences and is based on data obtained on white children in two regions of the United States. Average figures from other sources differ somewhat in detail but reveal basically the same patterns. For any one child the adolescent rate of rapid growth tends to be greater in amount and compacted into a shorter time than is revealed by this chart. The earlier termination of growth in girls than in boys, as revealed by the averages shown, does not hold for all children because of the variability in the speed of maturation.

Growth does not follow this general pattern in all parts or tissues. Growth of muscles follows it in general, but continues later into the adolescent period. Accumulation of fat in the subcutaneous tissues, on the other hand, tends to follow two cycles of gain followed by loss, one in infancy and the second in adolescence. The head grows very rapidly in fetal and infant life, and at a diminishing rate for the first 10 years after which essentially growth ceases. This corresponds with the growth of the nervous system as a whole. There is, on the other hand, very little change in the sex organs during the first decade, after which they grow rapidly and continue to enlarge late into adolescence even after growth in height has ceased. The lymphatic tissues grow rapidly in the first decade and then actually diminish in amount during the second.

These and other changes in the speed of over-all growth and in the characteristic differences in parts or systems of the body at successive age periods lead to different expectancies in respect to physical findings on examination, depending on the age of the child concerned. This makes it imperative that any child be related to his group in considering whether or not the findings on his physical examination are appropriate for him.

Although average values for populations of children, as presented in Figure 2 in terms of gains by years reveal general expectancies, the range of variability at each age must be appreciated. Figure 3 shows ranges or customary variabilities for boys in the actual values of measurements of heights and weights encountered at each age. Here again the norms have been derived from white children in the United States. The most extreme individuals to be expected in any group are not included in this range chart, the bottom dotted line at each age representing the third from the smallest and the top dotted line the third from the largest per 100 in the sample. The intervening lines give various percentile positions within the range for the boys studied. There is no fixed point within the range for any measurement at any age period below which or above which one may say the child is abnormal, the decision in any case being dependent upon his progress and upon associated clinical findings. The measurements of three boys studied by the writer are plotted in these percentile charts to show the extreme consistency in position *sometimes* held by individuals. Consistency in progress for the individual may express itself in other ways such as gradual change to a lower or higher position in the range due to relatively slow or fast progress or by change in rate from period to period. There is no reason to believe that the advanced child in this figure was a physically "healthier" or more "satisfactory" child than was the smaller one. He was clearly very different at every age and as a result undoubtedly had different needs. This must be borne in mind when considering any charts which compare children in this way. Consistent differences in level or speed of progress, or even changes in these from one age period to another commonly occur as apparently normal expressions of inherent potentialities. However, the more unusual or irregular the course which is followed the more justification there is for suspecting that some environmental factor or intrinsic abnormality may be interfering with appropriate progress. In such instances there is clear justification to search carefully for such possible causes. It must be noted that the range values in Figure 3, like the average values in Figure 2, are based upon studies of white children in the United States. Such norms differ somewhat from those derived from other geographic or national groups with different racial and socioeconomic compositions.

These contrasting characteristics of growth at successive age periods should be kept in mind while studying in more detail the physical and physiological characteristics and changes of each age period as presented in the following sections of this chapter. One should remember also that one period merges gradually into another and that individuals differ not only in the speed and extent of growth but in the timing in relation to age of the changes which do occur. In the following sections the major features of both growth and development are considered in more detail,

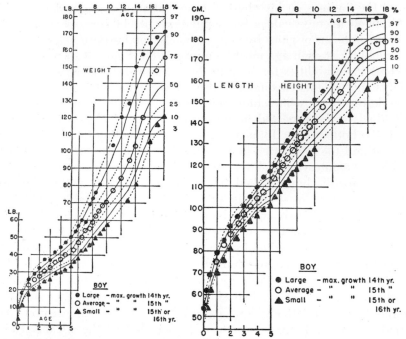

Figure 3. Growth curves of one large, one average, and one small boy, all showing consistent growth, as plotted against percentile norms for weight, length and height, by age[a]

Source: *Reproduced from H. C. Stuart, "The adolescent," Pediat. Clin. North America 1 (1954), 472.*

[a] Cases selected from Longitudinal Studies of Child Health and Development, Harvard School of Public Health.

PROGRESS DURING INFANCY
PAULINE G. STITT

THE NEONATE: BIRTH TO FOUR WEEKS

Good care is of the utmost importance for all babies during the neonatal period. It is especially decisive for those who are not completely normal at birth and have extra need for high quality care to enable them to surmount the ordinary hurdles of newborn adjustment plus their own particular handicaps.

From the standpoint of development the first 4 weeks following birth, the neonatal period, is the most important and critical age, for the infant is not only most immature and dependent but is changing most rapidly. During this crucial 4 week period — particularly the first 2 weeks — adverse conditions of environment and care are more likely than at any other time to have serious effects on immediate and future progress.

Appropriate care under close medical supervision and suitable environment during these 4 weeks, can also be decisive in respect to the outcome of many conditions which were initiated before, during, or immediately after birth. The fact that 60 per cent of infant mortality occurs during this period with half the deaths occurring during the first 24 hours emphasizes the importance to the infant of good prenatal care to prevent postnatal difficulties and of prompt and appropriate postnatal care when difficulties are present. On the one hand such care will often prevent neonatal problems from arising, and on the other it contributes to alertness in diagnosis, treatment, and individual care during the first postnatal weeks.

Many anatomic and physiologic changes must occur during the early days after the umbilical cord has been cut and the infant is no longer supported by the mother's circulation and body protection. Some of these special changes take place in a matter of moments; for example, the initiation of inspiration of air into the bronchi and the beginning expansion of the lung alveoli. Most of the adaptations to extrauterine existence are accomplished, although not necessarily fully, in a matter of days — for example, the fuller expansion of the lungs and the development of adequate pulmonary circulation. Until these changes have taken place it is normal for the baby to become cyanotic on crying or with exertion, and to have irregular breathing with momentary cessation followed by rapid, shallow breathing.

The flow of blood through the heart changes radically in these early days. The fetal flow from the right to the left side of the heart, bypassing the lungs through an opening between the auricles is now progressively discontinued and increasingly the neonate's blood is forced into the expanding pulmonary circulation until finally the opening between the auricles, no longer serving any useful purpose, closes. Other circulatory changes are associated with the cutting of the cord and discontinuance of the function of the umbilical vessels.

Gastrointestinal function does not proceed so rapidly but the healthy baby is born well supplied with nutrients to meet the needs of the first few days of life. Actually, however, the mechanisms are ready at birth for the taking, digestion, absorption, and evacuation of appropriate liquid foods. Sucking and swallowing reflexes manifest themselves immediately and meconium accumulated in the intestines may be expelled at any time. Somewhat more slowly, a series of physiologic, biochemical, and hematologic changes take place to permit appropriate utilization of all essential food nutrients and their conversion into needed tissue components for rapid body growth.

There tends to be a characteristic pattern for change in levels of biochemical substances in the blood with marked fluctuation in their levels during the early days when the infant is acquiring his ability to stabilize them. Stabilization of these levels of physiologic activities and biochemical substances becomes reasonably well established during the first month and tends to improve further throughout infancy.

During the early months the levels of amino acids, minerals, vitamins, and other components fluctuate greatly from day to day. They also vary from individual to individual and the various substances change according to their respective characteristic patterns. For example, the hemoglobin level and the red blood cell count are very high at birth, but fall rapidly during the early days and remain low until much later at from 6 to 9 months when they begin a gradual rise for the next year or two.

The kidneys begin to function shortly after birth but their ability to control water balance in the tissues and to dispose of waste substances is only gradually established, steady progress being made during the whole neonatal period.

Following birth, physical growth continues during the first month much as it progressed during late fetal life, except that there is some loss of weight during the first few days. Much of the loss, often as high as 10 per cent of body weight, is due to the readjustment of the water content of body tissue. This is considered physiologic and no attempt should be made to prevent it by haste in giving foods or fluids. Gain in weight after birth begins at very different times but usually is well started during the second week and birth weight is usually regained soon thereafter. After two or three weeks, if feedings are satisfactory, gain becomes increasingly rapid during the remainder of the neonatal period.

All the sensory mechanisms are capable of functioning at the time of birth but most do so at a primitive level. The response of the eyes to bright light and of the ears to loud noises can be elicited shortly after birth, but the tactile sense is the most highly developed particularly in the region of the mouth. The newborn's response to sensory stimulation of any kind is essentially a characteristic pattern of primitive body reflexes or over-all mass activity.

A clinically important finding in the newborn is Moro's reflex, otherwise referred to as the "startle" or "embracing" reflex. This occurs in response to a sensation of loss of support and can be elicited by almost any sudden change of body position. The usual method is to place the infant on his back on a firm flat surface then to strike that surface with the hand. The infant responds by throwing both arms laterally, opening his hands, spreading his fingers and then bringing both arms forward in an encircling, embracing movement. Simultaneously, the legs are usually drawn up and the child gives a sharp cry or looks startled. The same reflex can be elicited in various ways but all methods are based on creating a momentary startling stimulus or a sensation of loss of support. In the early newborn period this reflex occurs normally and its presence provides valuable information, for its absence or alteration is suggestive of damage to the nervous or skeletal system. Normally Moro's reflex is gradually lost during the second or third month.

Although the newborn's response to sensory stimulation is nonspecific and consists of over-all mass activity this mass response gradually disappears as neurologic development proceeds and specific response becomes possible. For example, whereas in the newborn stimulation of a foot evokes activity of the entire body the same stimulus a few weeks later will result in little or no general body activity but instead there will be purposeful withdrawal of the foot from the annoying stimulus. As maturation takes place the individual parts or members of the body become emancipated from the total reaction although still subject to integrated control. These liberating changes are based on the growth of new neural connections. Progress in this aspect of development proceeds in general from head to foot and from proximal to distal.

A survey of some of the specialized anatomical conditions peculiar to the neonatal period will be useful in establishing an understanding of later developments, normal or pathological.

The growth of the head is of particular importance during early infancy because it reflects the growth of the brain. It has been mentioned that relative to other parts head and brain grow very rapidly during fetal life and this continues throughout early infancy. The changes in the head during the neonatal period, however, are not due solely to growth but represent a correction of the temporary compression or molding which occurred during labor and delivery. The head at birth is usually somewhat misshapen, forced to fit the birth canal and to accommodate to the mother's pelvis. The flat bones which form the baby's skull are not fully ossified and are separated by lines of closure called sutures and by soft areas called fontanels. In the process of birth the skull bones are pressed together at the suture lines and sometimes they overlap making the head smaller in size. During the neonatal period these bones become separated again and are kept so by the pressure of the rapidly growing brain. One of the most serious types of birth injury, formerly common, results from the excessive molding of the skull due to a difficult or too rapid passage of a large head through a small or misshapen pelvis. This may result in hemorrhages within the brain or around it, causing a variety of injuries to brain centers or nerves and may lead to stillbirth or permanent neurological defects. The posterior fontanel usually may be palpated during the first month; the anterior is always palpably open and tends to increase in size during this period. The newborn face is round with the mandible less developed than the maxilla. The forehead is high and often appears to bulge.

Small ethmoid, maxillary, and sphenoid sinuses are present at birth although they are opaque to X rays as a result of being filled with mucous membrane linings. They are not often foci of serious infections in early infancy. The eustachian tubes, however, being short and wide and entering directly into the pharynx easily convey infection to the middle ear cavities and mastoid antra. The newborn eardrums are temporarily thickened.

The skin is covered with a greasy deposit, vernix caseosa, which appears to afford mechanical and antibacterial protection. Modern practice leaves this material on the baby's skin, and hospital reports indicate that the result is a reduction in the incidence of skin infections.

There is great variation in hair among the newborn. Some have thick mats of hair extending down on the forehead. Others are practically bald. Newborn hair is soon shed, and the original newborn hair status gives no clue as to the color, quantity, or other characteristics of future hair.

At birth much of a baby's skin is largely covered with a fine, downy hair called lanugo. This usually disappears by the end of the first week. For an additional week there is usually a fine, powdery desquamation of vernix and epidermis leaving the soft, healthy skin of early infancy.

From 50 to 75 per cent of the newborn infants show clusters of flat, rosy hemangiomas, consisting of excessive networks of fine blood vessels in the skin, especially under the occiput posteriorly, and between the eyebrows or over the bridge of the nose. Usually these fade, becoming practically invisible by 12 months without treatment. Sometimes less innocuous birthmarks may require treatment.

In most newborn the extraocular muscles, those controlling eyeball motion, are poorly coordinated, and may remain so for several months. A newborn cannot focus, but he reacts to bright lights and to objects before his face. The sclerae are bluish, and the iris gray-blue and unpigmented. The optic disk is somewhat gray. There is no tear secretion in the newborn and little develops until the baby is several weeks old, and even then the normally small nasolacrymal ducts may temporarily be too small to drain away the tears, giving the erroneous impression that there is excessive tearing.

The bridge of the nose is small or absent, and the nasal passages are small and easily blocked by normal secretion. Sneezing is vigorous from the start and often helps clear the narrow passages.

The sucking reflex and rooting reflex, both utilized in obtaining nourishment are present at birth. The former is manifest as sucking movements when the lips are touched. In the rooting reflex, when the cheek is touched, the face turns toward that side, and moves up and down with the mouth open as though searching for a nipple.

The frenum of the tongue is normally short and tight. This should be ignored since it is only temporary and does not interfere with feeding or talking.

The chest is rather circular, with the heart in a nearly horizontal position, the apex outside the left nipple-line in the third or fourth intercostal space. Complete lung expansion does not take place for at least several days, and audible rales may be normal throughout this period. Throughout the neonatal weeks breathing is principally diaphragmatic, with abdominal instead of chest expansion. The most conspicuous feature, however, is the irregularity of breathing, a normal phenomenon at this early stage. The thymus is relatively large at birth, a condition now recognized as normal and not as implicating the thymus as a cause for respiratory difficulty.

Some of the above and other clinical features which may be observed during the newborn period are given in the following list. An attempt has been made to indicate which of those features fall within physiologic limits and which suggest a pathologic condition.

Clinical Features of Importance in Recognizing Abnormalities in the Newborn

Posture and muscular tone. Slight tremors of variable intensity, especially of the extremities or mandible when handled, are within physiologic limits; that is, may be considered normal; severe coarse tremors, extreme flaccidity, failure to use all extremities in mass (motor) activity, e.g. arm, suggest a pathologic condition.

Respirations. Irregular but rather rhythmic respirations are within physiologic limits; otherwise irregular respirations suggest a pathologic condition.

Edema. In the early neonatal period slight edema in back, hands, feet, lower legs, and pubic area is within physiologic limits; any massive edema suggests a pathologic condition.

Cyanosis. Slight cyanosis (after crying), local cyanosis — particularly hands and feet for a few days after birth; or slight cyanosis of the presenting part is within physiologic limits. Constant or deepening cyanosis suggests a pathologic condition.

Skin. First day erythematous flush, light jaundice (starting second or third day and fading), slight desquamation, or white or light vernix are within physiologic limits; a deep or increasing jaundice (especially if present at birth), massive peeling or exfoliation, a bright or deep yellow vernix suggest a pathologic condition. Any evidence of infection is potentially serious.

Head. Molding (a form of "physiologic birth trauma" in which there is a temporary adaptive shifting and overriding of the bones of the skull) and caput succedaneum (local bruised swelling of the presenting head, usually present at birth, when it occurs) — subsiding within a few hours of birth or leaving temporary eccymosis are within physiological limits. Cephalhematoma — a hematoma (blood collection) beneath the cranial periosteum, usually caused by head having been pressed against a bony prominence of the mother's pelvis, is suspicious. If a portion necroses or if there is an associated fracture, it suggests a pathologic condition.

Eyes. A mild conjunctivitis (in response to the essential prophylactic medications) is within physiologic limits; a profuse purulent discharge suggests a pathologic condition.

Face. Mild moderate asymmetry of facial motion is within physiologic limits; extreme asymmetry of facial motion is suspicious.

Breasts. Engorgement without heat, redness, fluctuation, or regional lymph node enlargement is within physiologic limits; with heat, redness, fluctuation, or regional lymph node enlargement, engorgement suggests a pathologic condition.

Thorax. Retraction of lower sternal area — on crying is within physiologic limits — sustained retraction suggests a pathologic condition.

Navel. Purulent discharge, or any evidence of inflammation of the cord stump, or bleeding suggests a pathologic condition. A moist granulating surface for several days at the point of cord separation is within physiologic limits.

Genitalia. Edema is suspicious; moderate, transient edema is within physiologic limits; severe or lasting suggests a pathologic condition. Bloody vaginal discharge is suspicious.

THE PREMATURE INFANT

The types of necessary neonatal adjustments remain the same for all newborns, whether full-term or premature. In addition, premature infants have anatomic and physiologic handicaps based on the immaturity of the various systems which are not fully prepared to function. For these reasons, premature infants constitute a group of newborns at special risk.

About 400,000 of the total live births in the United States, or approximately 8 per cent, are prematurely born. Such a baby is a fetus, with the characteristics of his fetal age rather than those of a full-term newborn infant. Despite inadequate equipment he is obliged to make those adjustments which confront any newborn just separated from his mother's body and from the provisions it afforded him in terms of nutrition, respiratory exchange, temperature control, and blood circulation. In addition, there are usually further handicaps, the effects of the conditions causing the prematurity. Among these conditions may be faulty implantation, defective placenta, multiple births, poor nutrition of the mother, and illness or accidents of the mother, as well as many other possible handicaps including actual defects or disease.

While the physiologic adjustments required for independent existence are the same as for all newborn, they may be facilitated by modifying the environment. This approach constitutes an important aspect of early care and is based upon the infant's specific developmental inadequacies. As for the part played by whatever produced the prematurity, generalizations are of limited use. Factors vary from patient to patient and must be considered in order to understand the specific limitations of each premature infant.

The recognition of the premature infant as a fetus leads to an appreciation of the full significance of his individual physical characteristics. Since it is often difficult to determine duration of pregnancy, objective criteria are used to make the diagnosis of prematurity. The single criterion most generally used is a weight of 2500 grams (5 lb 8 oz) or less. Some prematures weigh more than this and some full-term infants weigh less, but it still is a reasonable basis for statistical analysis, and clinically is useful because it tends to provide one simple criterion to direct attention to a group of newborns for whom special care is indicated.

Although weight is the one criterion in common usage, others are also helpful when used in combination with one another or with gestational age. As examples, a crown to heel length of 47 cm ($18\frac{1}{2}$ in.) or less, or a head circumference of less than 33 cm (13 in.), probably indicate prematurity. Lack of breast engorgement is also a clue to prematurity for prematurely born infants do not have palpable mammary glands at birth, nor is there engorgement or lactation later in the neonatal period, as usually occurs in full-term infants.

Although smallness of size helps to identify premature babies, their problems are not of size but of function, each premature representing a stage of prenatal development. Since in fetal life the several parts of the organism do not proceed at the same rate, an interruption of the course of fetal development finds various organs and systems in different stages of maturity and competence. Thus, if one saw a newborn infant weighing less than 2500 grams at birth and having palpably engorged breasts, one would attach more significance to function than size and would conclude that despite the small size the infant was not born very prematurely.

Before the 28th week the condition of all organs and systems is ordinarily too immature to permit extrauterine existence; at full term (40 weeks) parts or organs are in variously higher stages of maturity, but the normal baby is well able to maintain extrauterine life. Between 28 weeks and full term, various intermediate degrees of organ development are present and varying degrees of fitness for extrauterine existence are attained. The greater the degree of prematurity, the greater is the need for special environment and care. The types of adjustment thus remain the same for all newborns, whether full-term or premature, but premature infants have additional anatomic and physiologic handicaps based on the immaturity of the various systems which are not fully prepared to function.

There are five major handicaps which the premature infant must overcome:

(1) The regulation of body temperature is handicapped by a large body surface in proportion to weight, with resultant heat loss by radiation, by lack of insulating subcutaneous fat, by feebleness of musculature with resultant low heat production, and by an incompletely developed sweating mechanism.

(2) Respiration is handicapped by incomplete capillary development in medullary brain centers and in the lungs, by incomplete alveolar development, by weakness of the respiratory muscles, by weakness of the thoracic cage, by feebleness of cough and gag reflexes, and by tendencies to regurgitate and aspirate stomach contents.

(3) Nutritional handicaps include the fact that the premature infant has the high nutritional needs of the fetus for rapid growth, that he is born with low stores of essential minerals and vitamins, that sucking and swallowing reflexes may be weak or absent, that small stomach capacity and feeble tone lead to a tendency to distention and regurgitation, that there is low gastric acidity, that absorption of fat is poor, that there is incomplete storage of calcium and ascorbic acid, and that the digestive enzyme system is even more incomplete than in the full-term infant.

(4) The premature is handicapped by increased chances of infections, due to its birth before the transfer of protective antibodies from the mother; premature loss of the placental barrier to infection; and the presence of new portals of infection through skin, mucous membranes, and respiratory and gastrointestinal tracts.

(5) The premature is handicapped by additional likelihood of injury to the central nervous system by frequent occurrence of anoxia, by capillary fragility, by prolonged prothrombin time, by tendency to breech presentation, by high proportion of multiple births, and by the vulnerability of delicate, immature tissue-structures to the mechanical stresses of labor.

In addition, every one of the handicaps enumerated above may be exaggerated or complicated by the nature of the specific factor which precipitated the premature delivery. These handicaps constitute special problems and require special care.

The basic consideration in the care of all premature infants is to du-

plicate or imitate, insofar as possible, the uterine environment, so that
the fetus can continue his fetal growth under propitious circumstances.

The growth and development of premature infants varies widely, depending on a multitude of factors, such as the fetal age at which the baby
was obliged to undertake his independent existence, the degree of damage which the fetus may have sustained from noxious factors leading to
the premature delivery, and the quality of care available to, and utilizable
by, the premature infant.

The multiple factors involved make prognosis of growth and development difficult in terms of schedule and timing. Practically all premature
infants are initially slow in establishing their weight gain. In addition,
there is delay in establishing the stability of their physiologic levels. One
can say, however, that in the absence of irreparable damage, the premature infant who survives the initial adjustment hazards goes through
the same subsequent stages of development through which all children
must pass, and in most instances ultimately reaches a point where, according to present-day methods of evaluation, he is indistinguishable in
size and function from infants who had their full quota of intrauterine
existence. The length of time necessary for these accomplishments varies
with the individual infant and the surrounding conditions.

Drillien,[1] discussing her own work and that of other observers in the
field concluded that "the differences found after the first few years of life
between prematurely born and full-term children, as regards height,
weight, and general development, are due largely to environmental factors, being the same adverse conditions as originally acted on the mothers
to produce the premature delivery."

In general, studies indicate that premature infants' physical development approximates that of term infants, if in the early months corrections
are made for gestational age, and most undamaged babies born prematurely catch up with full-term children between 1 and 2 years.

ONE MONTH TO ONE YEAR

As indicated in Chapter I, the periods one month to one year, and one
year to two years are somewhat arbitrarily defined as *infancy proper* and
late infancy. Despite striking individual differences between normal infants in all phases of their growth and development and in the timed
sequence of events, the preponderance of shared characteristics during
these two periods is such that they deserve separate consideration.

Both for full-term and prematurely born infants, the period of infancy
proper is characterized by changes in sharp contrast to those of the preceding months and to those of the year to follow. After the neonatal

period, chances of survival increase but infancy proper is, nevertheless, an important period since the child is still immature, dependent, and changing in many crucial ways.

Infancy proper and late infancy contrast interestingly in rate of growth, body position, and locomotion. During infancy proper, growth is extremely rapid but becomes much slower during late infancy. During most of the earlier period the child is recumbent, but later establishes an erect position. The early recumbence coincides with the primary growth or "body building" tasks of that period, whereas the subsequent erect posture permits the second year tasks of mastering the locomotion and motor control of that body. Another notable difference is that while during infancy proper a child tends to bring everything within reach toward himself, during late infancy with change of body position and development of motor controls, he tends to move toward his foci of interest. These outgoing activities usually begin near the first birthday, when locomotion begins to be possible. About that same time the child commences to use his forefinger to probe and investigate. These motor manifestations usher in the highly active exploratory periods of late infancy and the preschool periods, during which small children acquire further mastery of their bodies, and a beginning acquaintance with the surrounding world.

The physical tasks of infancy during the 2nd to 12th months are those of rapid growth and maturation, with increasing adequacy and stability of most physiologic processes, and with particularly rapid development of the nervous system.

Weight gain during the first three months averages approximately 1 oz daily, then the increments gradually lessen so that although birth weight is usually doubled by 5 months, it is only tripled by one year, and quadrupling is rarely achieved before 30 months. The plump appearance and firm, resilient feel characteristic of the latter half of the first year are due largely to the subcutaneous fat which increases up to 9 months but usually diminishes soon thereafter.

Growth in length continues at a swift but decelerating rate. Birth length is generally 18 to 21 inches. By 3 months the baby will have added 20 per cent to that length, and by 1 year, 50 per cent, thus a considerable proportion of adult height is attained in infancy.

Growth of the brain is extremely rapid during the first year, and by the first birthday the brain is approximately $2\frac{1}{2}$ times as large as at birth. Normally head dimensions enlarge accordingly to accommodate the growing brain. The average head circumference at birth is about 35 cm, and its gain during the first year about 11 or 12 cm, representing a 30 per cent increase. Measurement of head circumference routinely during this time provides a useful indicator of satisfactory progress, and may permit early detection of abnormality.

Vision develops rapidly throughout infancy, going from perception of light and of moving gross forms to color perception, all within the first few months. The short, shallow eyeball produces a normal farsightedness which lessens as the eyeball becomes deeper with advancing age. Extraocular movements begin to coordinate after the first few months of life and, for most babies are well coordinated by 8 or 9 months, about the same time that sitting balance is established and the baby can bend over and pull back to full independent sitting without losing his balance.

Nasal passages remain small and the available air space beneath the middle turbinates is quite limited. There is wide variation in different babies in the amount of mucous secretion present and in the efficiency of ventilation. Both antrums and the ethmoids grow rapidly during the first two years.

The Eustachian tubes remain wide. The canals are short and straight compared with those of older children or adults. Drums are pink in contrast to the pearl gray of later life.

Deciduous teeth are advanced in development at birth. At about 6 months of age they begin to erupt, usually starting with the two lower central incisors. There is a wide time range of variation in the first eruption of these, which occasionally may even go beyond the first birthday. Of the deciduous teeth, all but the four second molars usually appear between 6 and 18 months. In the well (and well nourished) child the teething process is usually without discomfort or signs of illness. However, even mild nutritional disturbances and intercurrent illnesses seem to aggravate and to be aggravated by this otherwise normal process.

The sacrococcygeal curve of the spine is present at birth, the rest of the spine being either a continuation of that curve or straight. The cervical curve begins to appear as head balance develops, and the dorsal curve develops later, after adoption of the upright posture. With standing and walking the lumbar curve becomes marked and remains so to a much later period.

All through the first year, while the baby has been growing at a tremendous rate, there has been simultaneous development of the various bodily systems and the beginning of their interrelated use. These interrelationships and resultant entire neuromotor response become established in specific ways for specific stimulating situations and are thus the first behavior patterns. The term "behavior" is used in this context not in the sense of conduct, but rather as that which a child does in action and response to stimulation. These patterns include not only all manner of relatively simple actions, such as standing, sitting, walking, and reaching, but also the more complicated performance involved in maintenance and change of posture.

Like other phenomena of growth and development, behavior patterns are highly individualistic, and yet have enough similarity among children at a given age to justify establishment of certain general criteria for use as developmental norms, helping to determine where a child is in his developmental journey and at what rate he is traveling. Human action systems are so complicated that behavior needs to be considered within several frames of reference. Of these, the four most commonly used have been described by Gesell [2] as *motor* behavior, *adaptive* behavior, *language* behavior, and *personal-social* behavior.

This categorization affords an orderly approach to study and comprehension of the patterns, even though the separateness of the categories is artificial. The baby himself and his action patterns are not compartmentalized. There is an interrelatedness in his behavior, so that practically anything he does may involve various proportions of motor, adaptive, language, and personal-social behavior, all at one time.

Motor behavior has particular neurological implications involving the maturity and integrity of all the neuromuscular controls, including gross and fine motor function, postural reactions, head balance, sitting, creeping, prehension, and manipulation of objects. *Adaptive behavior* is largely the utilization of the motor controls in the solution of problems. It is the use that the baby makes of whatever motor skills he has achieved. *Language behavior* also reveals the state of organization of the baby's nervous system. It includes all forms of communication which can be felt, seen, or heard — body tension or relaxation, postures, gestures, facial expressions, and all forms of vocal language. *Personal-social behavior* is the child's personal response to the culture that surrounds him. It includes not only the response to all the child care practices of the culture, but the interaction that occurs between the infant's personality and the personalities of those near him.

In all four of these frames of reference, the progress of development has orderly sequence. Each successive stage is the necessary precondition for the stages to come. The prime concepts are that behavior develops, and that in so doing, it follows characteristic patterns.

The developmental sequence for the first year may be summarized as follows: During the first 16 weeks the major developmental tasks are the neonatal adjustments, development of the ability to take and utilize food, and gaining control of the twelve extraocular muscles. The tonic-neck-reflex position channels visual fixation to the conveniently situated hand, and is the precursor of all the vital eye-hand-mouth patterns that emerge later in infancy. It is thought that the side to which the baby faces as he assumes this position is the side for which later handedness will develop. At 16 weeks head balance is usually steady, the baby assumes symmetrical postures, and his hands instead of remaining tightly closed are now predominantly open. He coos and laughs and smiles socially. He still reacts with total body response, so that at an interesting sight his total body moves excitedly, but he is gradually gaining command of his arms. They react noticeably at the sight of proffered objects and will shortly, within a week or two, reach out and contact objects. His eyes already establish such contact for they eagerly pursue a moving object and pause briefly on an article placed in his grasp.

Usually by 28 weeks trunk control has advanced enough to permit a baby to sit leaning forward on his hands. He enjoys bouncing up and down when supported in a standing position, and arm and hand command has advanced enough so he can grasp, transfer, and manipulate an object. When confronted with a cube or other small object, he reaches out, secures it with a palmar grasp, transfers it from hand to hand, and inspects it with eyes and mouth, thus revealing motor skill and developing coordination of eyes, hands, and mouth, as well as beginning acquaintance with texture, shape, and the characteristics of objects in relation to time, space, and gravity. He enjoys his own voice, crowing and squealing with delight, and he smiles at his mirror image.

At 40 weeks the infant usually has secure sitting balance, can creep, and pull himself to his feet in the play pen. He can bring 2 cubes together. He pokes and pries with his extended index finger in a way that suggests early awareness of the third dimension and of leverage. He tries to mimic sound, and may utter a sound, syllable, or word repeatedly. He also begins to imitate other actions and may play pat-a-cake or wave bye-bye.

From 40 to 52 weeks he gains increasing control of his arms and hands, and to a lesser extent, of legs and feet. He extends command to forefingers and thumbs, begins to master precise prehension and continues to poke, pluck, and pry.

Towards his first birthday the infant "cruises," hanging on to furniture, and walks when held by the hand. He usually has a vocabulary of two words by this time and he tries to help with his dressing. He cannot yet build a tower of two blocks, but he tries. He will relinquish a toy on request if one's hand is proffered and can voluntarily release a cube into a cup, thus combining the neuromotor complexities of release with his continuing explorations of the third dimension. The capacity for voluntary release of the cube alerts the observer to another capacity for voluntary release which tends to emerge at approximately the same time, or a little later — the release of the stool — although readiness for toilet training is not ordinarily attained until several months later.

In the second year the rate of growth declines markedly. The child actually loses subcutaneous fat during the year, and net gain in weight from month to month becomes small in striking contrast to the rapid weight gain of the preceding year. The rate of growth in length is reduced to about half in the second year, yet approximately half of adult height is reached by girls between 18 and 24 months, and by boys between 24 and 30 months. The striking progress of the second year is not in size increase but in voluntary motor activities and skillful use of the body. Walking without support is a gradual accomplishment. It usually begins between 13 and 15 months, and involves many mechanical and structural body adaptations.

When a child is preoccupied with mastery of motor skills he may appear to be making very little progress in other areas of development. For example, when busy learning to walk, he may slow down temporarily in learning to talk. These periods of concentrated effort toward motor mastery prove to be unrewarding times to attempt toilet training. This may be because an infant in the process of mastering complex neuromuscular performance, such as walking and maintenance of standing balance, has difficulty in achieving simultaneous mastery of another and different complex neuromuscular activity.

Voluntary control of bladder and bowel, which requires considerable development of the central nervous system, may or may not be acquired during this second year. The infant bladder has a powerful expulsive muscle but sphincter action is not yet under cerebral control. Anal sphincter control emerges earlier than bladder, but, even before it is present, stool catching can be gradually and successfully instituted as soon as solid sitting balance is established. Prior to the development of the capacity for voluntary (cerebral) control, attempts at toilet training are too fatiguing and frustrating to the child, and tend to delay his acceptance and conscious cooperation, even beyond the time when he acquires physical and neurological readiness.

Control of fine hand movements begins to be fairly dependable and comes into use in problem solving, such as fitting objects together. The skills acquired come more and more to be employed purposefully to accomplish some task rather than used just as activities satisfying in themselves.

There is considerable "casting" or dropping of toys from high chair, play pen, and crib, during which the child seems to enjoy the act of release, the resultant clatter, and the ensuing adult attention. He also uses these same activities to throw aside proffered food and toys in the negativistic conduct which characterizes his drive toward independence. Despite this behavior he increasingly involves adults in his play, bringing toys to them as means of contact, and even participates in a simple game of tossing the ball in an adult's direction, although true throwing or hurling come later.

Memory becomes evident and children retain concepts of objects even when those objects are no longer in view. For example, after a child has seen a toy in a certain place, he may go there to look for it and be puzzled if it is no longer there.

By 15 months, release of an object from the hand has come sufficiently under voluntary control to allow him to build a tower of two or more cubes. He also exhibits this newly found power of release by casting cubes to the floor and putting 5 or 6 cubes in the cup. Beyond this number his attention wanders and he begins to remove them from the cup. His sense of the third dimension becomes increasingly evident in his developing awareness of container and contained and this enables him to enjoy forms of play involving placement of small objects in larger receptacles.

He can imitate a simple crayon stroke on paper, imitating the motion of the stroke rather than copying what he sees on the paper.

In addition to his motor activities, he enjoys quiet times, possibly looking through picture books with his parents, turning the pages himself and patting and pointing at pictures.

Speech progresses from babble to jargon during this period and may be elaborate by 15 months. Jargon consists of vocalizations of consonants and vowels with inflections, distortedly reflecting the cadence and intonations of the particular adult speech to which the baby's ear is accustomed. There is increased understanding of words. He recognizes prohibitions now not only from tone of voice which he has understood for some time, but also from meaning of words themselves. He also recognizes the meaning of common words such as "toy," "dog," and "doll" and responds to such questions as "where is your nose?" and "where are your eyes?" Vocabulary size is variable, but he is likely to have 2 to 6 words — names of familiar people and objects, and expressions such as "hi!" He may be specific in his wants, signifying them by a word or by pointing.

From 15 months on, the child steadily improves in coordination in his play and in obtaining what he wants. He is no longer confined by crib or high chair, and spends much of his waking time in motion. He usually can walk rapidly and run, although stiffly, and instead of crawling upstairs, can go upright if he has a hand to hold. He enthusiastically attempts to climb furniture or whatever else he can find. He also shoves small furniture around the house and struggles determinedly to dislodge heavier objects.

The cephalocaudal order of the progression of development is plainly seen during this period. The child is much less skillful with his legs and feet than with his arms and hands. By 18 months he is usually able to throw a ball with fair accuracy but cannot kick as accurately until some months later. Hand preferences may become apparent by this time, but definite dominance may not be seen in ordinary activities. Foot preference is not clear and most eye dominance tests require more cooperation than can be elicited. He usually can seat himself cautiously on a small chair and can build a tower of 3 to 5 blocks. He plays at piling objects and knocking them down, showing as much pleasure in knocking down as in building up. He can imitate a crayon stroke and enjoys spontaneous scribbling on paper — or a wall.

Speech continues for the first half of the second year as busy jargon plus additional single words; there begins to be association of words not only with familiar objects but with their pictures. His new ability to relate verbal symbols to concrete objects enables him to follow simple directions, and by 18 months he can understand such requests as "put the cup on the table," showing a recognition of the meaning of "cup" and of "table" and an ability to follow verbal directions even without gestures.

By 18 months most children are interested in attempts at self feeding, and can manage to get spoon to mouth with little spilling. The amount of accomplishment, and the amount of interest in the process seems related to the family's willingness to let the child experiment when he is ready to do so. He likes to carry and fondle a doll and to trot about followed by a pull toy, especially if it can serve as a cart so that he can introduce, transport, and remove smaller objects. He also likes to play with magazines and blocks, and delights in pots and pans but throughout all this activity his attention span is short. He frequently interrupts himself to locate his mother and see what she is doing and likes to follow her about playing close to her heels.

He likes to dump objects and overturn things in general and enjoys emptying waste baskets and pouring liquids from containers. These activities, plus his rapidly increasing motor range, furniture shoving, climbing powers, and capacity to solve simple problems, introduce dangerous situations which make accident prevention a prime concern of the period.

In the last half of the second year changes in facial configuration, in body proportions, and distribution of subcutaneous fat, alter the child's appearance so that he begins to look like a young child rather than an infant. His motor development enables him to run with little falling, kick a ball, and go up and down stairs holding the railing. He climbs purposefully, moving furniture if necessary to reach for a wanted object. He can quickly alternate between standing and squatting and prefers the latter to sitting. He still likes to pile objects vertically. Fine motor control advances slowly, and he is usually near two years of age before he can make towers of 6 or 7 blocks. In the meantime, he develops interest in lining things up in the horizontal rather than only the vertical plane and can imitate a circular stroke with a crayon.

Play becomes increasingly elaborate late in the second year and involves imitation of activities observed around the house and neighborhood and a child likes to "help" adults do their tasks. He still requires frequent contact with adults and likes to bring them into his play, often pulling them to come and admire what he is doing or admire what he has created. His strongest relations are still with adults but interest is developing in other children though without real social exchange in a play situation. Toys are snatched from each other but there is some "parallel play," with children playing alongside each other for short periods of time. Imitations may include attempts to copy older brothers and sisters at play, even though he does not understand their games. Interest in pictures and books is expanding and usually he can turn pages, name pictures, and point to others named for him. The use of jargon diminishes toward the end of the second year, and he can communicate more effectively by combining words and gestures. His vocabulary usually includes 15 to 20 words and he begins to use these in 2 or 3 word phrases and short sentences. He becomes fairly consistent about telling when he needs to go to the toilet and able to follow simple instructions and retain them in mind so that he can sometimes carry out simple household errands. He can usually cope with spoon and cup and pull on simple garments. The extent to which he participates in feeding and dressing himself, however, depends considerably on his family's ability to let him experiment.

In the above descriptions of infants the terms "he" and "his" have been used repeatedly without intent to imply a sex difference. There is, however, a general tendency for girls collectively to be somewhat advanced over boys in the timing of most developmental steps.

THE PRESCHOOL CHILD: TWO TO SIX YEARS
PAULINE G. STITT

After the age of 2 the child gradually shifts emphasis in developmental progress from those aspects described for infancy. Growth progresses at a slower and more even year to year rate, while physical activities increase becoming broader and more strenuous. Further mastery and co-ordination of functions and motor mechanisms and rapid learning now play a more obvious part.

During the period from 2 to 6 weight usually increases at the relatively slow, steady rate of 4 to 5 pounds a year, although of course some children gain at a more rapid rate while others gain less rapidly. The child seems to grow relatively more in height than in other dimensions, appearing characteristically thinner. This is chiefly because he loses fat from his soft tissues. Obesity is seldom a problem at this stage.

Although change in size is slight, as compared with the tremendous growth rates of infancy, it must always be borne in mind that this growth takes place in an organism which is channeling its energies away from changes in size toward changes in function. Thus, even with relatively small size change, this is a costly period in energy outlay and calls for care to protect the child from undue stress and resulting fatigue. While awake, the preschool child is almost literally in perpetual motion. He is learning to coordinate motor mechanisms and functions previously developed. He has learned the elementary accomplishment of walking and talking, and is busy elaborating the more involved performances of those skills. His mind reaches with inexhaustible interest into the world about him, and in pursuit of these eager explorations his body is kept in almost continuous activity. The newness and unfamiliarity of this motor performance require an expenditure of energy greater than will be needed later, when experience permits greater efficiency.

The development of controls is at first somewhat faltering and the resultant uncertainty is as frustrating to the child as to the adults caring for him. Bladder control is a familiar example and most other controls are equally unpredictable. Like bladder control, the other new masteries are products of interrelated neuromuscular controls, and it is not surprising that consistent function requires considerable time. Thus, during the preschool period there tends to be wide fluctuation in the competence of performance of newly acquired functions. As new masteries emerge they tend to be precariously poised at first. Then, later on, temporary achievements become replaced by more adequate and lasting competence. During the period when reliability of performance is being established the new accomplishments react sensitively to stress or strain. Motor skills or sphincter controls may disappear temporarily in the course of even a minor illness, or under strain or fatigue. There is even noticeable diurnal variation, in that new controls which may seem firm when a child is rested and refreshed may disappear or be unreliable later in the day when he becomes tired. These are significant phenomena with meaning for parents and nursery school teachers, who learn from experience that intermittent function is to be expected in the preschool years, and that rest periods help in the achievement of dependable function.

Such rest periods need not be periods of inactivity, indeed the most refreshing rest seems to be a change to different and simpler activity. Provision of rest has other values, too, for fatigue manifests itself not only in loss of acquired motor skills but in emotional instability and perhaps an increased susceptibility to accidents. The latter is a grave consideration, for the combination of insatiable curiosity, eager but poorly coordinated motor activity, coupled with inexperience, lead to the high incidence of accidents characteristic of the period.

Some of the intermittence of early function is related to concurrent progress in another area of performance, just as at an earlier age we saw the way in which many children temporarily ceased talking while mastering some of the complexities of walking. Moreover, it is always well to remember throughout childhood that at times when a child seems most awkward, it may be a manifestation not only of a developmental phase but of development contingent upon practice and experience.

Body dynamics assume particular importance in the preschool period and subsequent early school years. In the normal course of events the preschool child gradually overcomes his infantile lordosis, walks on a narrow base, and loses the waddle of infancy. When a child first learns to stand and walk his feet usually toe out (are everted), roll inward medially (are pronated), and are held far apart. Knees are slightly flexed and the trunk leans somewhat forward over a tilted pelvis. These postural maneuvers help maintain balance by providing a wide base and low center of gravity. Body weight is thrown on the inner aspects of the pronated and relatively flexible feet, producing further pronation and stretching of the ligaments and muscles of the inner aspects of the feet and legs. As a result there is a combination of eversion and pronation of the feet with associated knock knees. This triad of normal conditions persists for a variable period of time, usually well into the early school years. As walking competence increases, the trunk is held erect with resultant deepening of the lumbar curve of the spine. As growth, strength, ligaments, and muscles progress, coordination and skill in bodily control advance, posture becomes more erect, the feet become better aligned, and balance becomes increasingly stable. Somewhat later the forward tilt of the pelvis decreases, with proportional reduction in the lumbar curve of the spine. Toward the end of the preschool years the toes point forward, the foot arches are maintained under weight bearing, the legs begin to straighten, the trunk is more directly over the thighs, and the lumbar curve of the spine is less conspicuous. These normal developmental changes in body mechanics proceed under the stimuli of the usual activities of childhood but at this period children should not be subjected to rigorous strain or fatigue. It is important in child health supervision to be aware of the normality of these body configurations during this growth period, so that appropriate changes are not mistakenly diagnosed as orthopedic abnormalities.

Postural defects and fatigue tend to reenforce each other, poor posture contributing to fatigue and vice versa. Both conditions are similarly linked with malnutrition, which is also frequently encountered in preschool children. The triad of poor body mechanics, malnutrition, and fatigue constitute a child health supervision challenge for these years and calls for attention to balanced physical activity, rest, and nutrition. Clinical appraisal of nutritional status is a particularly important part of the health supervision of children this age; it involves general inspections in addition to considering nutrition when surveying each of the body systems. General inspections should include appearance, vitality, and behavior at play which are informative to the accustomed observer. Detailed physical examination should pay especial attention to the eyes, skin, hair, mucocutaneous junctions, and mucous membranes, any of which may show signs suggestive of nutritional deficiencies.

Feeding of the preschool child is complicated by the factors just described and by his preoccupation with the fascinations of the world about him. These combine to lessen his interest in food. While this lessened interest is a normal characteristic it requires several precautions. There must be no forcing of unwanted food but reduced appetites make quality considerations paramount. However small the intake, there should be an assurance of adequate protein, minerals, vitamins, and sufficient calories.

Most of the primary teeth will have erupted before the preschool period, the second molars being those most likely to erupt after 2 years. Although these deciduous teeth are 12 fewer in number than the permanent teeth, they fill the jaws until about the fouth year and serve as space preservers and guides for the positioning of the permanent teeth. The deciduous second molars are of especial value and deserve attention, for if they decay early the permanent 6 year molars drift forward, crowding subsequent permanent teeth out of line.

Unfortunately, American children are extremely susceptible to dental caries particularly in certain areas such as New England. The lack of adequate fluoride in the water of the region is an important contributor to this high incidence. The highly refined carbohydrate content of the usual dietaries also is undoubtedly a factor. Carbohydrate operates chiefly by altering the bacterial flora of the mouth, particularly when it is lodged for a long period between teeth in pits and fissures. Therefore, lack of oral hygiene is another contributing factor. The primary teeth are extensively involved and many such teeth are lost prematurely due to neglect of developing caries.

As soon as the last primary teeth have erupted it is good practice to start periodic dental visits for inspections and appropriate care. In regions where there is insufficient fluoride in community water supplies it is best that this defect be corrected by adding it on a community basis because this is the safest, most natural and effective, cheapest, and surest method for protecting the teeth of all children. In the absence of community water supplies other methods have been attempted such as administration of fluoride with water or in vitamin preparations or having periodic topical applications, but all of these have important disadvantages, both risks and limitations. Child health supervision requires such services for dental preservation and protection of the child's general health.

Vision has a prime place in early development; visual behavior patterns are among the first and most complete to emerge. They precede much of body and limb function and are more closely correlated with total action system responses. When a young infant fixes his eyes on an object of interest almost continuous bodily motions tend to cease. He stops murmuring or fretting and may even tense his body or open his mouth in his rapt visual absorption.

The eyes, like the brain and the rest of the nervous system, are advanced in their growth throughout early childhood. The newborn eye has an antero-posterior diameter of 18 mm at birth, which is relatively close to the corresponding adult diameter of 25 mm, largely attained by the sixth year. The infant eye is farsighted as a result of being relatively broad and shallow. This hyperopia reaches its maximum at 6 to 8 years. Before growth of the eyeball ceases, the shape becomes more rounded and deeper, and the eye, therefore, less farsighted. In some cases there may even be nearsightedness or myopia, a tendency which increases as the school grades advance.

Whereas, side vision is present from a short time after birth, "straight" or central vision is low at first and develops gradually, reaching its adult level about the seventh year. The developmental processes involved are largely dependent on use, constant practice in seeing objects and focusing upon their finer details. The early preschool period constitutes a crucial time in this aspect of development. The eyes are constantly busy establishing effective working relations with rapidly changing motor equipment. These changes involve small muscles and delicate coordination as well as the large muscles of posture, locomotion, and gross coordination.

Many complex visual functions require binocular vision and stereopsis or depth-perception. One of the most important and intricate accomplishments in human development is the attainment of binocular vision, the capacity of the eyes to work together as an effective visual team. Under normal circumstances this combined learning and developmental process takes place automatically and equally in both eyes, so that in time their images are blended into combined, "binocular" vision. If something interferes with the delicate balance and cooperation between the eyes there is the dangerous possibility that the vision of one eye may be suppressed and visual development arrested. People with one eye learn to make compensations so that their monocular vision may serve for ordinary purposes, though it is inferior to binocular vision. The latter may be impaired or entirely lost if the eyes do not function together, in which case they work independently and produce two separate visual images or diplopia. The brain must reject double vision, so utilizes the visual image of one eye, while ignoring or suppressing the central image of the other eye. As a result, central keen vision develops only in the eye which is used constantly, whereas the visual acuity of the other eye fails to develop, or even deteriorates, so that that eye serves merely for indistinct noncentral vision. If an eye remains suppressed or unused during this critical developmental period it can never thereafter regain full function. The critical time seems to be late infancy and the preschool period. The resources of modern ophthalmology, if they are to salvage binocular vision, must be used during the first 3 or 4 years of life. Good response to treatment may be expected between the first and third birthdays. After the third birthday hopeful prospects lessen and after the fourth, even though obvious defects may be cosmetically corrected, full vision will not develop.

The extreme importance of early recognition is evident. Children with obvious defects, such as the muscle imbalance referred to as strabismus, should certainly be brought under ophthalmologic observation and care by the first birthday. There are, however, children in whom the lack of binocular vision will only be revealed on testing, so child health examinations should include, at least by the third birthday, provisions to see that each eye is tested separately. Any disparity between the vision of the two eyes should evoke suspicion and referral should be made for opthalmologic study. Proper treatment at an early age restores the possibilities of normal visual development.

Those interested in studying further on the development of the eyes will find it useful to refer to Gesell [3] and Keeney.[4]

Hearing is one of the primary means in which the child becomes related to his environment and is the foundation of much of normal development. With speech, it links children with their families and the rest of society, at all levels of activity.

Three "levels of hearing" are recognized, each contributing to normal behavior and development in infancy and childhood. At the most basic or *primitive* level, sound affords an awareness of movement and change in one's surroundings. In more complicated or *significative* behavior, noises and sounds come to characterize certain conditions, and in turn to evoke response: for example, the ring of the doorbell. Perhaps the most complex level of hearing is the *symbolic* level, related to hearing, comprehending, and reproducing language. The processes involved are based on interrelationships among auditory, visual, and muscular stimuli and responses, and on integrity of the sensory organs, and the peripheral and central nervous system.

Actual perception of sound is only a part of the hearing picture, for the resultant interchange with other minds is a major influence psychologically and socially on behavioral development.

In the preschool period hearing assumes new significance due to its effect on the establishment of speech patterns. The child steadily acquires these based on the speech he hears about him. If his hearing is faulty within the speech range, he acquires — and reproduces — faulty speech.

Through the second year the child experiments freely with sounds and sound combinations, and starts to reproduce the rhythm, form, and structure of the speech he hears. From then on through the preschool period his use of language moves rapidly, so that by age 8 or 9 the basic language pattern is fairly well established, a developmental achievement which is closely related to other forms of childhood behavior.

Child health supervision needs to include hearing appraisal. Testing methods are receiving much attention nowadays. Pure tone audiometry is of great diagnostic value in older age groups but is considered to have limited usefulness in preschool children. Some success is now attained with 3 year old children, by employing the principle of conditioned reflex, and attempts are being made to apply similar methods to 2 year olds. Objective audiometry, requiring no participation on the part of the child, is under investigation and through the use of a galvanic skin-resistance response with conditioned reflex, useful diagnostic information is available in preschool age children and even in infancy.

In summary, the primary concept of development in the preschool period is that though growth is slower, activity is greatly increased. It is a period of learning and adjustment, and a time of developing controls and coordination, so that the demands and tasks are fully as great as those of infancy. The developmental tasks of the period involve great physical activity which must be reimbursed through adequate rest and suitable food but adult judgment commonly undervalues the strength and stamina of the infant and overvalues the endurance of the preschool child. Because of these facts, the preschool period, contrary to much prevailing practice, is still a period for continuation of a substantial form of closely sustained child health supervision.

THE SCHOOL AGE CHILD: BOYS 6 TO 12 YEARS; GIRLS 6 TO 10 YEARS
HAROLD C. STUART

Physical growth during the years referred to as the school age period is characterized by rather slow, steady, year by year gain in most measurements, but with gains in height tending to diminish and those for weight progressively to increase. The skull and brain grow very slowly during this period and increase little in size thereafter. The trunk increases moderately in length, and the extremities become proportionately longer. The trunk broadens and deepens, with shoulders and hips developing similarly in each sex. The whole bony skeleton tends to become stockier. The muscles tend to accelerate their rate of growth, and they and the ligamentous structures become firmer and stronger. As a result, posture tends to improve further over that described for the preschool period, in the sense of becoming more appropriate for efficient upright stance and locomotion and for strength in use of arms and trunk. Toward the end of the school age period, there is also a tendency for the amount of fat in the soft tissues to increase moderately, although the extent of this change is dependent upon the individual's basic pattern of body build. The specific relationship between the comparatively increased rate of weight gain and the comparatively decreased rate of height gain also depends, to a considerable extent, upon developing body build. As a result, children differ more widely among themselves at the end of this period than they did at its beginning. Some individual changes, indeed, are striking. The kind of physique a child is to attain in adult life becomes increasingly apparent during these school years, and it is desirable to recognize the characteristics of each individual's type of body configuration as they begin to express themselves, particularly if they are extreme or unique. These characteristics usually become more and more apparent throughout adolescence but early recognition may help to explain associated characteristics of height-weight relationship, early or late maturation and important features of muscular, osseous, and ligamentous development.

There are three basic types of physique and most people show a mixture of all three, but usually the characteristics of one show some dominance. The types are variously named in different classifications, but the terms proposed by Sheldon,[5] now widely used, identify them as *endomorphy, mesomorphy,* and *ectomorphy.* Pronounced endomorphy is characterized by heavy trunk, thighs, and upper arms, with rounded, soft body contours, tapering forearms and legs, large amounts of fat in the subcutaneous tissues, predominance of feminine physical attributes, and large intestines and amounts of other endothelial tissues. Pronounced mesomorphy is characterized by heavy skeleton in body and extremities, broad rectangular shoulders, large strong muscles, athletic competence, and predominance of masculine attributes. Ectomorphy refers to preponderance of ectodermal tissues composing chiefly the skin and nervous systems, and is characterized by linear build, thin bones and muscles, and little fat in the soft tissues.

Being extreme in any one type of build tends to carry with it certain disadvantages. For example, endomorphs, particularly, but mesomorphs to a degree, tend readily to become obese, while ectomorphs are more likely to become underweight and to fatigue readily. During the school age period representatives of all types may be short, medium, or tall, but on the average mesomorphs are characterized by vigorous growth in height and endomorphs by increase in weight. Ectomorphs usually are the smallest during the school age period for they tend to be slow in their development and late in maturing. Because of these characteristics the extreme ectomorph appears physically inadequate during this period and this is often very disturbing to them and to their parents and causes problems of adjustment. After adolescent growth, however, they tend to be among the tallest of adults. They frequently change also from thin, angular, loose jointed, easily fatigued school children to physically strong individuals, having speed and endurance and being successful in sports which do not require weight. Sheldon and others have pointed out certain characteristics of physical functions and of temperament which tend to be associated with type of physique, but these associations are by no means universal. The ectomorph, for example, tends to be restless and active, and may have difficulty in digesting sufficient amounts of food to meet his nutritional requirements, which tend to be higher than the usual recommendations for age and body size. In contrast, the endomorph tends to be inactive and placid, to have large appetite, and to metabolize food readily.

The chief problem which type of build raises for the physician attempting to evaluate the health status and growth progress of school children is to estimate what is appropriate for each individual in these respects. Although all children should become more robust during the school age period, some may change relatively little, especially during the first 2 or 3 grades. This may be due to faulty nutrition, overactivity or lack of rest, or to recurrent illness or chronic disease. It may as well be due, however, to predominant ectomorphy and slow, late development, which results in extension into the school period of characteristics of the preschool period. Other children may gain weight more rapidly than seems appropriate for their size and age. If this represents advanced muscular and skeletal development or stocky build, it should cause no concern; but if it is due to progressive development of obesity it deserves attention in order to prevent the unfortunate consequences of this condition during adolescence as considered more fully below.

The average child shows no external manifestations of sex maturation during the school period as defined. However, the endocrine changes which lead to sex organ maturation and secondary sex character developments have progressed to such a degree in advanced children that they begin to appear in some during the last year or two. Because these changes begin about 2 years earlier in girls than in boys as stated in describing age periods girls of 10 to 12, still in the elementary school grades, usually manifest early pubescent changes comparable to those usually seen in boys in the first 2 high school grades. Only very advanced boys show these changes before 12 years of age. For these reasons the period between 10 and 12 is the one short period during which girls are likely to be taller and heavier, and gaining more rapidly, than boys. Their general advancement in physical development at this time is far more obvious than at any other.

Menstruation rarely occurs in girls before 10 years of age, and therefore it is an unusual occurrence during the period under consideration; but very advanced girls do reach menarche around 10 years of age so that it is important to be aware of a girl's advancement during the upper elementary school years and when recognized to prepare her for this event. These aspects of adolescence are considered more fully in the next section but occasionally they intrude upon the problems of the school age.

By the time children enter elementary school, physiologic processes in general have attained a stage of development which permits their maintenance under ordinary circumstances at stable levels and their ready adjustment to changing needs and stresses. For example, the pulse rate, which in repose at 6 months of age averages about 130 per minute, with a normal variation between 100 and 160, and which at 2 years averages 100, with variation between 80 and 120, at 6 years averages only 80, with normal range of 70 to 90. Similar improvements in efficiency of function in respect to rate of respiration, vital capacity, blood pressure, maintenance of blood sugar level, and the like, normally have been taking place before, but should continue further during the school years. These improved capacities and adaptations permit greater speed and effort in large motor activities, and coupled with larger, stronger muscles and greater efficiency and skill in their use, they permit much more prolonged and strenuous play without causing exhaustion. Therefore, a larger measure of physical activity should be expected and encouraged. It must not be overlooked, however, that the school child, even though he may be large and seem strong, is still a child and far from prepared for competitive athletics in the customary sense of the term.

Healthy school age children usually can indulge in activities of the types of their own choice without restrictions being imposed because of fear of harm from the activity itself. Prevention of accidents due to lack of judgment and experience is the important consideration and these may relate more importantly to the circumstances surrounding sport participation than to the sport itself. This is well exemplified by bicycle riding which is an excellent activity for this age group provided it can be carried out under safe circumstances. The range and extent of participation in sports should be determined initially and in large measure by the individual's readiness, as indicated by appropriate history and physical examination. Continuance of participation or modification in its type or amount can be determined more realistically by observing the effects of strenuous activity upon each of the children who have participated.

At the time of entrance to school a child may be expected to be proficient in climbing a jungle gym, hopping on one foot, skipping, and jumping. Many other abilities may have been acquired, depending upon the experience of the child. Most children can catch and throw a ball, but proficiency in these skills usually improves gradually throughout the school years. Gesell [6] has called attention to the coordination involved in these acts, including visual localization, stance, displacement of body mass, reaching, release, restoration of static equilibrium and, in connection with throwing, appropriate functioning of the fingers as well as the arm, trunk, head, and legs. Progress in development of coordination and patterned response in these skills is characteristic of this age period.

All growing children need some regular exercise. To assure that they take this, opportunities of various kinds should be afforded to provide satisfying experiences for those with various likes and aptitudes. The activities of choice for children during the elementary school grades and which probably reflect their needs and appear to be highly suitable for promotion of bodily coordination and development, include the following: running or chasing, skipping rope, swimming, roller skating, ice skating, and bicycle riding. The joy derived from the increasingly smooth, rhythmic, and efficient use of the body as a whole should be experienced and developed during the school years, because this conditions the child favorably toward regular physical activity.

Although children of school age naturally seek large motor outdoor activities of the kinds described, some soon withdraw from them for a variety of reasons. Recognizing their lack of skills, or feeling discomfort after exercise due to various physical factors, some of which have been mentioned, may spoil their pleasure. Failures in school adjustments or general emotional problems may also be factors of importance. Much can be done to help such children by seeking the possible causes and trying to eliminate them, and by offering alternative activities, both interesting to the child concerned and appropriate for him. Enforced participation in a rejected form of activity may generate dislike for all sports, whereas joy through physical activity is the foundation upon which continuing participation is built. It should be pointed out that abnormal physical inactivity not only leads to failure of optimum physical development or physical fitness but also to obesity. This state may lead *to* as well as *be* the result of emotional maladjustment. When a child fails to participate willingly or with satisfaction in any of the usual activities of his schoolmates search should be made for underlying physical or emotional difficulties.

Poor coordination, flabby muscles, excessive mobility of joints and poor posture may be factors leading to fatigue and poor performance. These frequent attributes of the preschool age may persist as handicaps throughout the school years.

Fatigue is difficult to identify with certainty and impossible to measure with accuracy because it manifests itself in such diverse ways, ranging from marked irritability or continuing overactivity to complete listlessness. A careful history of the child's routines, activities, appetite and moods, or changes in these may be helpful. Rapid pulse with slow return to normal after exercise, fleeting pallor, and other changes following strenuous or prolonged activity are characteristic. When these occur change to more moderate activities and more breaks for rest should be encouraged.

The question as to what competitive sports or athletics are appropriate for children in the elementary school grades has become of increasing importance, as highly organized programs are being developed for younger and younger children. The Committee on School Health of the American Academy of Pediatrics recently drew up a report respecting

Competitive Athletics for children during the elementary school years.[7] Among its recommendations the following selections are particularly pertinent:

At the elementary school level, programs of physical education should contain many non-competitive, non-athletic activities, such as games, stunts, hiking, nature studies, etc. as well as team sports in which all participate.

Athletic activities of elementary school children should be part of an over-all school program. Competent medical supervision of each child should be assured.

Athletic activities outside of the school program should be on an entirely voluntary basis, without undue emphasis on any special program or sport and without undue emphasis upon winning.

Competitive programs organized on school, neighborhood, and community levels will meet the needs of children 12 years of age and under. State, regional, and national tournaments, bowl, charity, and exhibition games, are not recommended for this age group. Commercial exploitation in any form is unequivocally condemned.

Body-contact sports, particularly tackle football, and boxing are considered to have no place in programs for children of this age.

Competition is an inherent characteristic of growing, developing children. Properly guided, it is beneficial and not harmful to their development.

Leadership for young children should be such that highly organized, highly competitive programs would be avoided. The primary consideration should be a diversity of wholesome childhood experiences which will aid in the proper physical and emotional development of the child into a secure and well integrated adult.

The problem of obesity in childhood is encountered most commonly during adolescence, but frequently it begins to develop during the elementary school years. It is difficult to bring about substantial loss of weight in the child or adolescent already obese, and particularly difficult to maintain any loss accomplished. Furthermore, it is questionable practice to attempt weight reduction during the period of rapid adolescent growth. Prevention, therefore, should be the primary objective in respect to childhood obesity and, if successful, should reduce the incidence and severity of this condition in later life. Since the obesity of infancy is usually transitory and relatively few children enter school markedly overweight, the school years provide the opportunity for recognition of the early stages of excessive weight gain and for correction of the faulty habits which lead to it. The three problems involved in the prevention of obesity in childhoood are: first, recognition of excessive gain in weight; second, discovery of the child's overeating calorically as well as being unduly inactive; and lastly, taking indicated steps for correction of the latter and for bringing about a balanced caloric intake.

The recognition of excessive gain is not as simple as some have been led to believe, because excessive weight for the individual refers to being above that appropriate for him, taking into account his body build and the rate of his development. Appropriate growth charts, with height and weight measurements periodically recorded upon them, can be most helpful; in fact they are indispensable for the early recognition of developing obesity. They may readily be made a part of the health service of any school. However, they should not be used as the sole criteria for making the diagnosis of excessive gain in weight, but only as a screening device to bring suspect children to the attention of the physician. The chart should be interpreted by the physician at the time of an examination, when the differentiation must be made between weight gain appropriate for an unusual child, and excessive accumulation of fat.

Discovery of the causes of overeating is essential to the continuing maintenance of a suitable diet. The causes include constitutional factors which predispose to ready accumulation of fat when more calories are consumed than are needed for maintenance. Since this basic characteristic cannot be changed the child must learn to live in accommodation with it. In other cases the cultural or family habits of eating and meal planning may encourage excess calorie consumption. The mother and father, being obese and liking food, often may set the pattern for calorically rich food consumption. Another factor is the poor adjustment of the child to home or school. The emotional disturbances resulting therefrom, often may lead to excessive interest in the satisfactions to be derived from eating. This same set of factors may lead also to withdrawal from the normal physical activities of the school child. Inactivity causes reduced caloric needs and hence may make excessive a diet which normally would be appropriate for the child concerned.

When the factors present in the given case have been recognized, the plan for changes in routine must be worked out in a manner acceptable to mother and child, and follow-up will be necessary to assure its adoption and continuance. Often it will be necessary to try various plans and to bring about many adjustments before success is attained. It should be remembered, however, that these efforts are directed toward improved mental and physical well-being of the child, for the future as well as for the moment, and not merely to control obesity.

The management of developing obesity involves the collaboration of the family, the school personnel, and the child's physician. The problem may be encountered at any age, but it has been considered in this section because its incidence begins to increase during the school age period and its prevention to be successful requires attention at this time.[8]

The problem of underweight, or failure to gain appropriately, arises during the school years as it does at all other ages of childhood. Its recognition and proper evaluation require the same use of measurements and clinical examinations as for obesity. Undernutrition is more commonly encountered during the preschool years but often persists into the early school years and is a fairly common finding at school entrance. Its background causes may be the same as in the preschool period but added school factors may be involved. Even the emotional factors which cause overeating by one child may cause undereating by another. Overactivity rather than physical inactivity is frequently involved, and fatigue may become chronic or recurrent. Either acute or chronic illness may contribute to its development. Its recognition and management by the child's family were considered in the preceding section but now they frequently involve the collaboration of the school personnel. Undernutrition and the accompanying state of chronic fatigue may first be recognized by the school teacher who carefully observes the appearance and behavior of the child throughout the daily school sessions.

The development of the teeth and jaws deserves further attention in a discussion of the progress of the school child. The teeth which usually erupt between 6 and 12 years are the first permanent molars, central incisors, lateral incisors, cuspids, first premolars, and maxillary second premolars, in that order. However, wide variations occur between individuals in the ages of eruption of the various permanent teeth. The individual deviations from the average age for both primary and secondary teeth tend to be in the same direction, that is if the primary teeth erupt early the secondary are likely to do so also.

Most children in the United States enter school with some missing and many decayed teeth. Unfortunately relatively few have previously received adequate dental attention. As was pointed out previously loss of primary teeth contributes to faulty growth of the jaws and may lead to crowding or malalignment of the secondary teeth. Carious teeth which are retained may become infected and require extraction or be painful and interfere with normal mastication. Therefore, the carryover of unfilled carious teeth from the preschool years adds greatly to the dental problems of the school period. In addition there is need for prompt attention to the correction of defects which appear in the newly erupted permanent teeth.

Much irregularity in alignment or crowding of the secondary teeth as they erupt may be outgrown as the dental arches enlarge and the pressures of mastication move displaced teeth into line. However, many complicated factors are involved and this improvement may not take place. Continuing progress of caries in the secondary teeth may further interfere with the development of the face and jaws. The first or 6 year molars are particularly important from this standpoint, and deserve prompt dental attention when caries begins.

When orthodontic treatment is required to avoid ultimate malocclusion or disfigurement, it is applied at different ages depending upon the nature of the defect but it may best start in most cases before the end of the school years and may have to be continued well into the adolescent period. Therefore, when malalignment or malocclusion are prominent periodic follow-up by an orthodontist is desirable during these years even though treatment may not be required.

It is appropriate to mention the growth of lymphatic tissues in the school age period because of the frequency with which problems of tonsils, adenoids, pharyngeal lymph follicles, and enlarged lymph nodes appear during these years. It must be appreciated by parents and physicians alike that lymphoid tissue, which is the basic component of these parts, increases steadily throughout the first decade of life. It becomes a much larger component of body tissues during the school years than it will be in later life, disappearing in considerable amount during adolescence. Hence, in the school child it is quite normal for tonsils to be relatively larger than at other ages. The respiratory infections and contagious diseases which occur so frequently during the preschool and early school years commonly involve the tonsils and other regional lymphatic tissues, however, and may lead to chronic infection in them. The physician must decide on the basis of clinical history and examination whether large tonsils and adenoids are simply large and will shrink with time, or are infected and a menace to health. The incidence and duration of respiratory illnesses may be expected to diminish throughout the school years.

The child should enter school with any visual defects known and as far as possible corrected. This emphasizes the need for early routine examination as recommended in discussion of the preschool years. This is particularly important in respect to unequal vision in the eyes causing failure in development of binocular vision.

Beginning school work imposes a new work load on the eyes, particularly for near reading, but also for blackboard distance observation. Assurance that both eyes are functioning satisfactorily at both distances is important for comfort and to permit normal school progress. Corrections to permit this should be made before difficulties arise rather than after, and this requires careful periodic testing for which simple procedures are now available. During the school years visual acuity may change in various ways, chiefly in progressive myopia among those who are essentially nearsighted. For this reason periodic retesting is desirable.

Good lighting and appropriate seating, posture, and book position in relation to the eyes is important for comfort, effective reading, and general health. However, not every child needs to have every visual defect fully corrected by glasses and natural accommodation may permit normal use without evidence of strain. Screening tests often detect defects accurately, and yet the ophthalmologist may not insist upon providing glasses, or glasses may be recommended for a time and then discarded. This represents one of the many situations in which the child's problem must be individualized, and in which cooperation and understanding of parent, teacher, and physician may be required.

The child may enter school deaf because of congenital factors, or because of damage to the auditory mechanism, most commonly in the middle ear and as a result of recurrent respiratory infections complicated by otitis media. The prevention of the latter is an important aspect of care during earlier years. Defective hearing may be of any degree and may involve only certain frequencies of the auditory range. The handicap thus differs greatly among individuals. Current practice calls for testing for hearing deficiencies periodically during the school years. This should be applied to each ear at each of several wave lengths. Hearing loss during these years may be progressive, or may be reversed, depending on cause. There is no recognized important change in acuity of hearing during these years among normal children. When defects are present and interfere with school adjustment or progress, suitable corrective or compensating procedures should be instituted promptly. The methods available for those with defects which cannot be corrected are the use of hearing aids and the teaching of speech reading.

THE ADOLESCENT
HAROLD C. STUART

The major accomplishments of adolescence are maturation of the reproductive system with resulting sex differentiations, development of adult capacities in physical and physiologic functions and advancement of mental, emotional, and social development and learning. Associated with these changes is an added cycle of rapid growth superimposed upon the diminishing rate of growth in the major body dimensions during the preceding years. The adolescent period, therefore, covers the years in which the individual "grows up," that is, changes from being a child to being a man or a woman. Some of the processes which bring about this transformation are in progress over a large portion of total childhood or beyond but the most rapid and striking changes occur within a much shorter middle period. For purposes of description, therefore, adolescence is here divided into three periods or stages referred to as: prepubescence, pubescence, and postpubescence. (The postpubescent period is more commonly thought of as youth than as a late period of adolescence but it is in fact the terminal phase of the broad adolescent cycle.) The ages to which these terms apply most clearly for average, early, and late maturing children are shown in Table 2 which lists also

Table 2. Approximate ages (years) and principal features
of the periods of adolescence

Maturation	Prepubescence		Pubescence		Postpubescence	
	Onset	End	Onset	End	Onset	End
Average:						
Girls	10	12	12	14	14	18
Boys	12	14	14	16	16	20
Early:						
Girls	8	10	10	12–	12–	15–16
Boys	10	12	12	14–	14–	17–18
Late:						
Girls	12	14	14	16	16	20–21
Boys	14	16	16	18	18	22–23
	Early endocrine and primary sex organ changes; increasing rate of gain in weight; changing from decreasing to increasing gain in height and other body measurements; broadening of shoulders in boys and hips in girls		Rapid acceleration followed by rapid deceleration in growth; development of pubic hair to full triangular shape; appearance of axillary hair; development of "primary" breast in girl; development of external genitalia in both boys and girls; further maturing of primary sex organs		Slowing terminal growth in height and weight; continuing muscle growth with filling out of skeleton; maturing of "true" breasts in girls; completion of growth and maturation of sex organs and secondary sex characters; completing sex differences in hair distribution and facial configuration	

a few of the characteristics of each which are to be discussed more fully in later sections dealing with the sexes separately. The ages given should be recognized as approximations which serve only as guides to general expectancy and it must be appreciated that some individuals differ from any of these maturation groups in the timing or the duration of the successive periods.

The developmental changes which occur during prepubescence are essentially precursors of the events to follow but are for the most part hidden and begin slowly so that the onset of this period is not usually recognized. Similarly, postpubescence is one of transition to adult maturity and diminishing rates of change so that it gradually fades off into the more subtle state of early adult maturity. The major recognizable events of adolescence occur for the most part during the central period of pubescence in which the sex organs are maturing rapidly, pubic and axillary hair, breasts and other secondary sex characters are developing, and rapid changes are taking place in body size and proportions. The characteristic changes in growth and physical development associated with pubescence receive principal attention in this chapter because they occur so rapidly and involve so many body structures and functions that they are prone to have disturbing effects upon either physical or emotional health.

It should be pointed out that because of the wide differences between the developmental stages attained by different children of the same chronological age very advanced boys may be expected to be ahead of very delayed girls of the same age. Since there are approximately 2 years difference between boys and girls on the average in age of attaining comparable stages of adolescent development, a girl 1 year delayed will be at approximately the same developmental level as a boy who is 1 year advanced.

During recent years interest has developed in the problems of the adolescent from widely different points of view and among different professional groups. Hence a variety of approaches to the study of adolescents has been adopted. In several studies repeated observations of the same individual were made and these have increased both knowledge of the customary sequence and timing of events and also the difference between age groups in these respects.[9, 10] Some more prolonged studies of individuals are uncompleted or their results unpublished, yet sufficient information has been obtained to dispel the notion that progress during adolescence is disorderly or entirely unpredictable. There is probably as much order and pattern in the progress of each individual during this period as at earlier ages although the differences in patterns among groups may be greater. Progress is characterized in the early years by gradual and moderate changes in growth and development, then by rather rapid and sometimes seemingly abrupt changes, followed again by moderate to gradual, terminal changes. Progress is also characterized by greater differences between individuals in the timing of these events on an age basis. Wherever the idea persists that all children of the same age should have reached the same stage of development some children will be misunderstood at any age but adolescence will be particularly subject to misunderstanding. These misconceptions more often result from thinking that normal variations are indications of pathology than from overlooking abnormalities at this period.

Differences between boys and girls in the average age at which each comparable aspect of growth and development occurs have been referred to in considering the young child but sex differences in ages of like occurrences prior to adolescence are relatively small. It was possible, therefore, to describe the patterns of growth and development by age periods for both sexes together in previous sections of this chapter. The great differences between boys and girls in the ages at which like changes take place during adolescence make it necessary to consider many aspects of both growth and development separately for the two sexes. Similar patterns or steps of progress still are followed by the two sexes in respect to many physical attributes but on a different time schedule in relation to age. Also, there tend to be more marked differences between the sexes in the magnitudes of the changes with growth at this period. As examples, one may generalize that girls mature earlier than boys, grow less rapidly, are shorter at maturity and have more fat in the subcutaneous tissues but less size and strength of muscles. These and other physical characteristics represent fundamental sex differences which are first strikingly manifest during adolescence. Among the latter are distribution of body hair, depth of voice, breadth of shoulders or hips, and ruggedness of facial structures.

In spite of the basic sex differences in the course of adolescent growth and development it must be appreciated that differences between individuals of the same sex may be greater than the average difference between the two sexes. Extreme femininity in boys and masculinity in girls can lead to close approximations between individuals of opposite sexes in many attributes. It is only in the primary sex organs which have developed differently since before birth and in the associated sex characters which are directly concerned with the reproductive process that normal boys and girls can in all cases be sharply distinguished. It is in these that developmental changes during adolescence are most profound.

The changing pattern of growth in height during adolescence provides a background of reference for consideration of other characteristic changes during each of its three phases, and their usual timing. This pattern is reflected in growth in most parts or dimensions, but with characteristic differences in the degree of expression of each. The progress of gain in weight must reflect the total of all gains which are appropriate results of growth; but it may also represent unsatisfactory gain due to an excessive or inadequate increase in body fat, poor muscle growth or loss of muscle tissue or abnormality in other tissue components. Hence, carefully-taken and suitably-recorded measurements of a child's height and weight at regular intervals throughout the period of adolescence may serve several useful purposes, but they contribute especially to an understanding of the orderliness of growth in general and the varieties of patterns followed by different groups and by individuals. The usual method of recording height and weight measurements is to plot them on charts against age. It is important that the charts used reflect the range of differences expected among children at each age, so that the child's consistency in progress *in his own part of the range* can be recognized, and not just how nearly he approximates the average. Figure 3 has already shown how consistently three boys followed by the writer grew in height and weight year by year, and how regularly they maintained their customary positions throughout the adolescent years in relation to the norms for the group studied. The consistency in the progress of each is considered to be more significant as an indication of health or appropriate growth than is the position each held within the range for either measurement. These boys were always very different in size but they were not as strikingly different in the year of age in which they attained their maximum rate of adolescent growth as were the groups presented in the next figure.

For purposes of study of the characteristics of growth at each period of adolescence it is more useful to consider the amounts gained or the increments of growth within fixed units of time. Figure 4 shows the gains in height during each year of age from 6 to 19 for 3 different groups of girls and of boys. The groups were selected retrospectively by Shuttleworth[9] on the basis of the age at which each made his largest gain. These are referred to as "early," "middle," and "late" maturing groups. This figure reveals for boys and for girls the changes in the rate of growth for each group, period by period, and also the characteristic differences in the magnitudes of these changes among early, middle, and late maturing groups.

In analysis of this figure, one may start with the *M* or middle-of-the-road group of boys. One notes that the gains by years have been declining slightly each year from 7 to 11 years. If this trend had continued the growth between 17 and 19 would presumably have been much as it turned out to be. However, something very different occurred in the 12th to 16th years. This is what is referred to as the adolescent cycle, or spurt, of growth. Remembering that for the middle-of-the-road boy 12 to 14 years represents *prepubescence*, it is clear that this period is *characterized by accelerating growth*. Taking 14 to 16 as representative of *pubescence*, one notes that the maximum rate of growth occurs during this period,

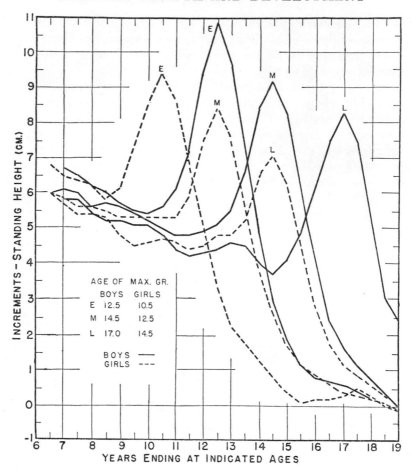

Figure 4. Average gains in height for three groups of boys and of girls (by year of age), each selected on the basis of age of maximum growth: E, early maximum growth; M, moderate group with maximum growth in middle period; L, late maximum growth.

Source: *Reproduced from N. Bayley and R. Tuddenham,*[10] *"Adolescent changes in body build," in* Adolescence, *Part I of the 43rd Yearbook of the National Society for the Study of Education (University of Chicago Press, Chicago, 1944), 41, redrafted from Shuttleworth.*[9]

but also that an abrupt change to a rapidly decelerating rate takes place during the latter half of it. Thus, pubescence is characterized by very rapid followed by abrupt change to much reduced rate of growth. Post-pubescence is characterized by slow and decelerating rate of growth until it ceases. Turning now to the *M* group of girls, one finds maximum growth occurring 2 years earlier than with the boys, in fact coinciding with the *E* or early maturing group of boys. This is the dominant sex difference in adolescent growth, and reflects the 2 year shorter period required to complete it by girls as compared with comparable groups of boys. This difference is seen to apply, essentially to the same degree, to all three maturity groups. The second feature of the girls' graphs is that the amount of increase in the growth rate was for each group considerably less than that for the boys. It is clear from consideration of these features that women tend to be shorter than men for two reasons: they average 2 years less in which to grow, and their adolescent spurt of rapid growth is considerably smaller in magnitude.

Two other features of Figure 4 deserve mention. It is clear that the later the occurrence of the adolescent spurt of growth, the less its magnitude. The late maturing boys actually had a smaller gain from their growth spurt than did the early maturing girls. The second feature is the wide difference in increments of growth among children of the same age. The late maturing girls had 4 years more in which to grow than did the early group but in comparison their adolescent spurt was a feeble one. The "late" boys in the 12th year gained about 4.5 cm, as against nearly 11 cm for the "early" boys. In the 14th year they gained about 4 cm as compared with over 9 cm for the "middle" boys. This, of course, has great practical importance when dealing with a developmentally mixed group of boys of 12 to 14 years in a class in school. It has much significance also for the mother who seeks satisfaction by comparing her son with the sons of her neighbors.

Figure 5 shows the growth in height and weight of 2 girls who differed chiefly in their speed of maturation, one being early and the other late in this respect. The growth curves of these girls correspond in all respects with the composite curves for groups of early and late maturing girls.

If one substitutes three groups of girls, based on reaching menarche "early" (i.e. before 12 years), "middle" and "late" (i.e. after 13 years), for the groups based upon age of maximum growth in Figure 4, one obtains three curves very much like those for girls in this figure. Similarly, if one substitutes three groups selected on the basis of "skeletal age," as assessed from radiographs of the hand, similar curves are produced for both boys and girls. All of these relationships hold to some extent for gains by year of age in body weight. The differences, however, are not as sharp or regular as for height because gains in weight reflect both general body growth and accumulations or losses of body fat due to nutritional factors.

In summary, the preceding figures show that there are regular and similar changes from period to period in the rate of growth of all the groups of children whose measurements are portrayed and that there are consistent differences among the early, middle, and late maturing

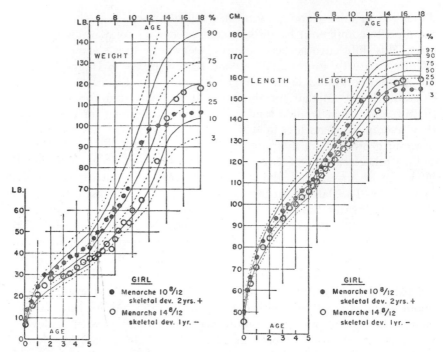

Figure 5. Curves for weight and height of one early and one late maturing girl (determined by age of menarche) plotted against normal distributions for these measurements[a]

Source: *Reproduced from H. C. Stuart, "The adolescent," Pediat. Clin. North America 1 (1954), 473.*

[a] The early maturing girl is seen to be larger in both measurements than the late maturing girl prior to her menarche but to fall behind her at 14 years of age in weight and at 15 in height. The two girls are furthest apart in their measurements at about 11 years, being quite near together at 5 and 14 years. Cases selected from Longitudinal Studies of Child Health and Development, Harvard School of Public Health.

groups for each sex. The progress of growth for all groups during adolescence is characterized by a cycle of acceleration followed by deceleration which interrupts for a period of 3 to 4 years the declining rate of growth which is characteristic of the preadolescent period.

There are several important reasons for attempting to recognize the time of occurrence of this period of rapid adolescent growth. One is because nutritional needs are very different when growth is rapid than when it is slow. Another is that this phase of rapid growth is highly correlated with all of the other changes of pubescence. When the change from slow to rapid growth occurs early, it may be assumed, that, similarly, the child is more advanced in other aspects of physical development than is the average child. When it occurs late, the contrary is probably true.

A few comments will suffice here to describe growth in the other dimensions or parts of the body. Almost all participate to some extent in the adolescent spurt of more rapid growth. The head does so to a very small extent, the small gain during adolescence probably representing chiefly the terminal stages of the earlier childhood cycle of growth. The face, however, and the jaws grow considerably in boys, but little in girls. The shoulders and chest of boys enlarge greatly, whereas it is chiefly in the pelvis and hips that enlargement takes place in girls. It is in these components of growth that the characteristics of the opposite sex may be highly expressed in some individuals and prove disturbing to them. The extremities grow relatively more rapidly during adolescence than does the spinal column, and more so in boys than in girls, so that the proportions of the body become altered. After the epiphyses of the long bones become fused as they mature, preventing any further growth in the lower extremities, the spinal column may continue to grow to a small extent, accounting for some of the late increase in stature. Finally, the continuing growth of skeletal muscle is an important feature of adolescence. This apparently continues, or may do so, long after growth in height has come to an end, or has become minimal. This is particularly a feature of adolescent growth in boys, and accounts for the greater muscularity of men. Although it has not been determined to what extent muscular growth is dependent upon or may be promoted among children with different genetic attributes by regular and adequate exercise it does appear that maximum attainment of muscular development is promoted by suitable activity. The size and shapes of muscle groups appear to be highly related to body build but their strength, endurance, and ability to avoid strain are clearly dependent to a great extent upon the regularity and appropriateness of their use. The most effective time to apply this use is probably when muscle growth is naturally most active. All indications are that the normal adolescent should be physically active and should indulge in a reasonable variety of physical activities to cultivate general and not localized muscle development. There is considerable evidence that faulty habits of activity constitute an important problem among many adolescents. Adequate rest in appropriate alternation with physical activity continues to be important and for some individuals requires attention. Adequate nutrition also is importantly related to muscular development.

It is during adolescence that marked differences in muscle strength develop between boys and girls. Starting with relatively little difference in prepubescent performance, under most tests for strength, this difference becomes very marked in postpubescence. The same increasing differences between the sexes as adolescence advances is observed in vital capacity, in average blood pressure reading, in blood cell counts and hemoglobin values, and other physiologic norms which have relationships to various physical capacities. Girls show quite marked changes in physiologic values between the premenarche and postmenarche periods, particularly showing increase in physiologic efficiency by lower heart rate and lower basal metabolic rate.

Knowledge of the endocrine mechanisms which account for the initiation of prepubescent changes is presently too limited to justify detailed consideration here. It may be said that the anterior pituitary gland increases the secretion of hormones which act upon the gonads, that is, the testes in boys and ovaries in girls, and thus stimulates their development. The testes in turn begin to secrete increasing amounts of androgens and the ovaries of estrogens. The pituitary also activates the cortex of the adrenal glands to secrete these or related hormones which contribute to the increased rate of growth and to the development of secondary sex characters. Concurrently the gonads enlarge and later develop their capacity to produce mature sperm and ova and in other ways to function as primary reproductive organs. Tanner, in a book listed as a general reference on adolescence, has recently reviewed the evidence which is as yet far from conclusive as to the roles of the endocrine glands and their respective hormones in the complex mechanisms involved in the development of the reproductive system in boys and in girls. These developments continue into late postpubescence. The appearance of the first menstrual period in midpubescence in girls is one stage in this long developmental process and it is a mistake to think of this as indicating sexual maturity and full reproductive competence.

Because of the complexities of pubescent development, and particularly of endocrine differences and their expressions in the patterns of development followed by individuals during this period, it is not uncommon to find both boys and girls being considered as abnormal who are simply late maturers or otherwise somewhat unusual in their pubescent progress. The vast majority of children referred to pediatric endocrine clinics for a study as to possible pathologic conditions are found to have no endocrine problem and to need no specific therapy.

With the exception of the testes, the reproductive organs are hidden and their growth cannot be evaluated at ordinary examinations. It is largely for this reason that clinical interest centers on following successive stages of maturing of the observable secondary sex characters. The events in the progress of each of these usually bear a close time relation to events in the others, to the stages of sex organ development, to skeletal development, and to the stages of growth in height. Thus, those familiar with the sequence and association of events can by recognizing the stage of development in one such attribute make a close approximation to the stages present in the others. These features and relations will be considered more fully in connection with the sexes separately.

Girls. An early change of prepubescence that may be recognized in girls is the broadening and rounding of the hips. Another is the first stage of breast development which usually is the earliest reliable sign of beginning sexual maturation. This manifests itself first when the areola surrounding the nipple becomes pigmented and enlarged. A little later it becomes elevated so that the nipple and areola together constitute a cone on a flat chest. This is commonly referred to as the "bud" stage, and is chiefly an occurrence of prepubescence. The second stage results from the deposition of fat under and surrounding the areola, which causes the latter to rest on a rounded base. This so-called "primary" breast usually develops during the pubescent period in association with accelerating growth and the early stages of pubic hair development. The third stage involves the development of the true breast tissue, which gradually incorporates the elevated areola, so that only the nipple remains elevated. This "mature" breast may be in its early stage of development at the time of menarche, but more commonly the breast is still in its "primary" phase and the mature breast develops for the most part during late pubescence and postpubescence.

Pubic hair usually first appears above the vulva, or centrally on the pubis, about the time that growth is becoming rapid and when the breast is in the "bud" stage. This occurrence is taken as the principal observable criterion of the beginning of pubescence proper. Hair continues to develop in the pubic area for about 2 years, changing from the characteristic sparse, straight, unpigmented hair to dense, curly, and pigmented hair, spreading from its original site of appearance to fill the triangle bounded above by the crest of the pubis and laterally by the folds of the groin.

Hair appears in the axillae somewhat later than at the pubis, and goes through somewhat the same stages of change. It usually begins to appear during the primary stage of breast development and is present to some extent at the time of menarche.

The ovaries probably begin to enlarge early in prepubescence, and they continue to grow and mature throughout adolescence, as do the uterus and vagina. Usually the first manifestation of these changes is the appearance of the first menstrual period at menarche, and some time later the gradual development of regular periods, and finally the demonstration of the capacity to become pregnant.

The age at which the first menstrual period occurs is a useful indicator of the developmental progress being made by the individual child.

Menarche usually occurs when adolescent growth is nearing its peak, or about the middle of puberty proper and one expects growth in height to decelerate rapidly after it has occurred. It may be delayed, or the first periods may be scant or irregular, without indicating that the ovaries are not developing satisfactorily, such irregularity suggesting only that the necessary hormonal balance had not become sufficiently stabilized.

The average age of menarche differs somewhat between populations, and apparently has changed by generations or centuries among the same populations. At the present time in the United States the average age of its occurrence is about 13 years. Within any comparable population group there are undoubtedly familial tendencies to be near average, advanced, or late in the appearance of this developmental landmark. Many of the differences in group averages, however, seem to relate to diet and nutrition, the incidence of chronic illness, and other environmental factors, which may have the effect of delaying growth and retarding associated aspects of development.

In discussing growth in height, Fig. 4 drawn by Shuttleworth[9] showed that a normal population of girls could be divided into three groups, reaching their maximum growth at approximate ages 10, 12, and 14 respectively. Simmons and Gruelich[11] have shown similarly that if girls are divided into three groups based on the age of menarche, three very similar curves are produced. They selected for their grouping: menarche occuring before 12 in their early group, between 12 and 13 in their middle group and between 13 and 15½ in their late group. These studies showed that except in girls reaching menarche very late, maximum growth and occurrence of the first menstrual period occur very closely together. Menarche also occurs most commonly when the breast development is in its "primary" stage, when pubic hair is dense but limited in area, and when axillary hair is still very sparse.

Boys. The later age of occurrence in boys than girls of the adolescent phase of rapid growth, and its greater magnitude, have been mentioned, as also the fact that muscular growth tends to be much greater, particularly during the postpubescent period. It is then that the facial contours, particularly the jaws, become more prominent, that the boy's entire skeleton tends to become more robust and angular, and that facial and body hair develop.

There is no recognizable event in the male which corresponds in time with menarche in the female, the sex organ functions of the boy beginning to operate in more gradual stages. Complete development of these organs, and reproductive functional adequacy, is a postpubescent phenomenon.

The first stage of breast development as described for the girl occurs to some extent in all boys, and affords useful evidence as to beginning adolescent changes. Sometimes this develops to the fullness of the "bud stage," and occasionally evidences of "primary" breast development are manifest. Broadening shoulders correspond to broadening hips in the girl as an early change.

Pubic hair proper, and axillary hair, develop in the boy as in the girl. It is the postpubescent appearance of facial, suprapubic, and general body hair, and the receding hairline lateral on the forehead, which distinguish the boy from the girl in hair distribution.

Associated with the development of pubic hair, and throughout much of postpubescence, is enlargement of the external genitalia, the testes, and the prostate. Greulich and his associates[12] have described the developmental sequence of these and other adolescent changes in boys.

In summary, the differences between boys and girls in their adolescent changes are not limited solely to their having different sex organs. The differences extend in varying degrees to most aspects of growth and development. Men are larger than women on the average because they grow during two additional years, and because their adolescent growth is more vigorous; they differ from women in body build because the rates of growth in different segments of the body reflect sex difference. It is interesting that at all ages girls tend to have more fat in their subcutaneous tissues than do boys, a feature which becomes more pronounced during adolescence. In general, the contours of girls' bodies are more rounded and the folds of subcutaneous tissue are thicker, a fact which mistakenly may be thought of as obesity. On the other hand boys become more muscular, a gain made chiefly during adolescence, when their bones also become more stocky and with sharper contours.

The timing of the developmental changes in the many different physical and physiologic aspects of development, and in growth, is highly coordinated. Recognition of advancement or delay in one may lead to appreciation that there is general advancement or delay in total maturation. The usefulness of observing growth in height as well as having evidence of skeletal development has already been discussed but the interpretation of these and differentiation between normal developmental individual differences and the rarer evidences of pathological development requires knowledge, experience, and usually follow-up studies.

The practical problems which arise during adolescence, and which are in some measure dependent upon the changes of growth and development, are numerous, but most of them are transitory and not intrinsically serious. The importance of their effects depends in large measure upon how successfully the individual adapts to them. This, in turn, depends upon many features of his own personality, and on his family and peer relationships. The incidence of diseases or defects which are fundamentally dependent upon faults in development, and which arise during adolescence, is very low. The total incidence of illness during this period has been shown in Chapter II to be considerably less than at earlier ages. The decline in the incidence of respiratory illnesses and allergic reactions is particularly striking.

The prevailing problems of adolescence might be referred to as those of health and development rather than of disease. Obesity constitutes a very important problem, in part because it is more common and more pronounced during these years than at earlier periods, and also because it has more profound effects upon the emotional and physical well-being of the individual. Since obesity usually develops during the school age period, the task during adolescence is usually that of dealing with an established obesity which is causing more and more unhappiness. The objectives now become those of avoiding progressive increase in weight, and securing self-acceptance of that degree of overweight which cannot be altered without undesirable consequences.[8]

Underweight is less common than overweight during adolescence, and the diagnostic differentiation between linear build or late maturing and undernutrition is a medical problem. When the thin adolescent loses weight or fails to gain in accordance with his rate of growth, the physician should seek for causes of this abnormal occurrence and attempt to adjust the individual's dietary habits and program of activities accordingly. Some adolescents drive themselves far beyond their physical capacities in connection with sports, social activities, homework, jobs, or most commonly because of a combination of these activities which in total means excess for them.

A common problem confronting the physician in connection with adolescence relates to the recognition of very early or very late onset or progress of adolescent development. Often the child and his parents are concerned by what amounts only to normal or very moderate advancement or delay. The extremes in either direction, however, are almost certain to create problems. Such situations call for careful explanation.

Because the adolescent becomes deeply concerned with himself and is especially interested in his physique and sexuality, he wishes above all to be assured that he is "normal" and like his peers. Much emotional distress is caused among early or late developers by mistaken judgments that their differences from their peers are evidences of abnormality which will persist into later life. The problem here is one of convincing them that they are normal despite their differences.

When the onset of pubescent changes is greatly delayed it is important for the physician to determine, if possible, when these changes will begin. It has been stated previously than an X-ray film of the hand can reveal, with reasonable accuracy, the developmental stage which the skeleton has attained, and from this one can generalize, within limits, as to when the successive stages of pubescence will occur. The time of onset of the accelerating growth of adolescence is not easily detected by watching weight alone, because weight gain has been accelerating year by year during the school years. It may be recognized more readily, however, when height has been measured periodically during the school years. The first sharp rise in the height increment is indicative of the beginning of the major changes of the pubescent period. So also is the first stage of breast development, or the first appearance of pubic hair.

Very slow onset of pubescent changes requires the physician to look for evidences of endocrine abnormality or developmental disease; but as stated before, these conditions will be rarely encountered. He must also consider the events of childhood and their possible delaying effect upon development. Any prolonged deficiency in diet, or any chronic disability which interferes substantially with the maintenance of normal nutrition, may greatly delay this development.

Highly sex-linked characters can be prominent in the opposite sex without the implication of abnormality or bisexuality. As examples, adolescent boys may have narrow shoulders, broad hips, rounded contours, or other feminine aspects of build. Girls, on the other hand, may have broad shoulders, narrow hips, considerable facial and body hair, deep voice, and the like. When these features of the opposite sex are prominent they may be very disturbing to the adolescent who manifests them, even though they are not pathological for him.

The intense concern of the adolescent with himself and his normality raises more difficult problems when he is in fact abnormal in any important way. Disfigurements, defects, and disabilities which formerly have been accepted may now take on new importance, often beyond that justified by their nature or extent. Patient and considerate help may be required at this time in order to permit healthy acceptance and adaptations.

The first menstrual periods in girls usually are quite irregular, often with several months being skipped between the first and second. Other irregularities relating to quantity of flow, duration, and discomfort are frequently observed. These are usually due to the immaturity of the sex organs and endocrine controls, and some such irregularities occur in most girls for a year or two following menarche. The very complicated interaction of various processes is understandably slow in achieving stability and coming to smooth function, just as other physiologic processes have been shown to be unstable and poorly regulated during infancy. It must be recognized, however, that nutritional deficiencies, illnesses, emotional tensions, and probably other factors may interfere with the functioning of this delicate mechanism in girls.

Aside from normal irregularity, as previously noted, periods which are prolonged, profuse, and painful are commonly associated with many subjective symptoms. They may be accompanied by headaches, nausea, incapacity for work or play, mood changes, and the like. These features are difficult to evaluate, but their causes are more likely to be related to general physical and emotional factors than to sex organ abnormalities. They are probably in part accounted for by temporary functional irregularities in developing endocrine mechanisms, possibly at times secondary to faulty dietary or activity habits. These occurrences should be investigated by a physician.

A problem which is commonly troublesome during adolescence is that of facial acne. This condition is due to overactivity of the sebaceous glands associated with the hair follicles of the skin, and results primarily from plugging of the orifices of these glands. It occurs during adolescence almost regularly, to some degree and at some time, although it tends to be more extensive and prolonged in boys. The normal skin changes of the period are probably brought about by increased amounts of circulating androgenic hormones. The sequence of events when these sebaceous glands become plugged is the formation of comedones, or "blackheads," which are prone to become congested or infected, leading to the formation of papules, pustules, indurated areas, and sometimes to permanent and deep scarring of the skin. The extreme activity of the sebaceous glands at this age causes marked oiliness, and calls for very frequent and thorough cleansing of the skin to avoid the sequence of events described. Unfortunately, the condition is difficult to control in early adolescence, particularly as there is commonly a contributory aversion to body cleanliness at that period. The early adolescent lack of interest in cleanliness often is manifested simultaneously by a high incidence of gingivitis, athlete's foot, and other evidences of neglect among children who previously have not exhibited these. At a somewhat later stage, and particularly among girls, interest in appearance seems to prevail but by this time much damage to the skin may already have occurred. The presence of chronic acne may be very disturbing, and it commonly appears to aggravate or be aggravated by psychological disturbances. This is an age at which the injudicious use of cosmetics or the excessive efforts to cure it may aggravate a moderate self-limited condition. The incidence of some degree of acne during the early pubescent period should be viewed as due to normal physiologic changes. Acne will usually disappear in the course of developing hormonal stabilization, as part of maturing, but it should be dealt with on the basis of control through particular attention to good facial hygiene. The basis for aggravation of acne by certain foods, such as chocolate, is not well established, but is so strongly suggested in individual cases as to justify careful consideration of individual eating habits and the elimination of suspected offending foods.

V

NUTRITION

INTRODUCTION

In many areas of the world nutrition ranks with sanitation as a major problem of public health and as one of the most promising approaches to the promotion of health and the prevention of disease. In countries such as the United States where sanitation is generally advanced and preventive control and treatment of many of the infectious diseases are well in hand, nutrition remains as perhaps the single most important environmental factor affecting health. This is especially true in all periods of growth and development when, because of additional demands upon the human organism, nutritional requirements are increased. Ignorance and poverty are the principal causative factors in inadequate nutrition. In this country, with respect to availability of food and financial means of procuring it, good nutrition is well within the grasp of the great majority of the population. Education of the public concerning the importance of good nutrition, nutritional needs, and the use of available food supplies to meet these requirements at various socioeconomic levels and different cultural backgrounds is important before satisfactory habits of food selection and consumption will be practiced by most people even if ample foods in all categories were available to all. And here all available health personnel must assume appropriate responsibility. Hence, nutrition education is essential for all medical personnel and others associated with them.

Several dietary standards are available for guidance in the planning and evaluation of educational programs concerning diets and food supplies of individuals and groups in the various areas of the world. The National Research Council's *Recommended Dietary Allowances*[1] is one such standard. It should be realized that the objectives sought by different food standards vary widely. In the use of any dietary standard it is important that its limitations be recognized and the standard correctly applied. The National Research Council's recommended allowances "are designed to maintain good nutrition in healthy persons in the United States under current conditions of living and to cover nearly all variations of requirements for nutrients in the population at large. They are meant to afford a margin of sufficiency above minimal requirements and are therefore planned to provide a buffer against the added needs of various stresses and to make possible other potential improvements of growth and function. The allowances are not to be considered adequate to meet the additional requirements associated with disease or for nutrient repletion in severely depleted persons. On the other hand, they may be more generous than would be practical for feeding large groups under conditions of limited food supply or economic stringency." "The title 'Recommended Dietary Allowances' was selected for this standard in the effort to make it clear that the levels of nutrient intake recommended were judgments . . . to avoid misinterpretation of the allowances as representing either minimal or optimal nutrient requirements." In interpreting these allowances it is important to keep in mind that nutritional needs vary widely among individuals, and in an individual who differs from the reference standard adjustments are necessary. These allowances are given in Table 3 and are referred to repeatedly.

MATERNAL NUTRITION DURING THE PERIOD OF LACTATION
BERTHA S. BURKE

The preparation of the mother for breast feeding and her success in breast feeding have two important aspects which may be referred to as psychological and physiological. Both are of sufficient importance to receive attention regularly as a part of prenatal and postpartum care until the infant is weaned. The essential aspects of the psychological preparation are to be sure that the mother understands what is involved for herself and her infant, that she is motivated to elect this method of feeding if there are no contraindications, and that she understands what is required of her to be successful. It is equally important that unjustified anxieties regarding it be dispelled, and that cultural factors which mitigate against breast feeding be dealt with appropriately.

The essential aspects of the physiological preparation of the mother are first that adequate medical care be given to assure that her general health and physiological processes are satisfactory, and second that adequate instructions be given her to assure that she is prepared nutritionally for continuing success in nursing. Attention in this section is devoted principally to dietary changes required and the reasons for them.

Attention has been given in Chapter III to the nutritional status and diet of the woman during pregnancy and before as an integral part of prenatal care. Consideration of these during the period of lactation is predicated on the belief that for infants, human milk is the desired source of nutrients. Breast feeding is particularly indicated during the first month of life when infants have difficulty in maintaining homeo-

Table 3. Recommended daily dietary allowances[a] designed for maintaining good nutrition in normally active, healthy persons in the U.S.A.

Group	Age (years)	Weight (kg)	Weight (lb)	Height (cm)	Height (in.)	Calories	Protein (gm)	Calcium (gm)	Iron (mg)	Vitamin A (I.U.)	Thiamine (mg)	Riboflavin (mg)	Niacin[b] (mg equiv.)	Ascorbic acid (mg)	Vitamin D (I.U.)
Men	25	70	(154)	175	(69)	3200[c]	70	0.8	10	5000	1.6	1.8	21	75	
	45	70	(154)	175	(69)	3000	70	0.8	10	5000	1.5	1.8	20	75	
	65	70	(154)	175	(69)	2550	70	0.8	10	5000	1.3	1.8	18	75	
Women	25	58	(128)	163	(64)	2300	58	0.8	12	5000	1.2	1.5	17	70	
	45	58	(128)	163	(64)	2200	58	0.8	12	5000	1.1	1.5	17	70	
	65	58	(128)	163	(64)	1800	58	0.8	12	5000	1.0	1.5	17	70	
Pregnant (second half)						+300	+20	1.5	15	6000	1.3	2.0	+3	100	400
Lactating (850 ml daily)						+1000	+40	2.0	15	8000	1.7	2.5	+2	150	400
Infants[d]	0–1/12 [d]						[d]								
	2/12–6/12	6	(13)	60	(24)	kg × 120		0.6	5	1500	0.4	0.5	6	30	400
	7/12–12/12	9	(20)	70	(28)	kg × 100		0.8	7	1500	0.5	0.8	7	30	400
Children	1– 3	12	(27)	87	(34)	1300	40	1.0	7	2000	0.7	1.0	8	35	400
	4– 6	18	(40)	109	(43)	1700	50	1.0	8	2500	0.9	1.3	11	50	400
	7– 9	27	(60)	129	(51)	2100	60	1.0	10	3500	1.1	1.5	14	60	400
	10–12	36	(79)	144	(57)	2500	70	1.2	12	4500	1.3	1.8	17	75	400
Boys	13–15	49	(108)	163	(64)	3100	85	1.4	15	5000	1.6	2.1	21	90	400
	16–19	63	(139)	175	(69)	3600	100	1.4	15	5000	1.8	2.5	25	100	400
Girls	13–15	49	(108)	160	(63)	2600	80	1.3	15	5000	1.3	2.0	17	80	400
	16–19	54	(120)	162	(64)	2400	75	1.3	15	5000	1.2	1.9	16	80	400

Source: Food and Nutrition Board, Recommended dietary allowances (Pub. 589, National Academy of Sciences — National Research Council, Washington, rev. ed., 1958).

[a] The allowance levels are intended to cover individual variations among most normal persons as they live in the United States under usual environmental stresses. The recommended allowances can be attained with a variety of common foods, providing other nutrients for which human requirements have been less well defined. See text for more detailed discussion of allowances and of nutrients not tabulated.

[b] Niacin equivalents include dietary sources of the preformed vitamin and the precursor, tryptophan (60 mg tryptophan equals 1 mg niacin).

[c] Calorie allowances apply to individuals usually engaged in moderate physical activity. For office workers or others in sedentary occupations they are excessive. Adjustments must be made for variations in body size, age, physical activity, and environmental temperature.

[d] See text for discussion of infant allowances. The Board recognizes that human milk is the natural food for infants and feels that breast feeding is the best and desired procedure for meeting nutrient requirements in the first months of life. No allowances are stated for the first month of life. Breast feeding is particularly indicated during the first month when infants show handicaps in homeostasis due to different rates of maturation of digestive, excretory, and endocrine functions. Recommendations as listed pertain to nutrient intake as afforded by cow's milk formulas and supplementary foods given the infant when breast feeding is terminated. Allowances are not given for protein during infancy.

stasis or physiological equilibrium due to different rates of maturation of digestive, excretory, and endocrine functions.[1] The Food and Nutrition Board in the 1958 revision of the recommended daily dietary allowances recognizes these facts and the dietary needs of the breast-fed infant are taken into account by additional allowances for the lactating mother (see Table 3).

The mother should know that it is no longer essential for her to nurse her infant if she feels strongly opposed or has difficulty with it, but the reasons for breast feeding are numerous and persuasive. Nursing at the breast is the natural method of feeding the offspring of all mammals. The composition of milk secreted by each species, including the human, is characteristic of that species and probably ideal for its young. Provided the mother's nutritional status and dietary intake are satisfactory, human milk more nearly meets the normal full-term infant's nutritional requirements than does any other food or probably any milk modification. After the initial supply of breast milk is established it is the simpler and easier method of infant feeding. Breast feeding avoids the necessity of periodic prescription of formula substitutes and also avoids errors which commonly occur in artificial feeding. Milk is an excellent culture medium and rigid sanitary precautions must be maintained in the preparation and storage of feeding mixtures to approximate the safety provided by breast feeding. Human milk is easily digested, ordinarily free from bacterial contamination and is ingested at body temperature. Furthermore, successful nursing helps to establish a satisfactory adjustment between mother and infant and gives to the infant that sense of security so necessary for future emotional stability.

The value to the newborn infant of the first secretion obtained from the breast, colostrum, is well recognized. It contains more total protein and has a higher proportion of euglobulin, the serum protein concerned with immunity, than does later breast milk. The newborn infant's blood contains virtually no euglobulin, but the quantity increases rapidly in infants who are breast-fed. The protective value of colostrum against infections for the human infant has not been proved, as it has been for the newborn calf, but the heightened resistance to infections exhibited during the latter part of the first year by breast-fed infants, even if they have been only partially breast-fed, is suggestive of the value of human colostrum. György[2] has reported that human milk contains a microbiological growth factor which differs from all known vitamins and growth factors. The amount of this factor in human milk is much greater than it is in cow's milk and is highest in human colostrum. This author believes that recognition of this specific growth factor in human milk, and its relation to the blood group substances, may represent a specific link with the whole field of immunological reactions, and may lead to an understanding of the higher resistance of the breast-fed infant. The vitamin A content of colostrum is high and rises to a peak on the third day of lactation when the average concentration is approximately three times the content of mature milk and four times that of cow's milk. The transfer of vitamin A and carotene across the placenta during pregnancy and the amount of vitamin A storage in the fetal liver have been investigated by several workers. "The general impression is one of wide variation in the infant's reserves at birth, but of rough parallelism between fetal stores and the maternal diet during pregnancy," and there is some reason to believe that the withdrawal of vitamin A from the liver to the rest of the body may be difficult after birth.[3] This, together with a possible relationship between deficiency of vitamin A and increased frequency and duration of infections, would seem to indicate further the importance of colostrum to the newborn infant. The preponderance of research data on infant morbidity and mortality support breast feeding rather conclusively and, except in cases of clear contraindications, it should be encouraged.

There is wide variation in the incidence of breast feeding. While in many cultures it is the natural and accepted procedure for the mother to nurse her infant, today the custom of breast feeding varies widely in different countries, within the same country, and even within the same environment. Bain,[4] reporting the incidence of breast feeding at the time of discharge from hospitals in various regions of the United States, showed the highest incidence in Alabama and South Carolina, where 60 per cent of the infants were completely breast-fed at discharge from the hospital, while in Connecticut and New Hampshire between 70 and 75 per cent were on bottle only at time of discharge. Macy,[5] in a study of 900 women in the Detroit area, found that all but 14 women in every 100 could, if they so chose, breast feed their infants.

It has been shown that approximately 90 per cent of mothers are physiologically able to breast feed their infants. If fewer do so, the reasons are mainly cultural, socioeconomic or emotional. Where cultural factors are the only contraindication, it is desirable that breast feeding be encouraged. A more favorable environment can be created if during the prenatal, lying-in, and neonatal periods, obstetric, pediatric and nursing attendants and others concerned give encouragement and specific advice until the supply of breast milk is well established, and the adjustment between mother and infant is a happy one.

Richardson[6] refers to Sedgwick who half a century ago listed the essentials for successful breast feeding as: (a) conviction on the part of the doctor as to its desirability; (b) conviction on the part of the mother as to her ability to succeed; (c) stimulation of the breasts at regular intervals; (d) complete emptying of the breasts, by the baby or by manual expression, after each feeding; and (e) patience and perseverance. He attributed the causes of nursing failure as a result of insufficient milk to one or more of the following factors: (a) failure to empty breasts; (b) poor nipples; (c) poor nursing by the baby; (d) fatigue; (e) irregular nursing; (f) poor diet; and (g) state of mind of nursing mother. The change in our culture and economy during the past half century has added new factors, for example, many working mothers are precluded from nursing their infants today. Current experience is that while most primiparae can be persuaded easily to inaugurate breast feeding, they are quickly dissuaded under the system of neonatal care which prevails in a majority of hospitals in the United States.

Another important factor in relation to breast feeding which has been little appreciated is the fact that the nutritional requirements for lactation are high, even greater than those of pregnancy. If a mother is to breast feed her infant successfully, postnatal care for her and her infant should include attention to her diet throughout the period of nursing. Instruction as to the mother's increased food needs during lactation should have preceded this as a part of prenatal care and during the lying-in period. During these successive periods she should acquire full knowledge of her food needs for lactation and how she can meet them under her own living conditions. To be motivated to do so the mother must realize why the recommended changes are important to her own health and the health and development of her baby.

The nutritional allowances suggested for the lactating woman may be studied in relation to the recommendations for the pregnant and for the nonpregnant woman. A comparison of the recommendations makes clear the added requirements of the mother for lactation which are proportional to the quantity of milk produced. For example, for the average woman an increase of 1000 calories is suggested above nonpregnant needs. A simple way of explaining the total caloric requirement of the lactating mother is to consider it made up of sufficient calories to meet the mother's ordinary daily energy requirements, plus sufficient calories to equal the energy value of the milk produced together with additional calories to include those used in the production of milk.

The amount of protein recommended for lactation is an additional 40 gm daily over the nonpregnant allowance. The value of a high protein diet during pregnancy as an important factor in successful lactation has been discussed. These increased protein needs are further elevated during lactation and are greatest during the period of highest milk yield. Macy's[7] nitrogen balance studies indicate that for every liter of milk produced 25 to 30 additional grams of protein are required, so that the mother has an increased protein need equal to one to two times the protein value of the milk produced. Since the protein stored during pregnancy is in part reserve stores for the high requirements of lactation, it follows that if a woman has been poorly nourished previous to or during pregnancy she probably has not stored protein in ideal amounts. If the mother's diet is deficient in calories and/or protein, the amount of milk secreted is usually reduced in an attempt to maintain a constant protein content in the milk produced.

The calcium content of human milk varies much more widely than is appreciated and probably reflects the maternal stores of this mineral as well as the calcium content of the diet which should be liberal.

The iron requirement during lactation probably is not increased over that of pregnancy. It may be even less since human milk is low in iron. A normal full-term infant born of a well-nourished mother should have iron stores sufficient to meet his needs throughout the early months of infancy.

The vitamin requirements of the lactating mother have not been as well determined as have her caloric, protein, and mineral needs. Since the infant's stores of vitamin A are low at birth, to maintain a desirable concentration of vitamin A in the mother's milk, the allowance of vitamin A recommended is liberal. The transfer of thiamine from the mother to breast milk is relatively poor, but the maternal diet has been shown to be the principal determinant of the amount transferred. Therefore, the maternal intake of thiamine should be relatively high. The quantity of riboflavin in breast milk appears also to vary with the intake of the mother. The need for riboflavin is related to body weight and the requirement is increased during lactation. The niacin allowance for lactation, expressed as niacin equivalents, is increased in accordance with recommended caloric intake. A diet containing an adequate intake of high quality protein will furnish adequate niacin. The allowance for ascorbic acid is high during lactation. The ascorbic acid content of human milk is much higher than that of cow's milk and the infant receives adequate amounts of this vitamin from a well-nourished mother, approximately 50 mg of ascorbic acid per liter of breast milk. The exact requirement for vitamin D during lactation is not known. Apparently it is not possible to increase the vitamin D content of human milk markedly by giving large doses of this vitamin to the mother. The recommendation for vitamin D is the same for the nursing mother as for the pregnant woman and probably serves an important role in the retention of calcium and phosphorus.

To insure an optimum diet throughout lactation the mother should be guided during late pregnancy and throughout the postpartum period in the adjustment of the diet which she followed during pregnancy to the higher nutritional demands of lactation. An additional pint of milk over the quart recommended for pregnancy will provide most of the increased needs for protein, calcium, phosphorus, riboflavin, thiamine, and niacin. If whole milk is used it will also take care of part of the increased need for vitamin A. Additional use of eggs, whole milk, cheese, butter, liver, and deep yellow and dark green leafy vegetables in the diet will furnish the rest. The amount of citrus fruit recommended for pregnancy together with liberal amounts of vegetables and other fruits (some raw such as cabbage and tomatoes) will supply the needed ascorbic acid. Additional calories may be necessary to adjust to individual needs. It may be easier and more pleasant for many women not accustomed to eating large amounts of food to eat four to six regularly spaced meals each day. Every effort should be made to see that the nutrients needed are available and that an educational program explains why the food is necessary and how it is to be obtained and used.

THE NUTRITION OF THE INFANT FROM BIRTH TO TWO YEARS

BERTHA S. BURKE AND HAROLD C. STUART

How a child is fed during infancy together with his nutritional status at birth, which includes the nutrient stores nature intended him to have when born under optimum conditions, may in no small measure influence what he is like at later stages of growth and development. While nutritional status and dietary intake are important at each stage, nutritional demands per unit of body weight are highest during the fetal period and the early months of infancy. Of course, there are many environmental factors other than nutrition which may affect an infant's ability to develop his inherited potentialities, but certainly nutrition is pivotal.

Following the provision of oxygen through the establishment of respiration at birth, food and water become the infant's basic physical needs. The need for love and security is another important consideration. The infant instinctively responds to the discomforts of hunger by crying and gratification by means of a comfortable feeding is one of the first pleasant extrauterine experiences contributing to his sense of security. If the food offered does not meet his nutritional needs, or if it is offered repeatedly in a manner which does not permit acceptance or utilization, much damage both emotional and physical may ensue. Whether the baby is breast-fed or bottle-fed, special care should be taken to insure that the total experience is satisfying. Thus not only the type of food but also the holding of the baby, and other mechanical and tactile aspects of the feeding process are involved. The general principles and practices of both breast and artificial feeding of infants are discussed in the following section of this chapter.

Nutritional Requirements During the First Year

For the early period of infancy human milk from a well-nourished mother is the food of choice, presupposing the amount and quality of the mother's milk to be adequate for the infant's needs except for vitamin D. For this reason the Food and Nutrition Board gives no allowances for infants for the first month of life. While breast feeding is most important during the early months an effort should be made to maintain it through the first six months of infancy. In this country breast feeding is rarely continued beyond the ninth month. When the baby is not breast-fed cow's milk is usually used in substitution. The recommended allowances (Table 3) for the remainder of infancy pertain to amounts of nutrients derived primarily from cow's milk and are intended for use when a cow's milk mixture or its equivalent is to be fed as the major source of nutrient intake. These values are given as a guide for use in artificial feeding and do not apply when an infant is fed human milk.

Total Fluids. The average breast-fed infant takes 2–3 oz of fluids per pound of body weight per day. Experimental calculations suggest that this is a reasonable fluid intake and clinically it seems adequate also for the artificially-fed infant. Fluid requirements for the artificially-fed infant are usually met by the dilution of the formula. In hot weather or in the presence of diarrhea or vomiting fluid requirements may be greatly increased. To insure opportunity for additional fluid intake plain water boiled and cooled should be offered at least twice daily to both breast- and artificially-fed infants. Thus the breast-fed infant early becomes accustomed to taking liquid from a bottle, should he suffer an acute illness or should it become necessary to wean him suddenly from the breast.

Energy Requirements. In the recent revision of the recommended allowances the caloric needs have been set at levels which reflect the general patterns of intake of healthy infants. They are 120 cal/kg of body weight (55 cal/lb) in the early months decreasing to 100 cal/kg (45 cal/lb) in the latter half of the first year, indicating the decrease in caloric need per unit of body weight as the infant grows. Because of the variability of different factors, such as size, activity, and rate of growth, which make up the energy requirement, the total caloric needs vary widely for different infants. The total amount of calories required daily should be estimated on the basis of an infant's expected weight for height and build. It is important that the caloric allocation be sufficient to allow for full activity in order that protein needed for growth and/or tissue repair is not burned to supply energy. The average breast-fed infant's daily caloric requirement is met by approximately 2.5 to 3 oz of milk per pound of body weight. In the case of the young artificially-fed infant the major portion of the caloric requirement is supplied by milk (20 cal/oz) which, in the early months is diluted with water as the pediatrician directs. The rest of the needed calories are supplied by added carbohydrate.

Protein. In early infancy human milk fully meets the full-term infant's needs for protein when fed at the breast and the process of lactation in the mother is not limited. The estimated protein intake of the breast-fed infant is about 1.5 to 2.5 gm/kg of body weight daily for the first six months. This assumes not only a well-nourished mother whose caloric and protein intakes are adequate and the diet well-balanced in other nutrients as well, but also an infant who is a good nurser, since the amount of milk produced adjusts quite rapidly to the infant's demands.

Acceptance of the concept, not irrefutably substantiated, that human milk is biologically superior to cow's milk has led to the common practice of supplying the artificially-fed infant with at least 50 per cent more protein in the cow's milk mixture than the breast-fed infant would receive. Such intakes provide good growth and performance and relatively high nitrogen retentions in artificially-fed infants. Babies who have been fed cow's milk mixtures have been shown to have more muscle than breast-fed infants. This difference disappears soon after the difference in diets ceases to exist.[8] Recent research on the essential amino acid composition of human milk and cow's milk shows that they are not very different.[9] It is no longer true that cow's milk is less easily digested than human milk because improved processing techniques have resulted in a finer curd, comparable to that of human milk. There is as yet no certainty or clear agreement as to whether or not the protein allowances formerly suggested for the artificially-fed infant are too high. However, infants on self-regulated feedings will often consume more protein than the 3.5 gm/kg of body weight previously recommended for early infancy. Several workers have pointed to the fact that generous allowances of protein and minerals create an additional demand for water, which is needed to excrete minerals and urea, and reduces the margin of safety against dehydration.[10]

Minerals. Calcium: Human milk supplies considerably less calcium than does cow's milk. However, the calcium in breast milk is better utilized than that in cow's milk and the infant's stores at birth are presumed to be adequate to meet this need in part. The total calcium retention from cow's milk is much greater because of the much higher intake. Linear growth of artificially-fed infants is related to the amount of calcium ingested. "On the other hand, the breast-fed infant has excellent linear growth despite a much lower calcium retention and grows at a rate definitely greater than that of the artificially-fed infant who has the same calcium retention." [8] The recommended allowance for calcium is 0.6 to 0.8 gm per day.

Iron and copper: The recommended allowance for iron of 0.8 mg./kg of body weight daily is not met by an all milk diet. However, iron made available by the breakdown of fetal hemoglobin will normally meet the infant's need for iron in the early months. The studies of Smith et al.[11] using radioactive iron suggest that utilization of dietary iron apparently does not occur during the first four to five months of life. For the later months of infancy additional iron is supplied by the introduction of other foods relatively rich in iron.

The copper requirement is small.[1] The copper content of human milk is considerably higher than that of cow's milk.

The requirements for other minerals are not known but there seems little likelihood that they will be deficient except possibly iodine which may need supplementation in a goiter zone.

Vitamins. The vitamin allowances for infants are based on available meager evidence from human and animal experiments and observations on the composition of human milk.

Human milk from a well-nourished mother apparently provides all the vitamins, with the exception of vitamin D, in amounts sufficient to supply the needs of the young infant though in some cases with a narrow margin of safety. Breast milk supplies considerably more vitamin A and ascorbic acid than does cow's milk. Breast milk is grossly deficient in vitamin D, as is cow's milk, and supplementation is necessary when either is used. Since the water-soluble vitamins are not stored to any extent in the mother, deficiencies are reflected in the milk which might not then provide adequately for the needs of the infant.[12]

Holt calls attention to the fact that in the case of the artificially-fed infant it is important to be sure that the vitamins whose requirements are reasonably well established are covered with a margin of safety. Ascorbic acid and vitamin D are both inadequately covered and should be provided for as supplements. A need for supplementation with vitamins A and the B-complex barring certain unusual circumstances has not been established.

For further information regarding nutrients not tabulated and for more details of those briefly discussed here the reader is referred to the full report of the Food and Nutrition Board.

Adjustment for Nutritional Needs During Late Infancy

The period between one and two years of age as far as nutritional needs are concerned is a transitional period. The major portion of the first year of life is a period of rapid growth and development in a healthy infant usually accompanied by a correspondingly large appetite and interest in food. Following this, growth rate decelerates, slowly at first. In some infants by nine months of age the decrease in rate of growth is sufficiently large to make the corresponding natural decrease in appetite marked. In other infants, who may have grown less rapidly in the earlier months, this decrease in appetite is delayed and may not occur to any great extent until one year of age, and in others it does not take place until the period between one and two years of age. Late infancy is then a period characterized by a natural decrease in appetite and as a result the nutritional needs per unit of body weight decrease. All mothers and others caring for infants and children should have this explained to them in advance of its taking place. Many feeding problems can be initiated through lack of understanding that a small appetite at this period is usual and should be respected. Many children apparently instinctively decrease their milk intake at this time; it is often helpful if the mother realizes this.

The recommended allowances for the period of late infancy and early childhood are given in Table 3. Although the child between one and two years of age is growing relatively slowly and his caloric and protein needs are decreased per unit of body weight, his total caloric and protein requirements increase because he continues to grow and the need for other nutrients increases correspondingly. In the Longitudinal Study of Child Health and Development, carried out by the Department of Maternal and Child Health of the Harvard School of Public Health the average caloric intake of boys between one and two years of age was 1287 and that for girls was 1273; the average protein intake for boys and girls respectively was 43.6 gm and 44.3 gm. Of interest is the wide range of variation from the average, for calories 800 to 1,700 for boys and 850 to 1,800 for girls in this age period; for protein 25 to 60 gm for boys and 32.5 to 57.5 gm per day for girls.[13]

Foods Commonly Used to Meet the Nutritional Needs of Infancy

Human milk is a thin bluish-white liquid; the caloric value averages 20 cal/oz, but varies with the fluctuating fat content. Its composition tends to follow a definite pattern in the individual woman, varying in different women and under varying conditions of diet and health. With successive pregnancies the amount secreted tends to be greater. Menstruation does not appreciably alter the milk supply; pregnancy decreases it. Certain drugs especially laxatives may be excreted into breast milk. Occasionally an infant may react to allergens in the mother's diet. Some food flavors such as onion, garlic, and leeks are transmitted in the milk.

The protein content of breast milk is highest in the early weeks of lactation and falls gradually from approximately 2 to 1.2 per cent at about six weeks after which it remains relatively constant. The protein content of mature human milk is less than half that of cow's milk. Breast milk has a higher percentage of carbohydrate (lactose) than does cow's milk, but the fat contents of the two milks are similar. The calcium and phosphorus contents of breast milk are much lower than those of cow's milk. Those who wish to compare in detail the average compositions of human milk and cow's milk are referred to publications of Macy[9] and Holt.[12]

Cow's milk in some form is the principal ingredient in almost all feeding mixtures. The exceptions in this country are almost entirely therapeutic feedings. In some countries substitutes are widely used owing to a shortage of cow's milk. The milk used should be of known and fairly constant composition, preferably pooled milk with a fat content between 3.5 and 4 per cent. It should be collected under sanitary conditions, by healthy persons, from healthy cows. Strict cleanliness and proper refrigeration are essential in the care of milk. All milk which is to be used should be boiled or pasteurized.

Evaporated cow's milk is used extensively. It is comparable to whole cow's milk in composition when diluted half and half with water. Milk modified in various ways, e.g., dried or partially skimmed, also may be used. It is important to know the composition of the milk used and to make any necessary adjustments in prescribing a formula. Various feeding mixtures are available in proprietary preparations. They are convenient but are an unnecessary expense. Under most circumstances, properly diluted evaporated milk or pasteurized whole cow's milk are the most satisfactory to use in feeding mixtures for healthy infants. Goat's milk may be used in place of cow's milk, especially if an infant is allergic to cow's milk. In many areas fresh, pasteurized goat's milk is available from the larger milk distributors; evaporated goat's milk may be purchased through drug and grocery stores. In either form it is expensive when compared to cow's milk.

In unusual circumstances when animal milk is contraindicated, usually because of a developed allergy to its protein, there are now available several canned substitutes using soy bean protein to replace milk protein. These are well tolerated and support normal growth when appropriately used under medical supervision.

Any clean, inexpensive form of carbohydrate is suitable, preferably a mixture of sugars which will ferment at their own different rates in the intestine and utilize small amounts of various digestive enzymes. Corn syrup and cane sugar are readily available and inexpensive. Dextrine and maltose preparations may be used.

Boiled water should be used for diluting the feeding mixture prescribed unless the formula preparation is to be sterilized terminally.

Water should be analyzed periodically by a public health laboratory unless it is from a community controlled supply.

Formula Preparation. The physician caring for an infant should always be the one to direct the feeding, prescribe the infant's formula, and the changes to be made in it from time to time, and direct the addition of foods other than milk. It should be understood that any method for determining the composition of feeding mixtures based upon weight provides only a procedure by which to approach the appropriate feeding for an individual infant. The physician is called upon to take many other factors into account in adjusting the feeding of an infant. Like all other infants, a malnourished infant should be fed according to his needs.

A feeding mixture in most instances in the early months is a simple mixture of cow's milk, sugar, and water. In the later months, as the physician directs, the amount of water added is reduced until the infant is taking whole milk or equal parts of evaporated milk and water. Following the introduction of other foods than milk the amount of sugar added to the formula is gradually reduced until the baby is taking plain whole milk.

A feeding mixture will be adequate if the recommended allowances already discussed are kept in mind when estimating the amounts of milk, carbohydrate, and water to be used. Cow's milk contains 1 gm of protein per oz. Consequently if the feeding mixture furnishes 1.5 to 2 oz of cow's milk per lb, the infant's daily requirement for protein will be generously supplied. This amount of milk also contains enough fat to supply the needed fatty acids and adequate minerals with the possible exception of iron and iodine in the goiter zones. The energy requirement is met by the addition of carbohydrate to supplement the calories provided by milk. The fluid requirements are generally met by dilution of the formula.

Unprocessed cow's milk forms tough curds which interfere with assimilation of protein and fat. To modify the curd, the protein must be denatured. This can be accomplished equally well by heating or by the addition of acid, or to some extent by other means. If evaporated milk is used it has already been denatured by the heat of the evaporating process. Homogenized milk forms curds similar to milk with denatured protein.

Additional Foods Other than Milk. The first supplements to the all milk diet of infants are usually vitamins added within the first two weeks of life. Additional vitamin D is needed by all babies whether breast- or bottle-fed. The bottle-fed baby also needs ascorbic acid (vitamin C). A water-soluble concentrate of vitamin D or a fish liver oil concentrate may be given in the amounts recommended by the physician. Some form of vitamin D should be taken daily until at least two years of age except in areas where exposure to the sun is adequate to make supplemental vitamin D unnecessary. Such exposure is not possible at all seasons in most areas within the United States. In prescribing vitamin D for the bottle-fed infant it is important to remember that most fresh cow's milk and evaporated milk supply approximately 400 I.U. of vitamin D per quart.

Ascorbic acid may during the first few months be given by simply adding the recommended amount in the form of a water-soluble concentrate to one of the feedings and mixing it thoroughly with it, or it may be placed on the tongue just prior to a feeding. Although citrus fruit juice in the required amount is usually well tolerated during the early months, its introduction may well be delayed until three months of age if ascorbic acid is contained in the vitamin concentrate prescribed. Thereafter both breast-fed and artificially-fed infants should learn to take strained orange juice or its equivalent. A good way to start is to give one teaspoonful of strained orange juice at first and increase as rapidly as well-taken until 2 to 3 oz are being taken daily.

Puréed foods may be offered in the early weeks of infancy although the value of such early introduction has not been established. If not readily taken, however, further attempts should be postponed until the baby's readiness for these foods is demonstrable. Commercial or home-prepared foods in any of the major categories may be fed to a healthy infant at almost any age without signs of ill effect. The very young infant may be offered such foods provided this is pleasurable to him and to the mother and is not interpreted by her as nutritionally essential. Conversely, the introduction of puréed foods can be delayed until eight or nine months of age without apparent ill effects except that iron deficiency may develop if no other source of this mineral is provided. Current conservative practice recommends the introduction of small amounts of simple puréed foods at about three months of age increasing the amount and adding to the variety so that the infant at six months is taking significant amounts of foods in all major categories. Supplementary solid foods wisely chosen and gradually added to the milk diet from about three to four months serve two important functions; i.e. they accustom the infant gradually to a variety of flavors and textures which is important in the development of good eating habits, and also supplement the milk diet with needed iron and B-vitamins. Each new food should be given in very small amounts, not more than "a taste" or $\frac{1}{2}$ teaspoon on the first three or four occasions, then, if all goes well, the amounts offered may be increased to meet the infant's desire. No specific order need be followed in introducing new foods, but only one food should be introduced at a time. For example, puréed fruit is often given at about three months, cereal at four months, strained vegetables and egg yolk at four to six months, scraped meat at the seventh or eighth month of age. Any food which is objectionable to the infant should be omitted from his diet for a sufficient period to allow him to forget his dislike for it. If the rejected food is nutritionally essential, substitution should be made for it.

The infant at five to six months usually has five or six meals a day consisting of his breast or bottle feedings and a variety of liquid and strained foods. By nine months of age the average infant will be on a three or four meal schedule. For the rest of the first year the changes consist in becoming acquainted with a large variety of solid foods. During the latter part of the first year the average infant should gradually get away from puréed or strained foods. The infant kept too long on these often develops feeding problems which could have been easily avoided had he been gradually accustomed to small amounts of less finely divided solids and foods from the family table. A variety of stewed fruits and vegetables may be offered. Bread, potato, scraped meat, raw fruit such as ripe banana, scraped apple, etc. may be incorporated into the diet. Butter may be used in small amounts on vegetables, potato, and bread. Simple puddings such as custards, tapioca cream, junket, and the like may be given.

Daily food for the one year old infant should include according to his needs and appetite approximately the following: milk, 3–4 cups (24–32 oz); an egg; lean meat, liver, poultry or fish, 2 tb or more (1 oz or more); potato, one small baked or boiled in the skin; cooked vegetables, 2 tb or more, dark green leafy or deep yellow often; fruit, citrus such as an orange or 2–3 oz unstrained orange juice, and another fruit is desirable; cereal, 2 tb or more, whole grain or enriched; bread, 1 slice or more; butter or fortified margarine, 1–3 tsp; vitamin D concentrate as the physician prescribes.

Helpful suggestions to mothers for the preparation of the formula, including sterilization, and the inclusion of foods other than milk in a young child's meals are given in The Children's Bureau Publication, "Infant Care." [14]

During the transitional period of late infancy (one to two years) the child learns to feed himself and usually gives up his bottle if he has not done so earlier. He learns to eat a wider variety of foods in kinds and consistency. Since this is a period when lifetime habits are being established, the handling of the child in this transitional period is as important as it was in early infancy. Failure to respect his natural appetite, his individual day to day preferences, his desire to feed himself, and his need to become acquainted with new foods and foods of different consistency may result in feeding problems. Children of this age enjoy plain, simple foods and usually prefer to have their food cooked the same way at each serving. For example, a child may refuse his cereal because it is poorly cooked and lumpy when he expects it to be smooth, or his meat because it is tough and he cannot chew it, or his egg because it is soft-cooked and he is used to and likes it hard-cooked. If the child is healthy and his natural appetite has not been interfered with his desire is for simple plain foods that meet his requirements, and unless tastes have been distorted by unwise feeding practices his natural appetite will help him to feed himself well.

PRINCIPLES AND PRACTICES OF INFANT FEEDING
PAULINE G. STITT

Breast Feeding

Since formula feeding is generally possible in the United States where safe milk is usually available, it is neither necessary nor wise to exert pressure upon a reluctant mother to nurse. However, the evidence presented makes it abundantly clear that breast feeding is the method of choice and is usually possible. The principal contraindications to breast feeding are: active tuberculosis, pertussis (whooping cough), chronic debilitating diseases, or dangerous psychoses. Commonly recognized relative contraindications are other acute infections, infected breasts, traumatized nipples, maternal malnutrition, grossly inadequate milk supply, emotional rejection of the nursing process, and an infant unable to suckle adequately. These and other rare circumstances account for a very small fraction of those who make no attempt to nurse or abandon it after a short token trial. Nursing enhances a mother's sense of well-being and general health more commonly than it affects it adversely. It is historically as well as currently obvious when viewed globally that the vast majority of women can nurse their babies successfully, but statistics based largely on hospital deliveries in the United States show that a small minority really do so. Success appears to depend in large measure upon its being undertaken optimistically and upon following simple procedures patiently during the first two or three weeks which are so often necessary to induce a fully adequate supply of breast milk.

The purpose of this rather explicit discussion of the process of breast feeding is to provide a broader and more adequate understanding both of what is needed for success and of the common causes of failure.

Breast feeding is always a physical partnership between mother and baby, and one which requires health and vigor in both partners. It requires that the baby be able to suck vigorously and that the mother have certain capacities. In animals, milk present in the gland is only partly available by ordinary milking methods if the animal is anesthetized or distracted. In normal animals it is made more fully available by an expulsion mechanism, an ejection or pumping reflex stimulated by milking and called "let-down." A similar process is an integral part of successful nursing by women.

It seems apparent that to facilitate more successful breast feeding in this country there is need for wider and more carefully applied knowledge of the mechanisms of nursing on the part of obstetricians and pediatricians and hospital nurses, particularly in respect to promoting or maintaining vigorous sucking and the avoidance of distracting factors which may inhibit the "let-down" reflex. It is of primary importance to have a realistic comprehension of what constitutes successful breast feeding. Present day mothers, and many professional workers attending them, abandon it too quickly because they are not sufficiently aware of individual differences among mothers to recognize when it is proceeding successfully, though possibly slowly in the early days. Many mothers expect almost immediate establishment of lactation, and become anxious during the normal, gradual establishment of the mother-baby nursing partnership. Unfortunately, professional attendants often attempt to relieve this in what seems the easiest or quickest way, that of weaning. Also they themselves frequently become unduly anxious about what appears to be slow establishment of gain in weight. There is ordinarily no need for haste in securing weight gain, in fact haste is not consonant with the realities of lactation. Mothers need to be told when they are succeeding or are likely to succeed because their ideas of what to expect may be unrealistic, and they may develop an unwarranted sense of failure and abandon a process that is really proceeding well. Women who have no adequate criteria to use in judging their personal competence to nurse are likely themselves to attach undue significance to the normal weight loss of the newborn or the infant's temporary failure to gain.

Adequate prenatal preparation for breast feeding, then, includes not only all the attributes of sound obstetrical care, with nutrition that anticipates the mother's needs for lactation, and the infant's needs for adequate stores during the period when lactation is being established, but requires the mother's gradual acquaintance with the facts that 4 or 5 days will elapse before the baby sucks efficiently, and that as much as 2 or 3 weeks may elapse before breast feeding is comfortably and effectively established. The comprehension of this gradual process is important to all women, but is particularly important in this country at present when we have almost universal hospital delivery, combined with early ambulation, and early hospital discharge. These practices, regardless of their obstetrical merits, result in some degree of emotional and physical stress, and certainly involve loss of personal professional support during the very days when the beginnings of lactation are most precarious and when the mother's physical stamina and general sense of maternal adequacy may be at a low ebb.

As soon as the mother and infant appear rested from the delivery, the infant is put to breast. This can be done whenever the mother feels ready, and is commonly done by 12 hours. The first contact is largely a gentle get-acquainted session, and the mother should not expect much of either the baby or herself. Some babies simply lie in deep sleep, some nuzzle a bit and make sucking motions but do not actually suck, and still others seize the areola and show effective vigor. The wide range of normal variation is impressive, and helps one see how misleading it is if one mother judges the normality of her baby by comparing it to a neighboring nursling. When the newborn is being established on breast feeding he is frequently allowed to suckle for from 2 to 5 minutes. The termination of the session should take place when the baby relaxes. By the 4th day of life sucking is fairly well established if the baby is normal. This is not synonymous with the milk being established, or the nursing process being completely launched, but it helps to launch the milk flow. The prime objective at this stage is to avoid or remove physical or psychological barriers to strong sucking on the infant's part and relaxed patience on the part of the mother. For want of strong sucking, milk may be lost; for want of milk, breast feeding may be lost; and for want of breast feeding, the mother's self-confidence and self-esteem may be weakened. In breast feeding, nothing succeeds like success.

Babies tend to fall asleep while nursing. During the first part of a feeding the baby may rest and rouse spontaneously. Toward the end of the feeding he may need a light touch to rouse. After a few such touches, the session may be regarded as finished. The sleep-eat and eat-sleep pattern is part of any infant feeding process, be it bottle or breast. However, the baby who gets too hungry between feedings because he is on an arbitrary and too wide feeding interval may be so exhausted that he falls asleep before finishing. Both the lusty eater and the feeble eater require and take rest periods interspersed through the feedings. The lusty eater goes at the breast with such vigor and gusto that he may exhaust himself and have to pause to get his breath while the feeble eater may tire even from languid effort. Nurses and physicians need to observe many nursing babies in order to acquire skill in recognizing the differences between successful though slow progress and unsatisfactory progress and in the latter to identify the causes.

Feeding intervals vary with custom in many lying-in situations. In general, the baby is put to breast at about 6 hour intervals during the first 24 to 48 hours, and this makes a workable regime. After the first 24 to 48 hours many infants tend to wake at approximately every 3 to

4 hours. This ushers in the era appropriate for "self-regulation." In situations where one can individualize care it is sometimes desirable to observe the baby and the mother and be guided by interactions between them. For the first month the baby will show considerable variation in the frequency of his feeding demands. Although he may be feeding as infrequently as every 4 hours in the hospital, it is not uncommon for him to increase the frequency even to every half-hour during the first days in his new home. This is a period when his needs are increasing, and when his mother's supply may still be small and even temporarily depressed by the first physical and psychic strains of homecoming and the consequent assumption of full care and responsibility. Little by little the over-all feeding intervals begin to widen, and a pattern begins to emerge. The baby should be regulating himself, and the pattern of his regulation tells the observant mother which particular schedule will work best for him. Whether the infant is breast-fed or bottle-fed, self-regulating feeding is the method of choice for a normal healthy infant. This is often somewhat erroneously called the "self-demand" method. In a study by Aldrich and Hewitt[15] 668 babies were put on a self-regulating regime in which the infants had free choice as to intervals of feeding and amount of food taken at each. The feeding intervals during the first month were irregular and frequent, for the most part, but thereafter the infants lengthened them gradually. In the first two months many preferred an interval of less than four hours, but by one year approximately 90 per cent had of their own volition adjusted to a three meals per day regime and had excellent appetites. Less than one per cent were considered problems in relation to appetite.

When infant feeding is conducted on a basis that encourages utilizing the baby's spontaneous sucking impulses, there are numerous advantages, most importantly that the baby is actually ready when put to breast. In general, most breast-fed babies soon become established on a 3 hour schedule during the day and as needed, ordinarily once or twice, during the night.

Time is a consideration not only in terms of interval between feedings, but of actual time at breast. The time interval between feedings largely determines the sucking time at breast. Where frequency of feeding is dictated by the baby's actual needs, the duration of sucking time tends to adjust itself automatically; the shorter the feeding interval, usually the shorter the time. The child who is on an arbitrary widely spaced feeding schedule tends to lengthen the sucking time at the individual breast feedings. This points to the need for feeding arrangements which permit flexibility in frequency, especially in the neonatal period aiming to keep the sucking time at breast brief enough to spare breast trauma, yet frequent and effective enough to stimulate milk flow and to empty the breasts, thus reducing the likelihood of engorgement. During the early days or weeks the use of *both breasts at each feeding* appears to be good for the breasts and helps in stimulating lactation. The first nursing sessions generally last from 3 to 5 minutes, and this time period gradually increases until, at the end of the first week or 10 days, the full nursing time of approximately 15 to 20 minutes has been reached. The baby ordinarily utilizes the effective milk flow within these time limits, and the breast is spared useless sucking, which only inflicts trauma and can well lead to abandonment of breast feeding because of such complications as fissured or excoriated nipples, or breasts too painful for nursing. During these early days protection of the vulnerable breasts is rewarding. Gentle care at this time may keep the breasts functionally fit for the time when milk flow is actually available. The best protection appears to be that of *frequency* of nursing as against long, unproductive, widely spaced, feeding sessions.

Consideration of the technics of breast feeding includes attention to the mother's physical position during nursing. Cultural patterns influence position, and so do individual preferences. Some women sit and hold the babies in their arms, some sit and bend over the babies on their laps. Some feel that they manage better lying down. It is found to be a help in breast feeding, and equally important in bottle feeding, to hold the infant for a little relaxation period immediately following feeding. Even in early infancy babies appear to enjoy the comfort and companionship of the feeding process as much as they do the actual ingestion of food.

Babies may have a "play period" of dawdling with the nipple before, during, or after feeding. Most successful and experienced nursing mothers recognize this as somehow being a normal part of breast feeding and let it proceed freely, or in many instances find ways of joining in the play. The uninitiated are sometimes frightened by the process, or at least regard it as an untimely interruption of what they consider serious business. Probably the commonest error in breast feeding is interfering. The primary goal is that of all well-child pediatric care — trying to understand what the baby is attempting to do, and then helping him to do it.

Breast feeding is not contraindicated in twins. It is common practice, however, when breast feeding is used with twins, to make up a full day's supply of formula sufficient for one child, and then alternate the babies between breast and bottle at each feeding.

A mother's desire to breast feed is no guarantee of immediate success in nursing. Scanty milk, awkwardly shaped breasts, sensitive nipples, and personal misgivings regarding her ability to nurse often delay it but need not necessarily prevent it.

Observations lead one to believe that flat or inverted nipples are a problem only when a baby sucks feebly because a vigorous baby tends to make such nipples accessible within a few days or even to nurse effectively on the occasional nipples which do not thus respond. Generally, when the baby is thus attempting to establish nursing, the nipple offered can be encouraged into an erectile state by the mother stroking and touching the nipple of her other breast. Many women who have worried beforehand because of infantile-appearing breasts are gratified to find that development occurs quickly as sucking and lactation are launched. Omitting emotional situations involving maternal attitudes toward nursing, failures in nursing appear to be less on the basis of anatomical or physiological aberration of the mother and more on the basis of inadequate stimulus from the baby.

There are many factors which may lie behind a baby's inability to suck, including particularly immaturity, neurologic damage, or simple fatigue. Because of these, an infant's reaction may be depressed to the point where he can neither function as a stimulator of lactation, nor participate in other aspects of the reciprocal dynamics that constitute the nursing partnership. Among babies who do not do well during the first days of feeding one may recognize irritability or lack of responsiveness such as to the cheek stroke. These may be manifestations of brain irritation but the physician watches for other evidences of central nervous system damage through neurological examinations. Many evidences of brain irritation are transient manifestations and may disappear within a few days. Sedation given the mother in connection with delivery may be another cause for the newborn infant to be inert. There is a definite distinction to be made between contentment in a baby, and lethargy or inertness. The characteristics of contentment are relaxed features that still maintain good body tone, good color, and a pleased, happy, general appearance. In contrast, the inert baby's characteristics are more those of a patient in surgical shock.

It is important to appreciate that newborn infants tire on manipulation. They do well when they are picked up frequently so that their clothes may be adjusted, their backs patted, and their positions changed, but they do poorly when subjected to extensive baths and other care performances by inept young mothers or overzealous attendants. After such ministrations the babies are often too tired to eat well. Babies respond better to gentle than clumsy or rough manipulations. Innumerable clues, such as pallor, flushing, or beads of perspiration may be silent testimony to the limited energy reserves of the postpartum woman. The easy fatigability of both partners demands simple child care routines, if the important practice of breast feeding is to succeed. The good reciprocal relationship between mother and nursing infant requires rest, freedom from excessive strains, both from social demands and work, and often privacy.

Since time immemorial, breast feeding has been a human practice transmitted as an art by members of the human family. Thus at any given moment, when breast feeding is thought of at all, it is not uncommon for the thought to represent strange and anachronistic components. These components are made up of fragments of contemporary science and the mother's own observations. Information acquired from her girl friends whose opinions, incidentally, are extraordinarily important to her, may add to her anxiety or discouragement at this stage. Woven through these acquired ideas about nursing often are the remnants of old wives' tales. This old lore combines, in many instances, the ancient wisdom of breast feeding with myths and superstitions, for some of the most startling myths were originally sage observations on situations which prevailed. The feeding beliefs of bygone days were not ridiculous because they were usually derived from ubiquitous occurrences. They deserve to be understood, so that today's women who believe these ancient observations are not challenged with the assertion that they are untrue, but rather are helped to see that they may have been true under conditions which have altered, at least in this country.

Anyone working with mothers and newborn infants in connection with breast feeding needs to be sure that he gets "clues" from successful breast feeders as well as from watching the unsuccessful. There are so many varieties of successful feeding that any one interested in the subject needs to observe successful women and babies carefully to acquire insight that may be helpful in working with those less successful. The most helpful role for the doctor and nurse in aiding breast feeding is probably in anticipatory guidance and in interpreting normal phenomena. The actual techniques of the nursing process may need to be observed and discussed. However, the physical presence of a doctor or nurse during the nursing process may be more of a deterrent than a help and should be as brief and private as possible and only as required for understanding any procedural errors in the techniques employed.

An infant born prematurely, or one born at term but small and immature, has special nutritional requirements which differ from those of a healthy full-term infant. For a full discussion of the nutritional handicaps of the premature infant the reader is referred to Dunham's *Premature Infants*.[16]

There are two different schools of thought in regard to the feeding of the premature infant. One group recommends human milk, which can be modified to meet the infant's needs. Others recommend cow's milk because of the high protein requirement of these infants. Because they do not absorb fat well, partially skimmed cow's milk can be used to advantage. Carbohydrate can be added to adjust the caloric requirement to meet the total amount needed daily in the neonatal period.

Obviously a physician well-trained in the feeding of premature infants should direct the feeding of such an infant, especially in the neonatal period, and at least until his feeding approaches that of a healthy, full-term infant.

Artificial Feeding

However great the advantages of breast feeding, they should be weighed against any individual contraindications to its continuance which may arise at any time. Early weaning for good cause should not be viewed as a failure to breast feed successfully. In discussing breast feeding it was recognized that there are a few contraindications to attempting it with the newborn infant, and that various developments may justify its early termination. It must be understood, therefore, that bottle, or so-called "artificial" feeding, may have to be introduced at the start and that mixed breast and bottle feedings may be necessary for a time during the neonatal period. Bottle feeding, although it may continue as a diminishing factor in the total feeding situation throughout some or all of the second year, is essentially a method applicable to the first year.

The goal of artificial feeding techniques is to introduce nutrients as required, in a manner that considers safety as well as mutual pleasure of the baby and the person doing the feeding. The latter is important because it influences the maternal-infant interrelationship. This goal involves establishing simple, clean, comfortable feeding activities, which are suitable for the baby's anatomical, neurological, and physiological development, and adaptable to changing needs as the baby grows and develops.

There can be no successful substitute for breast feeding of infants unless: (1) an ample supply of reliably pure cow's milk, or its modifications or substitutes, is readily available for the infant; (2) safe methods of storage of formula preparations are available and used, and (3) there is understanding and strict observance by each person concerned in regard to the precautions necessary to insure the purity and sterility of formula-preparation at the time of feeding.

Once a formula has been prescribed, the next consideration is when and how to offer it. This will depend in part upon whether feeding is to be fully artificial, or mixed — that is, complementing or supplementing the breast. Just as in breast feeding, the baby is the best clue to the most suitable schedule. It is well to be prepared for a 3 hour schedule, and to modify any arbitrary time span on the basis of the baby's performance; that is, if the baby wakes ahead of schedule, feed him and if he is sleeping, let him sleep. Watch the baby's feeding pattern for a week or two, charting it if that seems helpful to get the general pattern clearly in mind, and then set a feeding schedule on the basis of what the baby has revealed as being his most comfortable feeding interval. This mode of arriving at a feeding schedule is *self-regulation*. It quickly provides the convenience and predictability afforded by a regulated schedule, and yet takes its origin from the baby's comfort and expressed needs. In actual practice, during the first 2 weeks, feedings in the daytime may run a little closer than every 3 hours, but the baby soon stabilizes at approximately that interval, and by about 6 weeks widens out to approximately every 4 hours. One or 2 night feedings may be taken, but these gradually disappear except during periods of excessive demand, such as unusually rapid growth, extraordinary physical activity, or convalescence from an illness. Under such circumstances a baby seems to want and need night feedings, and may revert to them temporarily even though they had previously been dropped.

Not only should the baby provide the clues as to feeding interval, but he should also signal as to the quantity of each given feeding. Formulas are usually written to afford 2 or 3 ounces more per feeding than the infant's age in months. This gives a general idea of the total amount of formula to be prepared, but the actual amount offered is best made a little more than is usually taken. In this way the baby stops when satisfied and not for any other reason. This method has an additional value in that it requires watching the baby for clues as to care, and the habit of watching rather than blindly following arbitrary dicta soon permeates into other aspects of care with a most salutary effect.

The formula in such feeding regimes is usually fairly concentrated and the baby is offered boiled water at other times to assure that his fluid intake is adequate. This avoids the occasional possibility of the baby who drinks unnecessarily large quantities of feeding mixture in an effort to quench thirst.

The bottle itself should be fitted with a nipple which lets the milk flow freely in response to normal sucking but nipples should be watched carefully, for they tend to flow too freely as they get old. The length of the nipple should be considered because some babies with a low palate or short anteroposterior mouth space may gag or get palatal sores from a long one.

The general principles of a baby's performance in infant feedings are the same whether the baby is getting breast or bottle feedings. All the principles discussed in connection with breast feeding apply to bottle feeding.

The actual feeding of babies should be done in positions approximating those employed in breast feeding. A baby should not be left to feed as best he can with the bottle propped before him.

The comments on feeding vigor, made in connection with breast feeding, all apply here. All babies, lusty or otherwise, should have ample time to pause and rest if they want to do so during their feedings. The baby should provide the clues as to when pauses are appropriate. There are some infants who become so intent on the eating process that pauses only cause frustration. It seems best to let them carry on until they signify that they are ready to stop for breath.

Weaning from Breast and Bottle

If the baby is being breast fed, usually by the third month it is advisable to substitute 1 bottle feeding for 1 breast feeding. This accustoms the infant to taking a bottle, gives the mother more freedom, and makes eventual weaning easier by accustoming the infant to cow's milk. Ordinarily this does not interfere with breast milk supply nor should it lead to early weaning. Such mixed feeding may prove to be valuable, especially when emergency separation of mother and infant prevents nursing, and it facilitates weaning with a minimum of discomfort.

Contemporary weaning, in this country at least, is not a sudden transition to other methods of feeding and other foods. It is instead a gradual process that goes on almost imperceptibly over many months. It starts with the first vitamin drops and, later, orange juice, and goes gradually through the phases of introduction of foods of varying consistencies. Semi-solids and then solids are introduced little by little to give the baby some mouth and food experiences and to acquaint him with food consistencies, tastes, colors, and smells. This is best accomplished at a time when such feedings are not actually required for the baby's immediate nutritional purposes. These feedings are often of maximal usefulness from the third or fourth month on, when their introduction coincides with a high degree of mouth activity on the baby's part.

During these experiences the baby is as busy investigating the characteristics of his own mouth as he is in determining the attributes of the food, and he happily accomplishes repeated ejections of food by tongue thrusts and even by spitting. When parents understand that this is a definite, essential step in acquiring the ability to eat, and no longer interpret spitting, bubbling, and ejection as distaste and food refusal, they can relax and let the baby work happily through his specific stage of infant feeding.

The latter part of the first year or early months of the second are characterized by a change in feeding interest from breast or bottle to solids though the infant still maintains intermittent interest in the former. He tends increasingly to use solids or semi-solids and to drink milk from a cup, and uses the breast or bottle not so much for food as for comfort. When the baby gets casual about the bottle, taking a sip or two and then playing or simply chewing the nipple, it may be inferred that he no longer needs the bottle as his feeding mainstay. Such signs, therefore, are useful guides as to when to substitute the cup, which then may be used regularly at meals. The cup-fed baby should still be offered a bedtime bottle, but whenever he seems to lose interest in the bottle per se and shows that his real interest is in the holding and fondling, the bottle may be discontinued.

Breast weaning follows much the same pattern and clues as weaning from the bottle, and as babies enter the normal biting phase of their development, motivation to wean becomes strong. At this time a baby is ready for more chewing and biting on solids. These experiences should be provided, but simultaneously care should be exercised to see that the mother's breast is spared from trauma. This is not the time for abrupt weaning but should lead to a quiet withdrawal of the breast. The usual developments are that although the baby continues to bite the mother occasionally, he gradually begins to do vigorous biting on proffered solid foods and suitable toys. Simultaneously he begins to use the breast in a new way, a way that consists of a preliminary suck or two, followed by cuddling against the bared breast. These practices continue comfortably for some time, a few weeks for some babies, a few months for others. The breast milk now gradually diminishes and disappears. In most instances even after the milk has disappeared the infant goes through the sucking actions for a while at the start of his sociable sessions, but as time goes on he shows clearly that he is truly weaned and is getting his bodily nourishment from table food, and that he is using the holding and fondling for their emotional values.

When to begin terminal weaning depends, in part, upon such circumstances as the season of the year, the mother's inclination and competence to nurse, and the supply of breast milk. Observation of the baby himself often will guide the doctor and mother in regard to when, and how rapidly, to wean. There is individual variation in suckling needs, and some infants may resist direct weaning and cling to the breast or bottle until well into the second year. There is advantage in not starting to wean before 6 months, for after this time the baby can ordinarily be transferred to whole milk and semi-solid and solid foods, thus avoiding the preparation of feeding mixtures. Weaning is often accomplished by substitution of one bottle or cup feeding for one breast feeding every few days, or as rapidly as the infant will accept the change. When abrupt weaning is necessary, individual guidance is needed to make the experience as nontraumatic as possible for both mother and baby. It is always well to avoid weaning at the time of illness, hospitalization, or any other potentially traumatic emotional experience.

The transition from formula feeding to whole milk feeding, whether from bottle or cup, is made gradually as the total amount of whole milk in the formula approaches one quart and as other foods provide an increasing proportion of the total daily caloric requirements. It is well to try to establish certain habits early which facilitate this change later on, and thus avoid the resistance with which the infant sometimes meets changes in food mixtures or routine. This is best accomplished by gradual but early accustoming the infant to taking food in other ways than from a bottle.

Toward the end of the first year the normal infant becomes able to sit erect with ease and has developed facility in hand to mouth movements. At the same time, tooth eruption is proceeding. This is the ideal time for introduction of foods which the child can manipulate himself. He cannot do this readily with "junior" foods, but he can manage nicely such foods as a tough crust of bread, a large piece of carrot, string beans, or any smooth, well-cooked appropriate food. Lean meat adhering in shreds to its bone is often enjoyed. He can handle any of these with skill and pleasure. This kind of self-feeding precedes, and later accompanies, learning to use a spoon.

Many infants at one year of age take their milk wholly from a cup, while others are reluctant to give up the bottle entirely until much later. This wide range in behavior reflects the wide variations in maturation common in childhood, and if later emotional and feeding problems are to be avoided the cup should not be forced. However, failure to accept the cup may only be the result of lack of earlier conditioning. All such foods as cereals, vegetables, orange juice, and the like should be given unstrained — that is, rather finely divided, or mashed — unless the physician has directed otherwise. Infant feeding at this time concentrates on integrating child feeding into family feeding and maintaining high enough standards of family feeding to make that possible.

THE NUTRITION OF THE PRESCHOOL CHILD
BERTHA S. BURKE

The preschool years as compared with those of infancy are characterized by slower growth with an accompanying decrease in appetite. The child during this age period characteristically manifests a lessened interest in food along with his greater interest in the world around him; and is usually very active and relatively thin. However, the likelihood of malnutrition, which is more common to this period of childhood than to any other, should not be overlooked.

This age child characteristically also likes to express his independence by saying "No." Lack of appetite and refusal to take the food offered are common complaints during these years. It is important to appreciate and respect the natural loss of eagerness for meals which these children may manifest and to be aware that appetite and willingness to take foods offered may be impaired easily by unwise handling of the feeding situation.

Nutritional Requirements

The energy requirement per unit of body weight during the preschool years, although less than that of the infant, is still relatively high as compared to that of an adult. Until growth is completed the total caloric requirement increases each year, but not as rapidly as does body weight. Thus, the total caloric need will increase from infancy through adolescence, but the number of calories required per unit of body weight will decrease. For children one to six years of age the National Research Council's allowances approximate the average caloric intakes reported by different observers for children in this age range. The Longitudinal Studies of Child Health and Development conducted by the Department of Maternal and Child Health of the Harvard School of Public Health, to which reference has already been made, have included a careful evaluation of each child's average daily intake of nutrients from year to year. In the age range from one to six years the yearly increase in caloric intake averages approximately 100 calories per day for both boys and girls. However, the ranges show that within each age group there are wide departures from the averages; extreme variations of as much as 900 calories or more were found.[13] The child's appetite, his rate of growth, changes in the amount of his subcutaneous tissue, and his general health as appraised by a thorough physical examination at regular intervals should serve as guides to his caloric needs.

The protein allowances of the Food and Nutrition Board based on balance studies on healthy American children with relatively free access to common foods, while high compared to other standards for the preschool years, are below the average intakes reported recently by several study groups in various sections of the United States.[1] In our Longitudinal Study within this age range extreme variations were found where at least one child ate approximately twice or more the amount of protein consumed by another of the same chronological age. On the basis of protein intake expressed in terms of body weight there were children who ate a daily average of more than 5 gm/kg per day during the second year and children with an intake of less than 2 gm/kg per day during the sixth year. The average total protein intakes of this group of children are higher than the recommended allowances and are approximately the same for boys and for girls throughout the preschool years.

Stearns et al.[17] call attention to the need for a diet generous in protein for the preschool years. While growth in height and weight are slower in these years than in infancy, the rate of growth of muscle increases throughout the early years of childhood. Febrile illness tends to be highest in these years when immunity is being acquired. For these two reasons an optimum intake of protein during the preschool years is important.

Insufficient protein in the diets of young children leads to various degrees and manifestations of protein depletion, and this is probably more common in this country than is generally appreciated. In a group of young Boston children under the tenth percentile in height and/or weight, and whose "dwarfism" could not be explained medically, investigation disclosed relatively low protein intakes together with very inadequate caloric intakes as the probable cause of the "dwarfism." [18] In the preschool child whose appetite is small a deficit of even 100 calories could result in 25 gm of protein, more than half of the daily protein requirement, being burned for energy with resultant interference with growth. Macy[19] has shown that a difference in intake of as few as 10 cal/kg of body weight per day may spell success or failure in making satisfactory progress in growth. Since protein requirement and caloric intake must always be considered together an easy and practical way is to consider the protein intake as approximately 12 to 15 per cent of the child's caloric requirement.

In America ignorance and carelessness are more often the cause of malnutrition in children than is poverty, but feeding problems are also an important factor. Over the world, especially in the underdeveloped areas, severe protein malnutrition, usually diagnosed as *kwashiorkor* is the most common nutritional deficiency disease seen in children up to five years of age.[20] Kwashiorkor has been observed in the United States. In those countries where it is most common it is due primarily to lack of sufficient animal protein, and when accompanied by severe shortage of calories is more correctly referred to as *marasmus*.[21]

The recommended calcium allowance for this age period is 1.0 gm daily and for iron 7 to 8 mg per day. Under ordinary circumstances if the allowances for protein, calcium, and iron are met, other mineral requirements will be supplied in sufficient amounts with the possible exception of iodine in goiter zones.

The allowances for vitamins as recommended by the Food and Nutrition Board are given in Table 3. From a practical standpoint there is little likelihood that any of these will be deficient in a well balanced diet containing adequate amounts of calories, protein, calcium, and iron except possibly ascorbic acid (vitamin C), vitamin A, and vitamin D.

Thomson and Duncan in an excellent review article on "The diagnosis of malnutrition in man" point to the importance of good nutrition for the growing child. They state that scarcity of supply in nutrients which play a structural role will be met by economy of utilization, and the main manifestations will be in relation to growth and form. On this basis it is reasonable to expect that growth will be restricted to the rate permitted by the material in shortest supply, most probably protein and calcium. Since the organism must be healthy to grow satisfactorily, and since growth is the product of nutrition, growth measures the nutritional state. The authors add, "It is true that acute infections slow or arrest growth, but in the well-fed child such delays are rapidly and fully overtaken." [22]

The Diet

In planning meals for children of preschool age, as at other ages, the food should supply ample amounts of the essential nutrients for maintenance, replacement, and increase of tissues and sufficient sources of energy for full activity. Since appetite at this age particularly is frequently small and usually satisfied when the demands for energy are met regardless of other nutritional needs, it is necessary to have a plan of food selection which will insure that the necessary amounts of all the other dietary essentials go along with adequate calories. This food is best offered as a simple, well-balanced, varied diet in well-spaced meals so that natural appetite provides a desire to eat.

Between two and six years there is surprisingly little change in the construction of a suitable diet. Assuming the family diet to consist of simple, well-balanced meals, a child should be able to meet all his nutritional requirements from the family menu. In a family where there are several children the same meals may be served to all, the size of the serving portions being adapted to the needs of each child.

For the preschool age child the important foods are milk, whole, 3 cups (24 oz); an egg; lean meat, liver, poultry or fish, 1 to 2 oz; fruit, 2 servings ($\frac{1}{4}$ to $\frac{1}{2}$ cup each), one should be an orange or other rich source of ascorbic acid; vegetables, one potato, small to medium, and one to two servings of other vegetables, $\frac{1}{4}$ to $\frac{1}{2}$ cup, including deep yellow or dark leafy green vegetables; whole grain or enriched bread, $\frac{1}{2}$ to 1 slice per serving, or cereal, $\frac{1}{3}$ to $\frac{1}{2}$ cup portion, in all 2 to 3 servings daily; butter or fortified margarine, 1 tb. Either more of the above foods or additional foods of a child's own choice to meet the total daily energy needs may be necessary. The above listed foods are carefully selected for the proteins, minerals, and vitamins they furnish. A diet containing adequate amounts of these foods may be considered satisfactory for the daily needs of a healthy preschool child. If any of these foods are omitted or given in reduced amounts other foods of equivalent nutritional value should be substituted. Vitamin D should be taken daily to provide 400 I.U.

Table 4. A diet plan for the preschool age child

Breakfast	Lunch	Dinner	Supper
Citrus fruit or juice	Milk or fruit	Lean meat, liver, poultry, fish, or equivalent	Egg (may be given for breakfast in place of cereal, and cereal or a prepared main dish substituted here)
Cereal, preferably whole grain, cooked		Potato, preferably cooked in skin	Vegetable
Milk, whole		Vegetables	Bread, whole grain or enriched
Bread, whole grain or enriched		Bread, whole grain or enriched	Butter or fortified margarine
Butter or fortified margarine		Butter or fortified margarine	Milk, whole
		Milk, whole	Fruit, cooked or raw
		Dessert (simple puddings, custards, etc.)	

Importance of Formation of Good Eating Habits

If the young child eats foods which provide little but calories, his appetite and his energy needs may be satisfied before his structural needs for protein, minerals, and vitamins are met. For this reason the following foods are unsuitable for young children and should be avoided in planning diets for them.

Foods which interfere with normal appetites because of excessive sugar or excessive fat content. These include cakes, cookies, crackers, pies, doughnuts, fried foods, gravies, soft drinks, candy and the like. The child between one and three should not have these foods, except occasionally simple desserts at regular meals. Between three and six years of age, if these foods are used to any extent, they still will replace essential foods. Parents should realize that the child does not miss what he never has had and does not need.

The young child, just as the infant, should live a simple, well-regulated life in which he can feel secure and happy. His meals should be served at regular times and be planned in such a way that his nutritional requirements are met in three or four simple meals each day. Most young children do best with nothing between meals, but some children with small appetites do not take enough food in three meals and benefit by a midmorning or midafternoon lunch of milk or fruit. This lunch should be given at the same time each day and planned so that it does not interfere with normal appetite at the regular meal times. In some instances a bedtime snack may be given. This might well be a small sandwich with a protein-rich filling, together with a small glass of milk.

Many children who have established good eating habits lose these when they begin to eat with the family, sharing their meals and imitating their dietary practices. The problem here is one of education of parents and those in contact with young children. They should be given an understanding of which foods should be offered and which withheld, how the problems arising in connection with attitudes toward food should be handled, and the reasons for doing so. The preschool years are important from the standpoint of establishing desirable habits of eating, and proper attitudes toward food. Such habits tend to persist throughout life. It is far easier to prevent feeding problems than to correct them.

Prevention and Correction of Feeding Difficulties

Feeding problems are among the most common complaints about early childhood, and most children pass through periods of anorexia, or what the parents regard as poor appetite. Hunger is a set of reflex responses to physiologic states, such as low blood sugar. It is characterized by discomforts which are relieved by taking suitable foods. It reinforces or activates a natural and fundamental urge to eat which is called appetite. Hunger occurs intermittently, under special circumstances, whereas appetite recurs rhythmically and gives the incentive to eat a filling meal made of foodstuffs previously found acceptable. A healthy child eats well instinctively if an adequate selection of food is offered to him. The manifestations of appetite vary greatly in individual children, and from time to time in the same child. Appetite is initiated by hunger, and any factors which inhibit hunger are to be avoided.

Factors which Inhibit Hunger

Eating between meals. The child should be fed at sufficiently frequent intervals to satisfy his needs, but continuous "nibbling" inhibits hunger.

Hurry and emotional disturbances at meal times. These may completely inhibit hunger and divert attention from the food being offered.

Fatigue. A child worn out by too little sleep or by overactivity will not eat well. It is wise to have him rest or play quietly for a short time before each meal.

Excessive hunger. This also appears to destroy appetite, so that some children appear to have anorexia when there is too long a time span between meals. Too early a supper may indicate the need for bedtime nourishment if there is to be appetite for breakfast.

Illness. Loss of appetite may frequently be the first manifestation of acute illness in childhood, and is a usual accompaniment of chronic illness. A child showing anorexia deserves a careful physical examination in an effort to detect organic or functional disease.

Convalescence. Commonly the loss of appetite initiated by acute illness persists beyond the point of complete recovery in other aspects. This is best viewed as an expected and normal occurrence. Unfortunately, feeding pressures applied to the convalescent sometimes prolong anorexia.

Because of desire that a child be well-nourished, a mother often begins to force food, and feeding time becomes a battle between mother and child. When a mother forces some particularly disliked food upon a child he may learn to vomit this food, and will often extend his rebellion to other foods. A child soon learns that he can easily get attention by refusing to eat. This may be no hardship for him, for the tensions created may have already destroyed his appetite. Because of such unwise practices he often experiences frustration in what should have been his earliest experiences of satisfaction, and he develops an unhappy conditioning toward the taking of food. There is considerable evidence to show that these unfortunate early experiences often persist into adult life.

Certain suggestions are given here which if followed sensibly may largely avoid the creation of feeding problems:

Supply the child with a pleasant, quiet place in which to eat, with furniture and utensils adapted to his size and abilities.

Prepare and serve his food so that it is appetizing and attractive. Serve it in small portions to stimulate appetite and interest in self-feeding. Be sure the food is not too hot.

Avoid forcing him to eat; avoid any comment on his eating; avoid "rewards" for eating.

Set a well-balanced meal before him for a definite time — twenty minutes should be sufficient. At the end of this time excuse the child without comment.

If he shows a particular dislike for certain foods, avoid serving these for a time. Do not discuss or demonstrate food aversions in front of him.

Preferably have only one person supervise the child's feeding, one who maintains an attitude free of overconcern or oversolicitude.

Do not let him nibble between meals. If he becomes hungry at such times, he may be offered a small glass of milk or some fruit if it will not interfere with his appetite at the subsequent meal.

Prior to and during meals the atmosphere should be peaceful and tranquil.

THE NUTRITION OF THE SCHOOL AGE CHILD
BERTHA S. BURKE

The school age period, which for girls is six to ten years and for boys six to twelve, is one during which rate of growth in weight and certain dimensions increases while the rate of growth in height continues to diminish. In contrast to the slow growth of the preschool period for the majority of children, this is a period of more steady growth. Those children who grow more rapidly than others, or who become more active and muscular, may have displayed a marked increase in appetite even before the end of the preschool period; while others who grow more slowly, particularly if they are inactive in habit and late in physical development, may continue to progress in the way characteristic of the preschool period through a considerable part of the early school years and may show little, if any, inclination to eat more than they formerly did.

The nutritional requirements of the school age child are quantitatively distinctly different from those of adolescence which are high concomitant with accelerated growth. This is important in considering nutritional requirements and allocations during the latter part of this period since the chronological age at which a child enters the period of pubescence varies widely. For example, a very early maturing girl may be at the height of her adolescent growth spurt around ten years of age, which means that she will have been accelerating in growth rate and, therefore, have increased nutritional requirements during the last year or more of the school age period. Similarly, an early maturing boy entering his adolescent growth spurt before 12 years of age would have higher nutritional requirements than the recommended allowances for this age. When considering a child's nutritional requirements during these early years generalizations will not be applicable to children whose development has advanced to the adolescent stage. The only realistic way to evaluate an individual child's nutritional requirements during this period is in terms of his own growth pattern which requires recognition of his developmental age. It is also of interest that in our Longitudinal Studies of Health and Development[13] definite differences were observed in the average caloric and protein intakes of the boys and the girls in this period. In the National Research Council's allowances no distinction is made between the allowances for the two sexes until after the age of twelve.

The Diet During the School Age Period

The diet of a child in this period is essentially the same in type as during the preschool years. It is a basically simple diet. A natural increase in appetite and food intake is concomitant with increasing growth needs. At this time a child often increases his milk intake of his own volition, so that, if it is available to him and if he has not earlier developed aversion to milk, he will be taking approximately 1 quart daily. He may also increase his other protein-rich foods, if they are available. Ample protein in the diet throughout this period is as important as formerly although the requirement for protein per unit of body weight continues to decrease gradually. Again, the total amount of protein needed as well as other nutrients increases because the child is continually growing. In this period muscle mass grows somewhat faster than the body as a whole. In girls particularly it may approach adult proportions toward the end of this period. The total amount of protein provided by the diet should be sufficient to allow a child to attain his growth potential without depleting his body tissues. A sufficient intake of calories is also necessary to insure at all times that protein needed for muscle growth will not be burned for energy. The allowances recommended for all other nutrients are given in Table 3.

There is such a wide range of individual differences at any one age, and between the slow growing child of six years and the fast growing girl of ten or boy of twelve years, as already pointed out, that perhaps it is better to think of the diets of these children as varying on an individual basis somewhere between the type of diet described as suitable for a preschool child of five or six years and that for a girl or boy in the early adolescent years. A practical pamphlet available from the Children's Bureau, "Nutrition and Healthy Growth" will prove helpful in planning meals for children of various ages and with widely different problems.

Nutritional Problems

The nutrition of a child during this age period is important not only in respect to his growth and development at the time, but also in relation to the establishment of good lifetime food habits. Malnutrition may reduce a child's capacity to benefit from his educational opportunities. Attention to his nutritional status and food habits may result in improvement of his progress in school as well as in his health and development. In our Longitudinal Study of Health and Development, to which reference has been made, it is of interest that many of the children who had been difficult feeding problems in the preschool years outgrew their difficulties quite readily in the early school years. On the other hand some became problems during these years.

When a child goes to school there are several changes in his daily routine. He may have to get up earlier in order that there be sufficient time for him to have a good breakfast and not feel hurried. This will have to be planned; he needs help to start his day right. His lunch should be planned as an integral part of his total daily food intake whether he eats it at home, carries it to school, or receives it there.

The variety of foods eaten increases during these years, and the child usually eats as the family eats. Hence the quality of a child's diet is likely to depend to a large extent on the family pattern of eating. The choice of food to meet nutritional needs should be a part of a school's daily educational program. Classroom teaching in relation to health and growth at each grade level should be integrated with a school lunch program to provide a practical education in good food practices from a nutritional standpoint. At the same time an educational program is needed for parents and others who work with children, to explain nutritional needs in relation to growth, development, and health.

During the school age period many children consume excess calories and continue this excess each year. As a result they gain weight too rapidly. A tendency to accumulate even a few extra pounds over an expected gain in a given period should be watched for, and an attempt should be made to correct the child's eating habits before any amount of excess weight accumulates. This is important if one is to prevent some of the problems of obesity in adolescence. Children of this age who are underweight also need special nutritional guidance.

To deal most effectively with the health, growth, and nutritional status of individual children of school age, health examinations and progress records of each child's growth and health are indispensable, both to assure early recognition of the need for corrective measures and to adapt recommendations to meet changing individual needs. Children whose health or progress in growth suggests that nutrition may be unsatisfactory should be referred to a nutritionist for dietary study and advice.

THE NUTRITION OF THE ADOLESCENT
BERTHA S. BURKE

Nutritional Requirements

During adolescence nutritional needs are greatly increased concurrently with the rapid growth of this period. Maximum needs are related mainly to two aspects of the pubescent period, that is the middle period of adolescence; namely the age at which it occurs and the amount of gain or speed of growth during it. The two are usually related; that is, growth tends to be relatively rapid in an early maturing child, and relatively slow in a late maturing one. Because of the wide differences in rate of growth at any given chronological age, children differ greatly in nutritional needs at each age during adolescence. Their needs obviously are more highly correlated with their developmental than with their chronological age.

The majority of girls have their greatest nutritional requirements around twelve to fourteen years of developmental age. The greatest requirements usually immediately precede menarche; the requirements then decrease gradually to adult levels following menarche. The average boy experiences his highest nutritional needs about two years later than the average girl, i.e., at a developmental age of fourteen to sixteen years. In the recommended allowances, which are based on chronological age, the highest nutrient allocations for boys are for the age period sixteen to twenty years. The difficulty in estimating the nutritional requirements of an adolescent at any given chronological age is considerable. These requirements are largely controlled by factors related to developmental age, which during this period particularly are not closely related to chronological age. For example, the late maturing boy may develop so slowly that his needs may be less than the allowances indicate, but on the other hand his increased requirement while never perhaps as great for a short period of time as those of an early maturing boy, will increase steadily over a relatively longer period. Estimation of caloric needs is especially difficult because of the additional, variable activity. The extreme range of individual differences in habits of activity or sports participation, and the changing patterns for these among individuals in association with changing seasons, school grades, or part-time employment affect caloric requirements markedly. Natural increase in appetite, if the right kinds of food are available in sufficient quantity and there are no emotional or other deterrents, will provide not only for changing degrees of activity but also for naturally increasing growth, and thus permit attainment of appropriate adult size and build for the individual. Apparently, metabolic changes alter natural appetite in order to take care of growth needs. These inherent adaptive mechanisms can be relied upon, but only if there are no other factors interfering.

It is important that the increased nutritional requirements of adolescence be recognized, and that food intake be sufficient both in quality and quantity to meet the increased physiological requirements for growth. Since the health and development of the child in each succeeding period of life reflects the environmental factors of the preceding periods, together with inherited potentialities, these background factors must be given consideration in each individual case. The child who has been well nourished in the preceding years seems to have a spontaneous and relatively large natural increase in appetite during adolescence, taking a larger total quantity of food in terms of calories, protein, minerals, and vitamins. Spies[23] showed that by the time boys and girls with "nutritive failure" began to approach physical maturity, they had undergone a mean growth-lag of over two years as compared with controls. The mean growth-lag was somewhat greater in boys than in girls. Spies and his co-workers studied the degree to which this retardation in over-all body size and in skeletal maturity is reversible.[24] It appeared that the making up of these deficiencies is dependent primarily on the adequacy of the level of nutritional supplementation regardless of the age of the child.

Table 3 gives the recommended nutrient allowances for adolescence and reflects the very high dietary needs of children in this age group. After the age of twelve years allowances for boys and girls are given separately indicating the marked differences after this age between the sexes in their growth patterns and energy expenditure. The caloric needs of boys are higher than those of girls, because not only are boys more active but they expend more energy than do girls of the same age and body weight, because of a higher basal metabolic rate associated with a higher percentage of active tissue and possibly more extravagant use of muscle to accomplish the same work. Boys also attain on the average a larger final body size than do girls, which means that their total nutritional requirements as sexual maturity is reached are considerably higher than those of girls and the same is true also of average needs at the peak of their respective adolescent growth spurts.

The recommended protein allowances for girls are 75 to 80 gm as compared with 85 to 100 gm daily for boys. The need for protein is high during this period of rapid growth and development and continues to be high also in late adolescence because of rapid growth of muscle, particularly in boys, even after the growth in height has begun to slow. In order to allow for good nitrogen retention the caloric requirement must be adequate and about 15 per cent of the total caloric needs should be supplied by protein. If the protein intake previous to this period of rapid growth has been inadequate for normal skeletal and muscle growth the deficit must be made up before optimum storage and optimum growth can be attained.[25] If the demands for adequate calories and protein are not met, together with the accompanying increased needs for calcium and phosphorus, the body adjusts and equilibrium is attained at a lower level. Sexual maturity may be delayed, the extent depending in large measure upon the child's nutritional status and diet.

Beyond a certain point of nutritional inadequacy there may be failure to attain sexual maturity.[26]

The recommended allowances for calcium have been increased for the latter part of the adolescent period because of evidence that both girls and boys have ability to use increased calcium not only at the height of the adolescent growth spurt, but for a varying number of years following it.[1] The phosphorus needs in adolescence are also relatively high, but will usually be adequate in amount if protein and calcium are well supplied. Liberal amounts of calcium and phosphorus are as important as protein and calories in a well-balanced diet during adolescence, in order that optimum retention of these minerals may accompany optimum nitrogen retention. If for any reason calcium and/or phosphorus retentions in the years previous to adolescence have been low, the child's body will need an opportunity to make up these mineral deficits before optimum growth can be attained. For some children the requirement for vitamin D will also be increased in this period.

The iron requirements during adolescence are increased because of the growth spurt. The allowances recommended are 15 mg daily. The need for iodine may require attention during this period when growth is rapid. This is especially important in goiter zones.

At present there are insufficient data upon which the vitamin requirements of the adolescent can be established. The figures given by the Food and Nutrition Board are for the most part empirical and represent estimates. Waisman, Richmond, and Williams[27] have reviewed the existing literature and point to the need for studies of the vitamin requirements of adolescents, especially for the period of rapid growth.

Nutritional Problems

Despite his increasing self-sufficiency the adolescent still needs help in planning his diet so that his high nutritional needs will be met. He needs a good breakfast to supply approximately one-third of the day's nutritional allowances, and in addition plenty of time to eat it. A good noon meal, whether eaten at home, carried, or purchased, should be planned. The evening meal, usually the most leisurely and for many the main meal of the day, is of particular importance to this age boy or girl, and should be a planned part of the daily food intake. If additional food between meals is needed or desired, it should be included regularly in relation to the total daily nutritional requirements.

Many nutritional problems of adolescence are continuations of those noted for the earlier school years, but intensified by the higher nutritional requirements associated with a rapid growth-rate and increased activity. Problems that arise frequently, and make it difficult for an adolescent to have food which adequately supplies his nutritional requirements include:

(1) Failure of family groups to be aware of the high food requirements of this period. This is likely to occur because the adults themselves may need less food daily and because adults are likely to be weight, diet, and budget conscious.

(2) The tremendous appetites particularly of boys during the adolescent growth spurt, due to the need of possibly 2,000 more calories per day than men of the same size leading sedentary lives.

(3) The high food needs of girls and simultaneously a new figure-consciousness, finicky appetite, misinformation about food values, and willingness to skip meals, especially breakfast.

(4) Adolescents' interest in and need for group activities which may interfere with regular mealtimes.

(5) Many adolescents leave school to work, and often live under conditions not conducive to good health practices, including good food habits.

From the standpoint of nutrition the adolescent period despite its importance is one of the most neglected. There is an amazing lack of understanding by family groups of the relation of adequate food to health and growth. The adolescent and his family need to be educated in the special nutritional requirements of this period. The underweight or overweight adolescent boy or girl needs special medical attention, including an evaluation of his or her food habits and such dietary guidance as is indicated.

For girls good nutrition in this period is particularly important. The recent tendency to early marriage and parenthood has resulted in an increasing number of teen-age girls assuming the responsibilities of motherhood. Furthermore, illegitimate births occur commonly during these years. This creates additional nutritional problems, since pregnancy is not likely to be admitted until late in gestation, and therefore early prenatal care is not received. The Metropolitan Life Insurance Company[28] reports that about one-fourth of the mothers bearing a first child are less than 20 years old. There is evidence indicating a relatively high incidence of toxemia in this age group. Almost 6 per cent of the deaths among 18 and 19 year old girls in the insurance experience were due to pregnancy and childbirth.

The Diet of the Adolescent

In summary, the diet of the adolescent is one of relatively high nutritional needs associated with a further increase, especially in calories and protein, during the period of most rapid growth. This is followed by a decline to normal adult requirements. Natural appetite, if not interfered with, will serve as a guide to food needs.

To attempt to offer a suggested day's menu for either boys or girls of this age group seems impractical, since individual needs and eating habits vary so widely. However, there are certain foods which in our American culture are, from a practical standpoint, essential to a well-balanced diet. For the average boy or girl at the height of the adolescent growth spurt the nutritional requirements, other than calories may be safeguarded by the *daily inclusion* of the following foods: milk, 1–1½ qt; eggs, 1 or 2; lean meat, fish, poultry, or liver, or equivalent protein-rich foods, 4–8 oz; cereal, 1–2 cups, whole grain or enriched; bread, whole grain or enriched, 6–8 slices; potato, 1–2 medium (cooked in skin); at least one other cooked or raw vegetable daily, including deep yellow or dark leafy green vegetables, 2–3 servings each week; fruit, 2 medium oranges, or fresh, frozen, or canned orange juice, 8 oz or equivalent, and an additional fruit is desirable; butter or fortified margarine, 2 tb. The lower range more nearly represents the average girl's needs, except for calories, and the higher range will satisfy the average boy's nutritional requirements other than calories. Additional calories can be left to individual taste, but should be supplied in adequate amounts to meet growth and activity needs.

THE CHILD'S NUTRITIONAL STATE
HAROLD C. STUART

Taking required kinds and amounts of food is only the first of a series of processes which contribute to maintaining a satisfactory nutritional state. The food must be digested, assimilated, transported, stored or immediately utilized as fuel or building materials and the excess or waste products must be disposed of. The numerous mechanisms involved are complicated and it is not surprising that among immature individuals various kinds of nutritional problems arise more commonly than at later ages. The processes immediately involved may be classified as physiologic, biochemical, or anatomical but background factors may be of endocrine origin, metabolic, neurologic or psychologic. The determination of the functioning of these processes in the individual and of their appropriateness for age is primarily a task for the physician but involves at times assistance from others.

The first steps in the appraisal of nutritional status are to obtain a comprehensive clinical history and a thorough physical examination. The history should include careful analysis of foods customarily consumed, the functioning of digestive processes, weight changes, and behavior. The examination should be general in character but should devote special attention to hydration and turgor of skin, pallor, signs of fatigue, specific faults in the skin and mucous membranes, and importantly the amount of fat in subcutaneous tissues.

Laboratory tests such as hemoglobin concentration in the blood and at times biochemical blood studies help in diagnosis. Following the weight gain and comparing it with expectancy for age and body size or build are important parts of this assessment and make studies of a child's progress as well as of his status imperative for an accurate diagnosis in borderline cases.

In some countries where malnutrition is severe or chronic, or in sick infants or young children a prompt diagnosis can often be made clinically on brief examination. In this country malnutrition when present is more likely to be mild but chronic and therefore more commonly overlooked and less readily diagnosed.

The term malnutrition is frequently used incorrectly to refer solely to thinness or lack of the expected amount of soft tissue or of muscle development for age. These features may make a child appear malnourished and tire easily but they may actually represent an intrinsic type of build or slow pattern of development or a growth problem unrelated to nutrition. The unsatisfactory features of growth and development which may be due in whole or in part to long standing undernutrition relate chiefly to the muscles, subcutaneous tissue and structure of bones and teeth but defects in the blood, reflecting nutritional anemia, and in the skin or mucous membranes may add significantly to the evidence that malnutrition is involved in some degree. Specific nutritional diseases due to gross or long standing deficiencies in the consumption of particular nutrients are major problems in large areas of the world and continue to require attention in the United States but less and less frequently. Discussion of the clinical manifestations of these diseases is not appropriate for this book but the recognition of malnutrition and particularly the differentiation of nutritional state from other aspects of growth status constitutes an important task for the physician. The two closely related problems of underweight and overweight have been considered in various connections in Chapter IV in discussing growth and development by age. Obesity in adolescence has been given particular attention there as an important problem in this country which requires understanding and cooperation from many sources for its control. Factors related to malnutrition in infancy and the preschool period have been touched upon but are not given the attention here which they still deserve in large areas of the world. The problems differ so greatly between countries or regions, depending upon the kinds of foods in short supply, feeding practices and complicating chronic infections, that general discussion would be inadequate. Presently nutritional diseases and chronic malnutrition during early childhood are problems for medical and public health recognition and management at these ages. Attention to some aspects of these is required by health personnel in different fields but basically their role is to help in ways which present themselves to assure that every child is offered and encouraged to take an adequate diet for age and that children not doing so are quickly recognized. The background information which will assist all professional workers with families to contribute more effectively toward this end have been given primary attention in this chapter.

VI

BACKGROUND FACTORS RELATED
TO PSYCHO-SOCIAL DEVELOPMENT

SOME PHYSIOLOGICAL COMPONENTS OF HUMAN BEHAVIOR
STANLEY COBB

The anatomical and physiological aspects of emotion make up a rather new subject and one of extreme complexity. The anatomical basis of emotional behavior can be said to have had its origin in 1871, when Weigert's staining methods proved the continuity of the nerve cell and the axon. More convincing was Harrison's definitive demonstration in 1910 of the growth of axons out from nerve cells. The three essentials of the neuron theory then at last accepted by all anatomists were: (1) that each neuron consists of a cell body together with its protoplasmic outgrowths — axons and dendrites; (2) that transmission of impulses is in one direction only — dendrite to cell body to axon; and (3) that the neurons are the structural units of which the nervous system is composed, and that they stimulate each other by contact at the synapse.

Although recently there have been two main theories — chemical and electrical — concerning the transmission of the nerve impulse, the weight of present evidence points strongly toward the electrical theory as the more tenable. However, the too facile comparison of the nervous system to an electrical system has led to an unjustified belief that the nerve impulse is an electrical current. It is unlike such a current because the energy for the transmission of the impulse is derived from the nerve itself and not from the stimulus, and the nerve impulse is a discontinuous process, with a relatively slow rate of transmission. The discontinuity can be explained on the grounds that transmission of the impulse is the result of local electrical circuits flowing between inactive and active portions of the nerve, each local circuit acting as the exciting agent for the next adjacent segment of resting nerve. The nerve impulse is a reversible electrochemical reaction, in which the nerve fibers, within their membranes, behave like core conductors. The chemical change is in the differential concentration of potassium and sodium ions inside and outside the axon, the membrane of which is semipermeable. Sodium ions enter the fiber at the moment of excitation, and potassium leaks out.

Until the last 10 years or so the general concept of function within the nervous system was based on the image of the telephone exchange, input impulses flowing from sense organs along neuron lines to the central exchange, and out again along other neuron lines to the effector organs. It is now realized that this very inadequately schematizes the main afferent and efferent neuron systems, because the function of the short collateral neurons is not taken into consideration. These are far more numerous than the conspicuously larger nerve cells. A branch from an axon may play back upon the cell of origin, or more commonly, play upon several of the small internuncial cells through their axons, with secondary relays reaching the next efferent cell in the main chain. There are thus series of small nerve cells, beside the larger main tracts, with short collateral axons forming many synapses, circuits, and networks. These cause varied delays or inhibitions, as well as summations and facilitations, of the nerve impulses. That these reverberating circuit mechanisms in the brains of animals might provide a pattern for an electronic computing machine was quickly recognized by mathematicians, such as Wiener, and mathematically-minded physiologists, such as McCulloch.

It is perhaps not an exaggeration to term this new concept of the nervous system epoch-making. Memory had never been explained by any reasonable physiological theory until Wiener and his associates developed "cybernetics," using electronic calculating machines as the analogy to the new dynamic concept of the nervous system. The essential fact is that a neuron circuit can be set in action by an incoming single impulse, and that the circuit may go on reverberating as long as metabolism supports it, or until other incoming impulses change it. In the electronic computing machine one circuit is set to modify the behavior of the others in response to a certain signal; that is, the circuit stores the reaction. In the neuron circuit, on this analogy, essential past experiences are similarly stored, and constitute the equivalent of the setting manipulation of the electronic computer. The neuron circuit thus chooses the proper signal when it comes, rejecting all others, while the appropriate affirmative signal causes the circuit to act in the light of past experience.

All this depends upon "feedback." As applied to the nervous system, feedback means that the activity of the reverberating circuits is modified by the return of some of the output of the system as input. For example, when one reaches with the hand for an object, a series of signals flows back to the central mechanism, informing it through eye, touch, and proprioceptive receptors how far the hand is wide of its goal. The amount of error determines the return input, until the error becomes zero. Such a mechanism is called negative feedback, and accompanies every motor act. Similar mechanisms seem to be present in the auditory and visual cortical areas, and in fact all intelligent behavior might be explained in the same way — a goal is aspired to, and may be reached by means of a feedback into a reverberating circuit. In other words, choice means acting on the basis of stored past experience; a volitional act is the resultant of a primary impulse as modified by feedback influences.

Although there is as yet no proof that processes like those in computing machines actually take place in the brain, anatomical work indicates that nervous mechanisms exist which could act in this way, and so might explain at least one type of memory. There is good evidence for reverberating circuits and feedback mechanisms in the mammalian brain. Promising work now in progress may well soon clarify this important area of knowledge. Meanwhile the cybernetic concept of the nervous system illuminates hitherto dark places in the physiology of emotional behavior.

It is probable that activity in any part of the brain affects many other parts, if not all other parts of the brain. In this sense the brain acts as a whole, and the functions are so interdependent that, normally, no area acts alone. However, both histological and gross anatomical evidence is convincing as to the existence of cerebral differentiation, and physiological experiment indicates that, in a general way, the more differentiated areas have specialized functions. About 40 different types of cortex are recognizable in man, and topographical localization of function is rather well defined. In addition, however, there appears to be stratigraphical localization, with a distribution of different general functions in the different cell laminae throughout the cortex. Further, the cortical connections between nerve cells are radial. As a result of such complex interconnections, the plan of the brain provides the possibility of widespread association, and at the same time gives steadiness to the nervous discharges.

Studies along these lines, as well as a mass of clinicopathological data, indicate that local lesions cause specific neurological and psychological abnormalities. Certain areas are known to be concerned with visual and auditory memories, dream states, and the comparison of present perceptions with past experience. On the other hand it is impossible to localize the more abstract functions, those less obviously connected with the direct receiving stations of the cortex, or with the direct corticospinal motor mechanism. It is known, however, that lesions which injure both frontal lobes reduce the intellectual faculties, and while there is no qualitative loss of any one capacity, there is a quantitative reduction of restraint, judgment, ability to learn, initiative, and foresight, and the effect on mood is even more striking.

A clue to the nature of such mental attributes as memory and learning may lie in the mechanism that allows spread of impulses from one reflex level up and down to other segments, and thus also explain delay.

Short reflex arcs across the cord, medulla, or other lower centers give rapid automatic responses; but most impulses normally are shunted up the cord to higher levels. This allows for an enormous increase in association. The higher integration leads to delayed action and great spread of nerve impulses. This allows the past experience of the individual to affect his behavior. Surely the widespread activity of association paths is one of the essential phenomena of "mind."

There is considerable experimental evidence associating the visceral brain with emotional expression. A monkey after the removal of the uncus, amygdala, and anterior hippocampus, or the orbital and insular parts of the mesocortex, will be docile and devoid of fear, and will show sexual hyperexcitability and a strong tendency to explore everything with mouth and nose. Such behavior, produced in animals by brain operations, has far-reaching psychological implications. It connects the oral reflexes neurologically with sexual activity and passive behavior. It indicates that these reactions are not the result of early experiences, such as nursing, but are inborn behavior patterns older than the race. A possible teleological explanation is that the primates, being social animals which get their food by cooperation, connect oral behavior with docile, passive, and affectionate reactions.

Three Mechanisms of Emotion

There are at least 3 physiological mechanisms which are involved in the expression of an emotion. These are diagrammatically indicated in Fig. 6. One of these mechanisms is set off by the nervous impulses which pour into the thalamus from the external sense organs and from the muscles of the body. These are passed on from the thalamus to the neocortex of the cerebrum as shown in (c). From the cerebrum nerve impulses may reverberate back to the thalamus or to various other nerve centers of the cerebrospinal nervous system. In (b) is indicated the part played by the old visceral brain, which is stimulated directly by smell and has a close connection with all the viscera and the autonomic nervous system. This is called the archicortex and it discharges largely through the hypothalamus to the autonomic system and the vital organs of the body. The third mechanism, schematically drawn in (a) involves the glands of internal secretion, which alter their individual secretions of hormones in response to both external and internal stimuli, and add the slowest but most long-lasting part of the emotional reaction.

The visceral brain (b) while comprising a much smaller proportion of the brain in primates than in lower mammals, is far from vestigial, and seems to set the emotional background on which man functions intellectually. Closely connected with this visceral brain is the endocrine system, as shown in the connections between (a) and (b). The stimulation of the

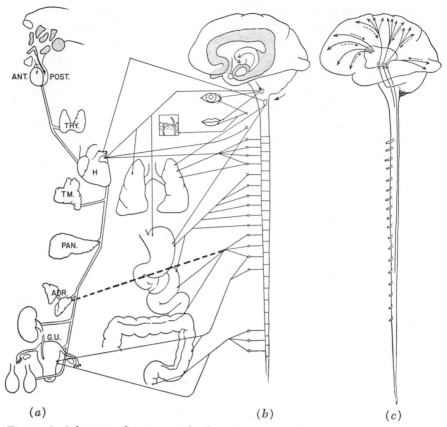

(a) (b) (c)

Figure 6. Schematic diagram of ductless glands and their relation to the central nervous system: (a) the glands from which the various hormones are derived, represented schematically (ANT. — anterior pituitary, POST. — posterior pituitary, THY. — thyroid, H — heart, TM. — thymus, PAN. — pancreas, ADR. — adrenals, G.U. — kidney, uterus, and gonads); (b) the hypothalamic-archicortical central nervous system, showing autonomic innervation of eye, lips, skin, and viscera; (c) the thalamo-neocortical central nervous system.

Source: S. *Cobb,* Emotions and clinical medicine (*Norton, New York, 1950*).

glands of internal secretion causes hormones to reach all parts of the body, including the brain, thus providing another feedback control system.

The part of the emotional reaction that is nearest to conscious awareness is carried out by the thalamus and neocortex (c). Stimuli from the outside world, and from muscles, joints, and the inner ear, are received in special sense organs, relayed to the thalamus, and thence relayed again to the neocortex of the cerebrum. Here pathways back to the thalamus are activated, and thus reverberating circuits are formed that relate the sensory functions of the thalamus to the highly discriminative functions of the neocortex. It may well be that it is the continuity of stimulation subserved by such reverberating circuits that gives to man what he recognizes as his "feelings." This is the part of emotion which is the private experience of everyone, but being entirely subjective it can be shared only through symbolic media — language, music, and the other arts. The disturbed physiological state set up by these feelings, however, can be seen, recorded, and often measured. This is the emotional *expression*, another part of the complex phenomenon called emotion.

The expression of an emotion is carried out by all three physiological mechanisms, the first of which is the private feeling, the affect that is felt by each individual but which must be interpreted if it is to be understood by anyone else. The second mechanism is the complex set of physiological changes set up in nerves, viscera, glands, and muscles. These make the characteristic stirred-up internal state. And third is the pattern of behavior which overtly expresses the stirred-up internal state.

Which mechanism starts first is probably a matter of what sort of stimulus began the reaction. Sensations of smell go directly to the hypothalamus without relay through the thalamus, and possibly that is why smells are so emotionally poignant. Things seen and heard stir up emotions by the more intellectual route of geniculate bodies to sensory neocortex (c) to associative cortex to thalamus and thus to hypothalamus and visceral (b) and endocrine expression (a). Shortcuts are possible, however, from subthalamus directly to hypothalamus.

Thus the full expression of emotion is activated by at least three separate but interconnected feedback systems.

Multiple Causation

All abnormal human behavior has a mixed etiology, combining two or more factors which may be genogenic, histogenic, chemogenic, or psychogenic.

Genogenic disorders of personality have their source mainly in heredity. The abnormal genes may or may not cause recognizable lesions or malformations of the nervous system.

Histogenic disorders of the personality are those that are largely due to nonhereditary lesions of the nervous system, such as those produced by inflammation, degeneration, asphyxia, toxin, trauma, or tumor.

Chemogenic disorders of personality come from the effects of chemical agents. These may be endogenous. Indeed the field of psychosomatic illness is largely concerned with the emotionally induced endogenous production of chemical substances.

Psychogenic disorders of personality are those that seem to arise largely because of disturbed interpersonal relations, social maladjustments, and the like.

For the most part histogenic disorders result in loss of function, except in the brief episodes where there is direct irritation of neurons. In psychogenic disorders, on the other hand, the most commonly expressed somatic effect is increased function in the autonomic nervous system and the endocrine system. The poorly adjusted individual reacts to another individual with increased irritability — that is, a lowering of the sensory threshold. Thus, the maladjusted person becomes the target of innumerable stimuli which begin by disturbing his autonomic equilibrium. His heart races or skips a beat, his breathing becomes labored or spasmodic, his hands and feet become cold and damp, he is "scared stiff," or his "mind went blank," or he was "struck dumb."

There is a large and growing body of evidence that emotional stress causes abnormal function, and that continued malfunction results in lesions. Vulnerability to stress is a phenomenon in which hereditary factors are probably important. As yet there is no very exact evidence concerning the role of heredity in the autonomic system, but the transmission of genes which lead to abnormal hormonal patterns is well substantiated. Probably it is correct to say that one inherits most of what one is. But the environment acting on this organism is equally important. In recent years there has been a great exaggeration of the environmental aspect, because, being subject to social manipulation, it is of so much practical interest. Interpersonal relations fall within the environmental part of our total potential. They are our personal responsibility, and the results depend on what we succeed in accomplishing with the organism handed us at birth.

THE INGREDIENTS OF PERSONALITY
ERICH LINDEMANN

Psychology can be defined as the study of the behavior of people for the purpose of description, understanding, explanation, and help. In community mental health work, since one wants to bring about constructive change, one wants to aid people to alter their behavior. In order to accomplish this, one has to know what behavior will be shown by what people and under what circumstances. One has to know to what degree one can predict a person's future behavior. It is necessary to keep in mind a number of essential ingredients of the individual, those factors which limit the possibilities of changes in behavior, and those factors which determine the persistence of certain kinds of behavior.

It is of interest that we are now culturally in a phase of scientific development in which hereditary and constitutional factors are no longer considered the most important determinants of behavior. They used to offer a convenient explanation as to why a person acted a certain way and could be expected again to act that way. It is true that there has been a recent recurrence of interest in hereditary factors, but it is no longer naively believed that a few physical determinants explain a person's personality or that there are simple hereditary laws controlling the transmission of feeble-mindedness, for example. The interest today is much more in terms of a very careful analysis of which traits are gene-transmitted and which are not. Of course there are some traits, especially certain pathological traits at the physiological level, which are very clearly gene-transmitted, such as hemophilia, or certain disturbances in metabolism which lead to defects like amaurotic idiocy. In other conditions the distinction between the contribution by genetic factors and by intrauterine illness of the child or birth trauma is much harder to make. In regard to mental illness, as Kallman,[1] has shown there is some indication that hereditary factors may play a role in the predisposition of the individual to the development of a particular type of psychosis. Many of the claims about heredity are still inadequately tested, however, even in the field of feeble-mindedness, and there is a certain danger that such claims may be transformed prematurely into legislative procedures. There is another aspect of gene-transmitted problems, namely, that of constitution. Is it possible from certain physical, anatomical, or bodily characteristics of an individual to make reliable inferences about his probable personality? This question really does not deal with gene-transmission alone but rather with the inspection of a person as a physical specimen. In internal medicine, as well as in psychiatry, much thought has been given to this subject. Draper[2] made a very careful study of the bodily configuration of selected patients, such as those with gastric ulcer. Kretschmer[3] tried to distinguish between those who had schizophrenia and those who had manic-depressive psychosis by describing their bodily characteristics, their muscular development, their fat-distribution, and their skeletal structure. Sheldon[4] has studied in great detail and with great care the somatotypes or physical profiles of a series of individuals in relation to certain personality traits.

In summing up the results of such research, it can be said that schizophrenia and manic-depressive psychosis are unfortunate categories to choose, because many people do not agree on the differential diagnosis. Taking certain forms of physical disease, such as ulcer, colitis, or arthritis, and relating these to certain characteristics of body structure, one finds that the disease conditions and the specific personalities observed under clinical circumstances do not appear to be related to a single factor. Any one of the above may of course have a physiological component and a body-build component. There are other factors involved, however, all operating in a very complex pattern of determinants. This inference can safely be drawn from available case studies. Each individual is a case, representing a complex individual in a multidetermined situation, showing certain disease manifestations. There apparently is something to the concept that there are relationships between physique and personality, but present knowledge is not sufficient to convince many that common or direct relationships have been established.

Thus, in attempting to apply the theories of heredity and constitution to the field of personality in a useful manner, we may say that an individual arrives in this world, not with finished traits, but with potentialities which are going to be accessible to environmental unfolding at suitable moments in the subsequent development. The opportunities which are available in the environment determine whether or not these gene-determined potentialities become realities in terms of traits of the personality. Good evidence along this line is available from the studies made by Alison Davis[5] and others who have been concerned with differences in intelligence quotients among different races. In the course of these investigations, it became plain that the argument for a different mean I.Q. from population to population was related to the range of the training opportunities and the school systems in which the children operated, as well as to the attitudes of the teachers, who expected different behavior from white and colored children. Rather than being something rigidly inherent in a person or in his capacity to learn, the I.Q. thus appears to be influenced by environmental factors which contribute to the bringing out of potential traits in terms of the basic capacity for learning and for unfolding of skills.

In regard to the understanding of behavior, there are at least three theoretical approaches which offer explanatory principles: the *reflex theory*, which treats behavior as a series of conditioned responses; the *field theory*, which conceptualizes behavior as motion in a field of force; and the *dynamic theory*, which is essentially psychoanalytic theory. Actually, all three theories may be useful in certain situations as explanatory principles, since some overlapping exists and, in addition, each theory fails to explain all aspects of behavior.

In the field of learning, the contribution of the reflex theory is extensive, helping to explain certain symptoms which are commonly seen at the clinic, such as phobias and avoidance reactions. Among these is the type of protracted avoidance reaction that a child might develop who has been unfortunately exposed to powerful anxiety during a bath scene. Subsequent encounters with water, in situations where other children are able to enjoy it, may then be responded to with an avoidance reaction. This avoidance reaction thus may be regarded as having become a conditioned response in the sense that whenever there is proximity to water an overwhelming anxiety response will occur. In this sense, an initial experience has provided powerful emotional stimulation and has established an obligatory, usually unconscious, bond between that experience and the emotional reaction.

How to form suitable conditioned reflexes in the learning process, forming such bonds that, in a special situation, the person will always find himself doing the appropriate thing, and how to avoid unfortunate bonds which sometimes come about through what analysts call "traumatic experiences," is the topic of a great deal of laboratory investigation. Much has been done with animals. It is unfortunate that the translation of results from the study of animal life to that of human life has been much more difficult than was formerly thought, at least at the level of behavior. Masserman[6] has made detailed studies of cats in various situations, combining disturbing stimuli, such as a blast of cold air, with the satisfaction of the food-intake response. In this way, conditioned responses have been formed artificially which prevent the cats from feeding because they are expecting, whenever they eat, to have cold air blown in their faces. Masserman tried various therapeutic methods to induce the cats to give up this response. He mapped out several kinds of behavior on the part of the therapist animal-trainer, who may try to comfort the animal or may use more forceful methods in an attempt to have it remain in the situation long enough to adjust to it. Masserman thinks of therapy as essentially similar to education, because education not only forms suitable new responses in auspicious situations, but also does the opposite, by undoing the kind of ties that have existed previously and that become obsolete at a later stage of development.

Kurt Lewin[7] has been the most important contributor to social psychology in the last 20 or 30 years. Lewin sees the human being as a reflection of the social forces around him. In common with the psychoanalytic theorist, he conceives of the individual not as reflex-oriented to a stimulus, but as being oriented toward goals, as having needs which have to be satisfied, together with driving or motivating forces which lead to goal-directed behavior. Certain interesting questions about a person then can be considered. How does he reach his goals? How does he get around barriers to such goal-directed behavior? How big a barrier can he master? How much does he get upset about barriers? The individual's goals are usually structured in terms of conscious wishes and described in terms of the power they have to motivate him to try to reach them. For example, if a child wants to get candy, one is interested in what kind of barrier may influence the movement of the child in the direction of the candy. When one studies individuals' goals and barriers, even in a geographical space, one may find different kinds of behavior according to the different shapes of the physical barrier. Real complexities occur when one translates the space concept into "life-space," the space which deals with social distance, with obstacles to social mobility, as for example in marrying a person from a different class, or getting a job which another person holds. Motion in social-space or life-space may proceed along a channel partially or completely blocked by other people or by rules and regulations. The child's reaction to punishment versus reward may be analyzed in terms of this theory.

Psychoanalysis takes as its starting point the assertion that behavior is a correlate of forces in the central nervous system. If these forces are interfered with by drugs or injury, there is not the same personality that there would be with an intact nervous system. A broad range of symptoms in psychoneurotic illness, however, cannot be accounted for by this explanation. Psychoanalysis started with the study of sick people, bringing to bear an historical perspective which explains present behavior in terms of previous experience. In doing this, Sigmund Freud ran across a number of reminiscences about childhood in psychoneurotic patients which he had not expected, and which startled many people: namely, that there are powerful emotional experiences, many of them involving passion and rage in the very early stages of childhood development. Adults who were well-meaning caretakers had handled these events in a way which appeared to have disturbed profoundly the growth process of the child. Psychoanalysis was thus a powerful stimulus to modern theory of emotional development.

How can these findings best apply to the problem of general psychology rather than clinical pathology? To make inferences from patients regarding the course of normal development is obviously risky. Of course, many normal people have been analyzed lately, especially candidates for psychiatry and social work. However, the inferences made from retrospective accounts are scientifically quite precarious until they can be compared with another body of data which is collected by direct observation of children. Such knowledge has been growing slowly, starting with Susan Isaacs,[8] Piaget,[9] Robert and Pauline Sears.[10] Particularly important are the studies of war orphans by Anna Freud,[11] and such observations as Rene Spitz[12, 13] made with orphans in the hospitals in New York.

A number, though not by any means all, of Freud's hypotheses have been substantiated by such studies, and psychiatrists today feel reasonably sure of certain principles for understanding the behavior encountered in individuals. One of these principles relates to the "mature" or "immature" handling of basic needs. Personality is usually viewed by us in terms of our own values. If a person does not fit in with these values we call him a "deviant" person, and classify him as "psychoneurotic," "psychotic," or just "immature."

The implication of 'immaturity" is that there is a process of development reaching an optimal point, at which we call a person mature, and that in certain adults this process may not be completed. This has very little to do with the biological maturation to which we referred above. Biological maturity is reached by the growth processes of bone development, organ development, and changes in the configuration of the body and also by successive stages of intellectual capacity. It is possible that there is an inherent biological maturation process involving emotional maturity, so that, quite apart from specific environmental influences, the progress from being emotionally immature to being emotionally mature might go through a sequence of steps typical for various age levels. Psychoanalysis, however, is primarily concerned with the study of the effects of environmental influences.

A child is permitted, during infancy, to carry on without interference his essential functions, those which have to be executed in order to satisfy his needs. A state of pleasure is expected to accompany the opportunity for need-satisfaction without regulation. In all cultures it is demanded of adults that the satisfaction of basic needs be put into a time-space system in such a way that need-satisfaction occurs at certain times and in certain places only. An individual, then, in order to be mature, would certainly have to come to be able to control his need-satisfactions, his impulses, and emotions.

The basic needs, according to psychoanalysis, fall into two groups. The first consists of those related to self-preservation, like food-intake, elimination, and having a reasonable amount of security and shelter; the second group of needs includes those ultimately having to do with procreation, which are initially satisfied by close contact with nurturing adults. The child cannot satisfy most of his needs without help from other people, with the result that he is extremely dependent. Consequently, one of the qualities which many people include in assessing maturity is that of independence, the implication being that the individual does not need anyone outside, or that he can supply all his needs himself. Of course this is an illusion. There are still plenty of dependent needs in adult life, but for satisfaction they are distributed among quite a number of people. Dependence in an adult becomes conspicuous when the need-satisfaction is mediated by one person or two persons only. A mature person, then, has to have learned to satisfy his basic needs by satisfaction mediators, properly placed in space and time, and properly used. They have to be kept friendly. The child soon has to learn, in order to grow up and mature, that he has to arrange his need-satisfaction to suit his mother and other significant adults.

Expectations of the child's behavior at different stages of his development vary in different cultures. Some people have felt lately that it would be important to make a comparative study of different cultures and see the effect of various ways of interfering with need-satisfactions. Such interference of course rises from the socialization process which forces the child to give up the breast, to have proper bowel control, to be increasingly independent, and to keep his affectionate needs under control. It is possible that child-rearing practices and their variations may be the crucial factor determining the degree of maturity which a person will attain later as he grows up. Considerably more investigation on a cross-cultural basis, such as that carried on by Whiting and his associates,[14] is necessary before final conclusions can be drawn.

Psychoanalytic theory recognizes that maturity, as it is defined in the Western world, might not be the same thing which people in Samoa, for example, call maturity. What is demanded there of an adult, a mature person, may be quite different. Hence child-rearing methods must be understood in terms of the culture for which they are designed. However, maturity implies essentially that people should be able to postpone need-satisfaction. They must be able to map out a program of steps leading to ultimate satisfaction, by taking a number of dissatisfying intermediary steps. They have to be people who have learned to control their emotions in a very special way, not repressing them so that they disappear altogether, but using them and having them available in the proper time-space context.

The two most striking emotions which usually wreak havoc with the supposedly mature person are those related to his sexual and aggressive drives. It is true that special modes of control are required. The emotions connected with these needs should not appear at inconvenient moments. Religious idealism sometimes seems to require that one never be angry or feel hostile, but such a degree of control appears incompatible with healthy adjustment, in our culture at least.

Parallel attitudes exist in the sexual field. Many parents do not like any sexual manifestations at all in the growing child. They do not recognize that, at a certain level of maturity, such manifestations may be quite an acceptable expression of the child's developing instinctual life. In any case, cultural values demand that sexual behavior disappear during long periods of development. Later, when the boy or girl gets married he or she must have available just the right amount of sexual response to have a happy marriage afterwards. Parents often suppose that this response will suddenly come from nowhere. The truth is that such appropriate sexual behavior is the result of a complicated process of development. The task which is put before the maturing person is indeed challenging, for he must design an arrangement whereby he can have the proper emotions at the proper time. To become mature in this sense is a difficult job which faces young people in a special way in our society.

What tools does society provide to help the child to develop control? Certainly there is an important degree of learning by precept, by being taught at home and in school by adults. The kind of learning which has become much more significant to those who are interested in dynamic psychology, however, is what is called "social learning." This process involves learning social skills by witnessing and emulating another person who serves as a model for identification.

This problem of acquiring skills, manners, and equipment in human relations by emulating models represents an indispensable part of growing up to become a mature person. Some workers in the psychoanalytic field go so far as to say that one may assume that the models with whom one has lived, and the configuration they make when internalized as part of one's own ways of behaving, are the very essence of individual personality patterning.

In clinical work we have a tendency to distinguish rich personalities from impoverished or rigid ones, the latter term referring to individuals who had a very limited number of exclusive models. The "overprotected" child is usually distinguished from other children by the fact that he has had access to fewer people who could be models for him. A mother who wishes the child to have the "right" manners may hope to achieve this by rigidly excluding those models from "bad" company, who might bring about other sets of manners in the child. If such exclusion is carried to an extreme, the child is thus deprived of the opportunity to acquire, by at first copying street boys and girls, a kind of behavior which can then, by differentiation, be assigned to the proper place to use it. There occur different life-occasions for which such behavior may be suitable. One varies one's behavior to suit different kinds of company. A highly respected person, a professor of Sanskrit, for example, although adequate in certain circles, may be severely handicapped in many human relationships, such as with his child or with the man in the street. His range of social skills appropriate for different levels of human relations may not have been developed. The social rewards of the family, and of some institutions of learning, have been such that there is a tremendous premium on top performance in a limited sector at the expense of the acquisition of social skills in other areas. The professor in question, for example, when confronted with a labor union, would probably feel very shy and might try to get out of the situation as fast as he could. Being deficient in suitable social skills, he may be called "immature," because he cannot control his emotions in such situations.

In other words, there is a very complex interplay between the arsenal of social skills in a variety of situations acquired by copying other individuals, authoritative figures, or peers, and the areas in subsequent adult life in which one can operate without having to appear immature because anxiety, tensions, or depressions are mobilized. Hence the problem of providing suitable models to the growing population is important in any mental health program.

There are some special versions of this process of identification which are important in considering personality development. One version, which often appears in the clinic, is the cross-sex identification: a boy identifies with his mother, a girl with her father, and the identification is so strong that the masculine traits in the girl or the feminine traits in the boy become conspicuous. In our culture there is great pressure against this, although it is not so great in some other cultures. Here the boy who has feminine traits is extremely uncomfortable, and frequently develops reaction-formations to protect himself against the injuries and emotional insults to which he may be exposed. Yet there is great likelihood that a certain percentage of the population makes such a cross-sex identification because often the cross-sex parent happens to be a more suitable model, and happens to have qualities which mobilize those psychological processes which lead to preferring a person as a model. How does one choose a model? How does one find oneself acting like somebody else against one's own expectations? The answer is that determinants of choice are principally unconscious, as Miller and Dollard [15] have pointed out in their studies of social learning.

One other instance of identification with another person which may color one's subsequent personality appears in the study of bereaved persons. Following the loss of another person with whom one has interacted at a high level of intensity, a number of people find themselves acting like the person who has died. In such instances, there seems to be a forced or involuntary and unconscious psychological incorporation of the image of the deceased, with the result that sudden, unexplained personality changes occur in such individuals requiring psychiatric treatment.

Copying the ways which other people have developed to manage their emotional growth is thus one important resource for emotional growth, however hazardous it may be. Another aspect of social learning concerns the differentiation of role behavior and the development of flexibility with regard to role taking. There are some people who, at any cost, have to maneuver themselves into situations where they are the unquestioned boss or know more than anybody else. There are other individuals who have had little opportunity in the growing period to practice what is so valued in our culture — what we might call "constructive" or "cooperative" competition, or as someone lately has said, "antagonistic cooperation." A person who misses the experience of getting along with another, even though he may be a rival or has "beaten him up," or the challenge of getting along with a group even though he has to be an inferior member for a while, is likely later to find himself handicapped in occupational situations which require subordination. There are different kinds of social skills required in different roles: the initiation rate, for example, is decidedly different. Certain personality types have quite characteristic ways of dealing with different dimensions in the social system; other personality types may be impoverished or rigid in that they operate well only at one spot in the social system. For example, there is the typical clinical picture of "promotion depression" which befalls people who, once they get to the top, do not know how to behave. They have nobody to criticize them any more, and it may be discovered that they feel utterly lonely because the relationship to a person at a higher level of the social hierarchy, to the boss or authority, or as the analysts would say, to a father-surrogate, is necessary in order for them to have secure control of their emotional expression. In this way also, then, personalities may be rich or impoverished.

Another dimension of personality which it might be useful to consider is that of the "system of defenses." For instance, there is the type of person who has acquired a great number of the ingredients which are highly suitable for the mature personality, but has overdone it a little: the obsessive-compulsive person. With excessive perfectionism and cumbersome interest in details, such a person often finds it hard to make up his mind what course of action to take. He can be very useful at certain levels of research, in fact-gathering, or in ordering of facts, but difficulties may arise if that person is promoted or is put in a position where he has to make decisions. In other words, certain kinds of personality organization are reflected in certain traits which are suitable for certain places but highly unsuitable for other places in the social system, especially if the traits border on psychoneurosis.

Another personality type, the hysterical, is represented by the individual who has marked "blind spots," one who has used to excess the device of "repression" in his growing up, making it possible for him not to have undesirable emotions at inconvenient moments. Mastery of emotional control has been replaced by over-strenuous repression, a forceful putting of these things out of one's mind. Such individuals do not mind "stepping where angels fear to tread." They can step into many difficult situations with conscious ease because the emotional implications do not bother them, but at certain times they may quite suddenly and apparently inexplicably break down with symptoms, representing a breakthrough of repressed but unsolved conflicts and emotions.

In both the instances cited, the individuals concerned have unconsciously "preferred" a specific kind of defense against their emotions and against the impact of the educative process. This defense may be quite suitable and convenient at a given time, but may at other times be a handicap. In the obsessive-compulsive person the defense of reaction formation against any sort of sloppiness and perhaps dirtiness has been carried too far; in the hysterical person, the defense of repression in the face of powerful temptation or stimulation may block the normal reactions when they should occur. The system of defense which a person has devised in his process of development offers, then, another approach to the description of his personality.

The application to growth and development of this way of thinking could be summarized in this way. Many students of personality believe that past experiences, including early childhood experiences, are significant though not exclusive determinants of later personality in terms of what they like to call "adjustment." Adjustment in this sense means balancing the outer pressures with the satisfaction of one's desires; protection from unpleasant emotions is required on the one hand, balanced against the environmental demands on the other hand. In the psychoanalytic view, the adjustments habitually made, in terms of a compromise between the two forces, describe an essential aspect of a person. The kind of defenses he has utilized, the way of operating in life situations which he has designed, are referred to as part of his "ego." The ego checks what is going on outside, and has a system of devices available either to handle situations or, if necessary, to avoid getting into them. The mature person thus makes adjustments in terms of an arsenal of adjustment tools which are collectively called the ego, supplemented by the conscience or superego, and he has a reasonable awareness of and control over his id, or those forces which he has to accept as his emotional self.

People of course differ emotionally; their needs for social interaction vary both quantitatively and qualitatively. It is important that individuals have some insight about themselves, and know pretty well the measure of their emotional needs. If a person knows this about himself, we think that a good deal of his id is known to his ego, and this is important for maturity. Psychoanalytic work reveals many people who, extremely unacquainted with their own emotional needs, often and even repetitively put themselves into situations where they do not quite fit and where they are frustrated; the balance of frustration versus satisfaction becomes heavy on the side of frustration, and the individual is chronically dissatisfied. Unfortunately many people, even in our privileged society, do not have this sort of self-knowledge.

Dynamic psychology thus distinguishes mature persons from immature persons, and identifies a variety of impairments of maturity. It appears reasonably certain that the sequence and constellation of early experiences determine largely the path along which the basic modes of one's defense system are developed. These defenses are assumed to have developed by the time the child enters school; fortunately, however, they appear to be open to later modifications. More detailed knowledge in this field will be a prerequisite for the further development of the application of a preventive approach to mental health.

THE ORIGINS OF BEHAVIOR IN THE NEWBORN INFANT
DANE G. PRUGH

The Influence of Heredity

If one searches for the origins of behavior one logically reaches backward in time beyond the point of birth, since the newborn infant already possesses inherent though rudimentary equipment with which to meet the challenge of his environment. Much research has been devoted to the question of the influence upon emotional and personality development of inherited or genetic factors. At the present time, however, the sum total of exact knowledge in this area is extremely small.

Like all living organisms the human infant possesses at birth certain biologically determined characteristics — the manifestation of spontaneous activity which is apparent in growth, development, and various physiologic processes; the capacity, within limits, to become able to adapt to his environment and to obtain from his environment the basic elements necessary for survival; and the ultimate capacity to reproduce his species. However, all of these basically biological attributes can be influenced in various ways by environmental stimuli. In common with others of his species, the human infant is equipped with a central nervous system which, in contrast with all other species, is capable of developing great complexity of response and adaptation, including the use of abstract and symbolic reasoning and communication processes. Because of the wide developmental span between young and adult forms, human young have much greater possibility of responding to environmental influence, and of the acquisition of learned behavior, than is the case in the lower animals, in which biologically determined, unlearned patterns or instincts predominate in behavior. With the greater plasticity in the behavior of the young, however, comes greater need for care and education by some form of family unit. It calls for a longer period of dependence upon such care-taking figures than is the case with lower species. There is also, at the same time, greater vulnerability to distortion of personality development as the result of exceedingly complex social and emotional stimuli. Recently, Bowlby[16] drawing upon the studies of ethologists such as Lorenz,[17] has suggested that the human infant may possess certain inborn patterns of response, such as those appearing later in the face of separation from the mother.

In addition to these broader characteristics, the human infant possesses certain inherited potentialities for growth and development which are more specifically determined by his individual family and ancestral background. Anthropological research has long since determined the essential similarity of inherited potentialities, other than those related to physical appearance, among members of different races. It remains an unsettled question as to whether children are born with potentialities for particular types of personality development. Recent research involving identical twins would support the possibility that, within very broad limits, some such potentiality does exist. Susceptibilities to certain types of mental illness are known to occur more strikingly in certain families than in others, as indicated by the work of Kallman[18] and others. Differences in basic intellectual capacity and in certain talents, such as for musical creativity, certainly are influenced by genetic factors, as are particular physical attributes and a few diseases. There is also some evidence, from a variety of sources, that differences in motor capacities or "congenital activity types" are present in human infants from birth, ranging from very active to relatively inactive characteristics of motor behavior.[19] Recent psychosomatic research, dealing with monozygotic and dizygotic twins, suggests further that differences in the potential degree and nature of physiologic activity, particularly the functioning of the autonomic or involuntarily innervated portions of the central nervous system may have a large portion of their roots in inherited sources.[20]

Most of these inherited potentialities appear to be susceptible to environmental influence. Indeed, appropriately positive stimuli from the environment are as necessary for the full development of intelligence in a potentially outstanding intellect as are noxious stimuli for the development of mental illness in a strongly susceptible child. Thus the above material is not presented as a case for the inherited basis of human behavior. Some statement of these few available facts seems indicated, however, in order to achieve a balance between the extremes of point of view which have been entertained by workers in the children's field over a number of years.

Before the rise of modern science and current scientific methods of study, even professional people in Western society were inclined, with some notable exceptions, to lean heavily upon heredity as an explanation for deviant behavior as well as for healthy emotional or personality development. With the increasing results of psychological and, particularly, psychoanalytic investigation in the area of child development during the past 50 years, however, a swing in the pendulum of opinion has occurred, finding its extreme expression in the views of Watson[21] in the 1930's that environment and education could produce any desired result in any child. The success of Western scientific method and industrialization in altering the physical environment may have contributed to the seductiveness of the view that heredity had very little if anything to do with later development. Although the "nature vs nurture" controversy has abated considerably, many workers in the fields of psychiatry, psychology, and social work still tend to disregard or at least to regard lightly the influence of biologic factors in child behavior, feeling that the newborn infant represents a veritable "tabula rasa" and consequently arriving at times at unrealistic child-rearing or treatment goals and overly narrow theoretical concepts of the casuality of disturbances in behavior.

Instincts and Emotions

It was mentioned earlier that instinctive or unlearned behavior predominated in lower animals. The human infant at birth is also equipped with potential patterns of unlearned behavior. The use of the term *instinct* to describe this behavior as well as other aspects of human functioning has led to much confusion and even controversy among varying schools of psychological and psychoanalytic thought. In this area, as in many others, more than one point of view has some validity. Perhaps the broadest and most inclusive definition is that of Engel [22] who regards "an instinct as an internal force which acts as an impctus to some action involving the external world." This concept transcends the classification of instincts as bits of unlearned behavior, such as the nest-building patterns of birds or the core of specific sexual behavior in the human being. In such behavior, a number of reflex patterns, the simplest form of organismal response to stimuli, are of course involved.

Instincts thus can range from such relatively simple phenomena as the need to find water to satisfy thirst, to the complicated needs involved in sexual satisfaction in adults. The energy for such instinctual forces or "drives" comes from within the organism, with a predominantly physiologic source. The expression of instinctual drives in human beings, however, can be delayed or diverted by the action of the central nervous system in the service of adaptation, in contrast to the lower animals, and much learned behavior may be involved in this process of "long-circuiting" an immediately perceived need of this nature.

From a psychological point of view, the principal instinctual drives which are perceived by the developing child, and which are accompanied by an intrapsychic or subjective emotion, are the *sexual* and the *aggressive*. As Freud[23] pointed out, the sexual drives include others related to the goal of reproduction of the species, while aggressive drives relate broadly to self-preservation and the mastery of the environment, often with competitive connotations. The emotion or affect most intimately experienced in relation to the sexual drive is that of love, the polarizing force for later marriage and sexual union; that most closely bound up with the aggressive drive is the emotion of anger, hostility, or hate, ordinarily aroused when drives toward mastery or competition are frustrated, as they frequently must be. Appropriate control of the emotions associated with these drives is, of course, demanded of every child in human society, although the particular form of control and of behavioral expression of these emotions may vary from culture to culture. Obviously, some successful fusion of these two opposite emotions is necessary also, as for example, in the somewhat aggressive competition with others of the same sex, commonly exhibited by the adolescent or adult to win the affections of a potential mate. To some extent there is a potential ambivalence or two-sided quality to every human relationship, as in the situation when a child feels angry at a loved parent because of jealousy of attentions shown a sibling.

Just as the body exhibits a kind of automatic internal regulation of processes and needs, called "homeostasis" by Cannon,[24] so the developing child must utilize his potential mental apparatus to regulate and delay, or long-circuit, his emotional fluctuations in order to achieve a balanced but steadily expanding adaptation to and mastery of his environment. Obvious parallels as well as interrelations between physiological and emotional regulation exist, and these will be described later in relation to differing stages of development.

No attempt will be made here to classify the emotions beyond the polarities of love and hate, with all the constellatory emotions, such as admiration and tenderness or anger and hostility, which may be grouped around each pole. Perhaps a better metaphor would be that of a continuum, with gradations of positive and negative emotions distributed between the two ends of the continuum. Each subjective emotional state can be conscious or unconscious, carrying with it in either case the physiologic concomitants and the behavioral expression mentioned earlier. Biological or developmental phenomena may influence emotions as the result of fluctuations of instinctual drives in addition to environmental stimuli. Examples of the former are the increased sexual drives during puberty.

Prenatal Influences

During the prenatal or intrauterine period, the fetus undergoes sweeping maturational changes in a relatively short time. Any damage to the fetus resulting from disease or poor nutritional state of the mother or abnormalities in embryonic development, or other such causes, can of course produce later effects upon the child's adaptive capacity. Such effects may operate as limitations in intellectual powers, defects in motor behavior, or abnormalities in physical appearance, all of which pose a challenge in adaptation for both the child and his parents.

Although the influences of physical factors upon the growth and development of the fetus are becoming increasingly clear as the result of the work of Warkany,[25] Ingalls,[26] and others, any possible influences of this physical phase upon the infant's future emotional development are much less fully understood. In Chapter III, the psychological implications of pregnancy for the mother in relation to her unborn fetus were discussed and it appears clear that the emotional climate of the family is the most significant factor at the time of delivery. There remains the recently recognized possibility, however, that the intrauterine existence and functioning of the fetus may be affected by the passage across the placental barrier of certain hormonal substances. Recent research has suggested the likelihood that the outpouring of such hormones may be affected by the mother's emotional state. The empirical observation has been made[27] that severe anxiety states or extreme fatigue in the mother during the last trimester of pregnancy have been associated with increased and prolonged muscular activity of the infant *in utero*. Other observed changes in the later activity of the newborn infant's gastrointestinal system and the state of fat-storage at the time of birth are less clearly the result of this type of influence. There does seem to be a rough correlation, however, between the degree of motor activity of the fetus *in utero* and that demonstrated following birth. Certain experiments[27] have indicated the possibility of conditioning the fetal heart rate and startle reaction by means of external vibrators placed on the mother's abdominal wall. The exact mechanisms by which a mother's disturbed emotional state might produce alterations in her neurohormonal balance, with consequent physiologic stimulation of the fetus and thus possible predisposition to states of tension following birth, have not been fully elucidated as yet because of various methodological and other difficulties.

At the present time the extent of our knowledge in this area is minimal. Future longitudinal research may lead to enhanced theoretical understanding of possible predisposition to anxiety or tension, and perhaps to preventive implications. For the present it remains essential for clinical workers to concentrate upon understanding the reaction of the mother to the meaning of pregnancy and its management, her perception of the reaction to her pregnancy by her husband and family (and by society, if the pregnancy should be unsanctioned), as well as the consequent effects, for better or for worse, of such factors upon herself and her husband in their approach to the rearing of this particular child.

The Birth Experience

With the advent of birth the physiologic aspects of the parasitic existence of the fetus come to an end. It is obvious, however, that in an emotional sense a parasitic relationship of the infant to the mother continues to some extent beyond this point. The human infant is helpless at birth, equipped only with a few reflex patterns, such as crying capacities, "rooting" and sucking reflexes, and startle responses. It has long been known that the birth experience can influence the capacity of the infant to exercise even these rudimentary abilities. No attempt will be made here to summarize the possible influence of birth traumata, including cerebral hemorrhage, anoxia resulting from respiratory difficulties, or the effects of obstetrical anesthetic or analgesic agents, upon the infant's immediate or later functioning and adaptive capacities. Suffice it to say that, from the moment of birth, even in relatively healthy infants there appear to be differences in the rapidity of crying, in the strength of sucking reflexes, in activity patterns, and other modalities of function. In spite of certain claims there is no clear indication that mild brain damage necessarily predisposes in and of itself to the development of serious disturbances in behavior.

Much has been written by certain psychologists and psychiatrists, particularly Rank,[28] about the psychological aspects of the birth trauma. At the present time there is no available evidence to indicate that the impact of birth — the sudden transition from a relatively quiet intrauterine existence to an uncertain state in a world full of new stimuli — is responsible for lasting emotional imprints. The fact that the newborn infant operates largely at a subcortical level of behavior would alone indicate the unlikelihood of such a subjective response. As Greene[29] has suggested, it is possible that the intrauterine world may not be such a quiet one, in view of the varying stimuli, from spontaneous uterine contractions, respiratory and vascular rhythms, which may impinge upon the fetus. It is conceivable, however, as certain workers[30] have pointed out, that the length or degree of difficulty of the birth process might exert an effect upon the infant which could result in the sensitization of an embarrassed respiratory or cardiovascular apparatus to later stimuli of varying nature, including emotional ones, with possible influences upon later symptomatic pictures. No incontrovertible evidence of this sort exists at the present moment, however. Perhaps the most one can say, as Freud did,[23] is that the birth experience and the first cry may represent the physiological prototype of later anxiety attacks, setting the pattern for such a response, but exerting no perceptible causal effect.

In summary, heredity, instinctual capacities, prenatal influences, and the birth experiences all may contribute, in varying measures, to the nature and the degree of intactness of the biological equipment which the infant carries with him at the time of his entry into the extrauterine world. The interaction of this equipment, as it unfolds during the process of development, with environmental influences and opportunities appears to be more important than the equipment itself, within broad limits, in determining the ultimate success or failure of adaptation and the attainment of maturity.

THE ROOTS OF HUMAN RELATIONSHIPS:
MOTHER AND INFANT
GERALD CAPLAN

One of our most significant new insights during the past few years has been the importance we have come to ascribe to the emotional milieu as a critical factor in the child's total development. The quality of the interpersonal relationships in the family circle not only has a potent effect in molding the child's emotional unfolding, but it also exerts an influence on his capacity to make use of his intellectual endowment, as well as on his general physical growth and development.

During the first year of life the family's effect on the child is ordinarily conveyed via the mother. Her relationship with the infant is his key to the social world. She is the first "other" in his awareness, through whom he makes the first steps in developing a recognition of his own self-identity, the basis for all subsequent personality development. The emotional atmosphere and the day to day happenings in the family circle affect the mother's relationship with her infant, with these indirect influences representing at first his principal contact with other family members. Towards the end of the first year the child begins to develop significant relationships not only with his mother, but also with his father, and during the second year with the siblings and with other family members. To begin with, these new links are patterned by him in accordance with his primary bond with his mother, and it is not probably till later that other people are perceived and dealt with in their own right.

In thinking about mother-infant interactions, it is important to realize that these take place in a relationship between two people, even though in early infancy one of the people manifests little active, recognizable personality. Nevertheless, the baby has some individuality at this stage, which is expressed in his physical shape and appearance, and in the sensitivity of his reactions to stimuli, as well as in his general pattern of responses as regards activity and passivity. Although these phenomena are not consciously intended by the baby as communications, they are nevertheless perceived by the mother and reacted to almost as though they were. Her own behavior to the baby is modified by them, and her behavior in turn affects the baby's reactions.

The interchange at this stage between mother and infant must, therefore, be conceived of as a circular system, which is in constant dynamic flux. It is in effect a reverberating circular system, and we must take care that in calling it a "mother-child relationship" we are not misled into conceiving of it as a unidirectional static factor which is not being constantly influenced by the actual happenings taking place between mother and child, and child and mother.

It is also important to realize that although there is some over-all stability of the patterning of this relationship, a stability which is dependent on the mother's more or less unchanging personality, the child who is the other element of the equation is in a state of continuous change, especially marked in his earliest years. A basic theme of this book is that a child is not a little adult, but that he passes through successive phases of development which are qualitatively different from the adult state. This means that over a time continuum the mother-child relationship must be expected to show parallel successive changes in its pattern. In practice this is found to be true. A mother who may feel happy and relaxed in her relationship with her child at one stage of his development, may experience tension and difficulties at a successive stage. This may occur for a variety of reasons, which may include not only her involvement with other problems in her emotional milieu at that time, but also the revival inside her of unsolved problems from her childhood and her interactions with her own mother, stimulated by her day to day contact with the manifestations of the same phase of development in her child. Thus a mother may feel quite secure in handling her baby's feeding problems; but when she begins to deal with toilet-training this may stimulate and revive unconscious and unresolved difficulties from her childhood battles with her own mother. Her upset may then interfere with her management of her child. On the other hand, just as in pregnancy, when old problems are revived, new and better solutions become possible, and this explains the personality maturation which often takes place as a result of the life experience of motherhood. Such maturation often occurs spontaneously, but nurses and physicians may well accept a responsibility for encouraging it by the specific support they give to the mother as she wrestles with her problems.

In our efforts to help mothers solve their problems with their children we need to have some practical clinical yardstick with which to assess the state of the mother-child relationship at any time. This will help us to decide when to intervene and in what degree, or when to adopt a policy of watchful inactivity while the mother makes her own attempts at solution. The important thing to realize is that we must assess the relationship on the basis of our observations of what is going on currently between the mother and child, and not wait for unfortunate results in the child's development. Such results may take months or years to appear, and when they do it will probably be too late for simple remedies.

Since the mother-child relationship has been conceived of here as a circular reverberating system of forces altering dynamically over a time continuum, and influenced constantly by developmental changes in the child as well as by changes in the emotional milieu of the family and in the social environment, it is difficult to think of a way of crystallizing it at any moment so that it can be rated as healthy or unhealthy, i.e., promotive of mental health in the child or hindering it. Yet experience in well-baby centers with mothers and infants who manifest healthy relationships, as well as clinical experience in child guidance clinics with mothers who have disturbed relationships with their children, has in the last few years provided us with a working definition of a healthy, as compared with a potentially pathogenic, mother-child relationship, which can be used as a rough guide by nurses and physicians.

A healthy mother-child relationship can be defined as one in which the mother reacts to the child *primarily* on the basis of her perception of the child's needs as a person in his own right, her respect for those needs, and an attempt to satisfy them to the best of her ability, in line with the accepted practices of her culture and society. This is contrasted with an *unhealthy* or *potentially pathogenic* relationship, in which the mother perceives and reacts to her child *primarily on the basis of her own needs* and attempts to satisfy these, by means of her behavior, through the child. He is not perceived by her as a person in his own right, and even if he is so perceived his needs are not respected.

Clearly this definition is not independent of cultural factors, since the perception of a child as a person in his own right, whose needs are worthy of respect, may not fit into the role pattern and value system of certain societies. Nevertheless, such a definition does appear to hold for our western culture at the present day.

Stress must also be laid on the word *primarily* in these definitions. A healthy mother-child relationship involves reciprocal gratification of mother and child, and the mother certainly satisfies her own needs to be motherly, protecting, nurturing, and comforting when she relates to her baby. The goal of these needs, however, is the baby's welfare, and the mother's gratification is consequent upon the satisfaction of the baby's wishes. This is to be contrasted with an unhealthy relationship, where the mother uses the child for gratification of such nonmotherly needs as personal ambition, need to be loved and the solution of problems of marital disharmony. The mother who comforts her son when she perceives that *he* feels lonely and forlorn derives motherly satisfaction from helping the child. She is to be contrasted with the woman who, herself feeling lonely and forlorn at the time, comforts *herself* by hugging and fondling her child without regard to whether he feels the same way, or whether in fact she is interrupting some satisfying game in which he is at the moment absorbed.

It is important to note that the definition of a healthy mother-child relationship, which is based on the mother's perception of the child as an individual in his own right, implies the gradual psychological separation of the child from the mother. During the past few years we have been very much impressed by the evidence adduced by Bowlby[31] and others regarding the harmful effects of prolonged geographical separation of mother and child, without an adequate mother-substitute, during the first few years of life. Such extreme deprivation of maternal care interferes significantly with the personality development of the child. It is therefore a little difficult to realize that a certain degree of psychological separation of mother and child is essential to healthy development. This point has been recently very well made by Allen.[32]

In this connection it is well to remember that although physical separation of mother and child occurs when the umbilical cord is cut after birth, in some cases psychological separation does not spontaneously occur at the same time. In the section on the emotional implications of pregnancy, it was pointed out that many women develop, with varying intensity, emotional relationships to the fetus or to the fantasied babies which may be equally parts of themselves. The baby after birth experiences the carryover of these relationships. In these cases, the earliest stages of the mother-child relationship appear to be in large part narcissistic and symbiotic, i.e., the mother is relating to the child symbolically as part of herself. She identifies the baby with herself and she identifies herself with the baby. This means that she is very sensitive to the expressions of the baby's needs, which she experiences, as it were, subjectively rather than by objective perception. This is especially noticeable in the breast feeding situation, which, if all goes well, gives the impression of a symbiotic unity rather than of interaction between two separate people. Middlemore[33] has used the term "the nursing couple" in order to stress this point.

This attitude of the mother towards the child as a psychological extension of herself during the early weeks or months of his life is mirrored by the lack of differentiation of a feeling of self in the child at that stage. As such differentiation begins to take place, however, it is essential that the mother's attitude should change. If she continues to relate towards the child as an extension of herself, the child on his part will have difficulty in developing the concept of his own identity, and this may well lead to fundamental disorders in his personality makeup.

Much research is still needed in order to chart the time relations of this basic development in mother-child relationships, from the symbiotic pattern of mother-child unity to that of two separate individuals. The latter is the so-called "anaclitic" pattern, named from the Greek words meaning "leaning against." The idea expressed here is that the child leans against the mother for help and protection, rather than being inextricably intertwined with her. Spitz[34] has recently suggested that if we are considering the relationship from the point of view of the mother we should call it "diatrophic," meaning "supportive," rather than anaclitic, to make clear that the mother is presenting herself for the child to "lean against" rather than the other way round. It is likely that there is a fairly wide range of individual variation in the rate of this changeover from symbiotic to supportive relationships. It is usually not a sudden change, and some symbiotic features may persist into the second year, and in certain cultures much later. In most normal cases, however, the change appears to start about 3 months after birth and to be reasonably complete before the end of the first year. There is evidence that cultural factors, particularly the educational efforts of such caretaking agents as doctors and nurses, may exert an important effect on this process. Much of the parent-education in well-baby clinics may be conceived of as an attempt to help the mother to "get to know" her baby, i.e., to separate herself from him so that she observes his behavior from a distance with some objectivity, in order to realize his individuality and therefore perceive his needs. It may be as well to emphasize that this process is not accomplished by giving the mother intellectual information about babies in general, although this is undoubtedly of value in other connections, but by the nurse or doctor reporting personal observations of *this* baby and affording the mother the opportunity of identifying with this procedure. The doctor, as it were, lends his eyes and ears to the mother during the consultation, so that by identifying with him she can step back and look at her baby as a separate individual.

Such assistance in promoting an optimal degree of mother-child separation has to be based on the needs of each individual case. In most instances it will not be especially needed, although it is not likely to do any harm. In certain cases the doctor will already have been warned during pregnancy, by an especially strong relationship between the expectant mother and her fetus, that she will very likely have a strongly marked symbiotic relationship to her baby. If his observations during the early months after birth confirm this, and if the pattern shows no signs of altering spontaneously as the months pass, he will be well advised to focus his efforts in his well-baby care upon encouraging separation.

It should be mentioned that a significant proportion of mothers do not appear to pass through the stage of a symbiotic relationship to their babies, and the first relationship they develop after the baby's birth is already diatrophic or supportive. These are the mothers who during pregnancy had little or no feeling towards the fetus, and after birth often have a fairly long lag before developing maternal feeling. To these mothers their babies are "little strangers" at birth, and they have to "get to know" them before developing a relationship. Such women often have difficulty in understanding their babies' needs in the early stages, and especially with their first babies they consequently have more than usual difficulty in breast-feeding and other early nursing procedures.

The task of the nurses and doctors in such cases is to reduce the psychological distance between mother and child in the first few weeks, rather than to aim at future psychological separation. Here again the caretaking agent may act as a model, or may encourage contact with a grandmother or friend with well-developed maternal attitudes, with whom the young mother may identify. Much more active support is needed by such mothers in the early weeks, and more advice and direction in regard to details of nursing care, than in the case of mothers with symbiotic relationships. On the other hand, once these mothers have been helped to relate to their babies in a warm way, they usually have little trouble subsequently in allowing them to develop towards self-differentiation because they do not have to change from a symbiotic to a supportive pattern. It may also be as well to emphasize that although a closer relationship to the child should be actively but subtly encouraged, these mothers should not be rushed, especially if, as described below, they show signs of special fears of small babies. The goal should be the development of a warm relationship by 3 to 5 months, but in cases with special difficulty a few months longer can safely be allowed. If no progress is made during this time the possibility of deeper trouble should be suspected, and referral to a psychiatrist for preventive intervention considered.

In supervising the mother-child relationship, as in other aspects of well-child care, the rhythm of development of the individual case is a prime diagnostic consideration. This is why it is so important to try to arrange for continuity of care from pregnancy on, and if possible from one child to the next.

We have so far considered factors influencing the mother-child relationship which originate primarily in the mother, and we must now turn to a consideration of some which originate in the child. The first year of life can be somewhat arbitrarily divided into three periods, in relation to psychological developmental processes in the infant, which exert a major influence on the mother-child relationship.

The first period is from birth to 2 to 3 months. The second stretches from then till 7 to 8 months. The third occupies the rest of the first year. Naturally, this timetable is very rough and there are individual variations from one baby to the next.

The first period is characterized by the relative lack of manifest "personality" as compared with older infants. During it the infant is a relatively helpless bundle of instincts, with little voluntary control over its physiological or psychological processes and probably no real awareness of its environment, and no power of communication, although of course it does have means of expression. It is mostly dependent upon its mother for the maintenance of life, and although her efforts in this connection bring obvious results, the baby can give no verbal thanks to the mother for these efforts.

Many mothers, especially those who experience a well-marked maternal feeling, are positively stimulated by the helpless condition of the baby in this stage. It evokes in them the full flow of their protective, comforting, nurturant feelings, and they derive satisfaction from the gratification of the baby's needs by their identification with the baby. They do not need special interpersonal communication from the baby any more than they need conscious messages from their own limbs or bodily organs.

A few mothers, however, are quite frightened by the baby at this stage, primarily because they see in it an example of primitive instinctuality which is uncontrolled. If they have problems in regard to their capacity to control their own instinctual impulses, close contact with this situation is likely to stimulate deep fears. These usually show themselves in one of two ways. Either the mother reacts irrationally to the baby, as though he were a dangerous object who would do her some harm — as though he were full of uncontrollable hostility — or she feels the uncontrollable hostility inside herself, and fears to go near the baby lest she take advantage of his helplessness and harm him. In extreme cases the mother may actually do harm to the baby, but such cases are rare. More common are those instances in which this mechanism is present to the extent that it obtrudes between mother and child, and prevents or delays the building up of a relationship between them till after this stage has passed. The doctor who has taken care of these mothers during pregnancy will probably already have been warned to expect such a situation, because they will either have voiced explicit fears of small babies, or will have talked about fantasies of their babies-to-be in terms which have pointedly excluded infants under 3 or 4 months.

The management of this type of situation should focus upon reassurance regarding the harmlessness of close contact between mother and child, but there is no point in pushing the child into the mother's arms faster than she can bear it. Apart from the fact that such an approach would be ineffective and would very likely make her more frightened, we know that the stimuli coming from the child will change within a few months and the pattern is likely then to alter spontaneously.

Another source of difficulty during this first stage is caused by the infant's lack of a capacity to communicate. This worries most mothers, as evidenced by the universal joy on the occasion of the infant's first smile. The developmental importance of this is instinctively understood by most mothers. The very young infant manifests gratification only passively, e.g. through his appearance of flushed and relaxed contentment after a successful feeding. He is at peace with himself and isolated from the world, a picture contrasting pleasantly with his state of half an hour previously, when he was screaming with hunger. With his first smile to his mother, however, he seems to emerge from himself and actively enter the world. He seems to be telling his mother that he appreciates what she has done for him, and that he is thankful to her personally. The former relaxed content was merely a *sign* of the baby's satisfaction; the smile to the mother is a *communication*. It symbolizes that the baby has become capable of appreciating the source of his gratification, and that he acknowledges his thankfulness to his mother. It is this message of appreciation which the mother so eagerly awaits.

Although the majority of mothers give evidence of dissatisfaction that their babies cannot respond to them in the early stages, they are able to put up with this, often compensating by imaginary happy conversations with the baby. Some mothers, however, especially those who are young and inexperienced and have feelings of unworthiness or self-depreciation, cannot comfort themselves in this way. If they were to have imaginary conversations, their babies would be accusing them of not doing enough for them. They pass through agonies of doubt as to their capacities for motherhood, they suspect that their milk is too weak or is insufficient in quantity, they are afraid of their clumsiness in handling the baby, etc. Moreover, they feel that they are constantly called upon to give, give, give. They must dance attendance on the baby for 24 hours a day and 7 days a week. And they see no return. They get no thanks, no reassurance from the baby that they are doing the right thing. True, every now and again they can get an approving word from the doctor, or they can weigh the baby and gain reassurance from the weight chart. They are in need of more frequent and immediate communications, however, and they are especially in need of the emotional supplies which the baby will later inject into the circular system of the relationship, once he starts actively to communicate.

Physicians and nurses can be especially helpful to such mothers during this preliminary phase by continual and unstinting support and reassurance, by helping them learn the behavioral cues in the baby which can be used instead of communication to determine that all is progressing well, and by mobilizing the sources of love and affection for the mother in her circle of family and friends. Pediatricians are sometimes rather worried by the burden of satisfying the apparently insatiable dependent needs of such mothers at this time. They may feel that a mother should be helped to stand on her own feet as soon as possible, and with the constant demands of a busy practice it is hard to keep constantly at the telephone answering the apparently childish questions of an overanxious young mother. The experienced pediatrician will, however, realize that patiently satisfying the mother's needs at this time of crisis will have a far-reaching effect in increasing her self-esteem, so that when the baby does begin to communicate with her she will already have gained the confidence in her own worth which will promote a positive basis for the developing relationship. Just as a baby with a constitutionally intense need to suck, who has this need fully satisfied in the early months, may be expected to get over this period without difficulty, but if he is not satisfied may remain a thumbsucker till late childhood, so these mothers, if their heightened needs are respected and satisfied in the first 3 months, will later develop spontaneously an increased independence and maturity in their motherhood.

In our consideration of the patterns of mother-child relationship of the first year we now come to the smoothest and happiest phase, namely, from about 3 months to about 7 months. This is the phase of the "perfect baby." He begins to develop an obvious "personality" and shows signs of recognition of, and love for, his mother. He has usually adapted to extrauterine life and to the feeding situation. His development is exciting and rapid, and very obvious, yet it does not involve him in creating a "nuisance." He lies happily in his crib, most of his waking hours, fascinated by his play with such simple things as his fingers and toes, or the sights around him. He begins to babble and vocalize and play with sounds in a way which delights the heart of any mother. In fact, he fits easily into most mothers' stereotype of the ideal, trouble-free baby. Although he is still dependent on his mother, she sees that he is rapidly developing control over his functioning, and his demands on her are not continuous and insistent, so that she can get a rest from her mothering duties whenever she so desires.

Difficulties are common during this period in the baby's sleeping habits. Mothers may need pediatric help in regulating the baby's rhythm, so that he sleeps at night and is awake during the day. This regulation may occasionally be interfered with in unapparent ways, as for example by sexual problems between the parents, when worry about the wakefulness of the baby may be used vicariously by a mother to avoid working through the difficulties with her husband which would otherwise emerge at night. Such a situation is a sample of the main difficulties which occur during this period. The mother may have no serious complaints about the child — quite the contrary — but since his own needs are at this time not obtrusive, there is the possibility that he may be woven more easily into a vicarious solution of some nonmaternal problem of his mother. The results of this process in distorting the mother-child relationship may not be obvious till later.

On the whole, however, this period is one which is conducive to the laying down of a confident, relaxed type of reciprocal relationship in which neither party is making undue demands, and in which both can experience and express their gratification and thus produce a benign reverberation.

The only real danger of this phase is associated with this very gratification. If the mother for some personality reason, or because of emotional deprivation in other current relationships, cannot handle the frustrations of the succeeding stages, she may become fixated at this second phase, and may either try to prevent the child moving out of the "perfect baby" state or may react with excessive disappointment and feelings of rejection when he starts growing away from her at the end of the first year.

The latter process is the main characteristic of the third phase of the first year. During it, many signs appear, indicating that the baby is developing a "will of his own," and this may not be entirely in line with his mother's wishes. His capacity for aggressive expression begins to develop. Pleasant sucking at the breast comes to an end and teeth appear. Neuromuscular development allows him to stand on his own, and usually by the end of the year he takes his first steps. These are greeted by most mothers with delight, but they soon realize that these are the first steps the baby is taking away from them. Similarly, the baby's beginning control over defecation and, later, urination, are signs of growing independence, leading, however, to the inevitable conflicts of socialization. The mother is overjoyed when her baby develops the capacity for verbal communication, but the word "no" appears fairly early in the second year!

The third phase of the first year is therefore a period of transition between the dependent "trouble-free" infant and the young toddler, who is still dependent, but showing already the signs of his future independence. This is the stage when the stimuli from the child increase the pressure towards the diatrophic or supportive and away from the symbiotic type of relationship; at this time, the mother first really faces the necessity of striking an appropriate balance between control and gratification of the child's impulses, as well as satisfaction of his dependent needs and provision of freedom for independent expression. These are essential parts of the task of parenthood.

At this stage, too, the child begins to build up relationships with others besides his mother, and if she has in the past been unable to come to terms with rivalry situations she may have difficulty in accepting this. The good-humored arguments as to whether baby learns to say "mama" before "dada" may symbolize deeper jealousies. This is the time when maternal overpossessiveness may first be seen, and, if recognized, it may be most appropriately dealt with by the educational efforts of pediatricians and nurses.

The details of later development will be considered in the next chapter. In succeeding stages, the child's increasing activity, his curiosity, the development of expression of his aggressive impulses, the nagging quality of his expressions of love, his interests in his excretory functions and products, and the other manifestations of his growth and development, all feed their messages into the developing relationship between him and his mother. They have their effect on the pattern of that relationship mainly through the meaning they gain for the mother by virtue of her personality, of her cultural values, her current satisfactions, and of her past experiences, particularly at the corresponding phases of her own childhood.

VII

PERSONALITY DEVELOPMENT
THROUGHOUT CHILDHOOD

INTRODUCTION

The terms "psychological development," "emotional development," and "personality development" are employed somewhat loosely throughout the literature dealing with the studies of various professional workers in this general area. The concept of personality refers to all aspects of the functioning behavior of a human being — his intellectual capacities, physical attributes, and patterns of social behavior, as well as his inner mental and emotional experiences and his awareness of himself as an individual. Physical patterns of development are dealt with in Chapter IV. Social behavior and development in the setting of family and community is considered broadly in Chapter VIII, while Chapter IX devotes itself more directly to the description of intellectual development as influenced by formal education.

Of the four major areas of personality development, intellectual, physical, emotional, and social, all but emotional are considered separately. Emotional development cannot be considered in a vacuum, however, and in this chapter other aspects of over-all personality development will be sketched in concurrently with the discussion of emotions and their motivating influence upon behavior. To some extent personality development continues, or should continue, throughout the life of the individual. Unlike the physical components of the organism, personality attributes need not degenerate seriously with advancing age. The childhood foundation upon which an individual's personality structure is erected is generally accepted today as the major, although not the single determinant, of the nature and degree of his mental and emotional health in later life.

INFANCY
DANE G. PRUGH

THE FIRST THREE MONTHS: UNDIFFERENTIATED PHASE

During the neonatal period and for 2 to 3 months thereafter, the infant shows a fairly characteristic type of behavior. Mention has been made in

Chapter VI of the principally reflex nature of the infant's responses immediately after birth. His complete dependence upon his environment is another outstanding feature, with crying as the only initial means of expressing his urgently arising needs.

In this early phase, the infant's needs relate largely to the satisfaction of hunger. The state of tension which is set up in the infant by the perception of hunger brooks no delay and soon produces fretting or crying, diffuse motor activity, sucking movements of the mouth and, frequently, attempts to suck the whole hand. Coordinated sucking of the thumb or fingers is not possible, except on an accidental basis, until the hand-to-mouth reflex develops at some time around the third month. If feeding satisfaction is not forthcoming after a reasonable period of time, the infant ordinarily works himself up into an emotional state overtly resembling rage, with intense and uncoordinated motor activity, "strangled" crying (frequently including breathholding), redness of the face and often the body, and, in many infants, emptying of the bladder or rectum, vomiting, and other signs of participation by the various organ systems in this diffuse emotional response.

There is no evidence to indicate that a subjective component to this intense emotional behavior as yet exists. Indeed, in the first few weeks, with subcortical behavior predominating, this is most unlikely. The state of apparent satisfaction which follows feeding and satiation is well known. Observation of these facts has led most students of infant behavior to conclude that there are two major types of emotional response available to the newborn infant, a state of pleasure and one of "unpleasure," with some gradations between these poles. Pleasure, principally induced by satiety after feeding, appears to lead rapidly to sleep, an apparently "ideal" state resembling, in some ways, the intrauterine existence. Unpleasant stimuli, such as hunger, cold or pain, awaken the infant and, if not relieved, induce an unpleasurable response of the type indicated.

The purpose of this description of infant behavior is simply to point out the fact that, at this stage, the human organism operates in a most undifferentiated fashion in its emotional response to stimuli of various types from within, as the result of sensations arising from bodily processes, or from without, deriving from contacts with the environment and, principally, the mother-figure. It is furthermore apparent that instinctual needs, which relate largely at this stage to the satisfaction of hunger and of the needs for warmth and for tactile and rhythmic experience, are not capable of delay at this point. The infant operates on the basis of what has been called the *pleasure principle,* with as yet no capacity for postponing gratifications in accordance with a *reality principle* which must later develop if the child is to become a social being.

Modern physiological and psychosomatic research has contributed data which cast considerable light on the significance of this early phase for later development. It appears, for example, that the immediacy of the needs of the infant stem largely from two principal sources. One of these is the aforementioned lack of development of the inhibitory functions of the cerebral cortex, which can delay or "long-circuit" the satisfaction of such needs in accordance with an adaptively appropriate goal, as opposed to "short-circuited" or principally reflex expressions of needs immediately following their perception. An additional source of this immediacy of needs is the relatively ineffective physiologic homeostatic functioning of the infant at this point. Certain potentially automatic bodily processes which operate predominately at a subcortical level, such as those involved in the relatively steady maintenance of the body temperature or of blood sugar as a result of the integrative activity of the autonomic nervous system, do not function smoothly as yet. Gastrointestinal peristaltic activity is also quite irregular in the first several months of life. As a result of these and other factors, hunger appears to occur at variable intervals in the very young infant, and the infant's reserve supply is exceedingly small, rendering his needs for nutriment immediate and intense. Related to this variability of physiologic functioning is the concept that as yet the infant has failed to develop a steadily effective "stimulus barrier" in the central nervous system. These stimuli of varying nature, from within or from without, apparently cannot yet be dampened down in such a way as to maintain a relatively steady and balanced inflow, with the result that the infant may be overwhelmed by such stimuli, producing tension which must be discharged or alleviated with great urgency.

Techniques of Infant Care

Observations such as those just cited, among other influences, have recently led many professional persons working with parents to recommend flexible feeding schedules, which are in accordance with the irregularity and immediacy of the infant's needs, as well as his incapacity to wait for satisfaction. This current approach is in contrast to an earlier one, during the years following the turn of the century, involving the practice of feeding young infants on a schedule of clock-like regularity. It is of course true that mothers have always intuitively fed babies in the more flexible fashion, and it now seems clear that a flexible schedule, the self-demand or self-regulation approach, meets the infant's needs during this phase in a more appropriately physiologic and emotional sense. If fed in this fashion, most infants will move spontaneously toward a more regular schedule by two or three months of age, thus finding a feeding rhythm which is a more truly individual one than one which is arbitrarily imposed. Many mothers are able, if permitted or encouraged by physicians to follow this approach, to carry through effectively and happily. Some mothers, however, appear to have greater needs for regularity and predictability for themselves than is available to them on such a basis. Having read the latest literature regarding self-demand, they may feel guilty over being unable to follow their intellectual convictions without inner conflict. Others may need help in determining when the baby is hungry and not over-tired, since not all mothers in urban society today have an intuitive capacity to judge this from the quality of the baby's cry.

At the present time there is no buttressed evidence which indicates that babies fed on a flexible schedule necessarily develop more healthily from an emotional standpoint, although Holway's work would support this possibility.[1] Several careful longitudinal studies of the influence of this variable are going on, however, and answers should be forthcoming. Currently it seems clear at least that this approach, if successful, can increase the mutual pleasure of mother and infant in the feeding process, and perhaps can increase the confidence of the infant in regard to the likelihood of prompt satisfaction of his needs. However, it seems also evident that an approach of this kind, if followed grimly by a mother who is only partially convinced of its wisdom or necessity, can be less satisfying to both persons than a more regular schedule. The obvious answer to this situation, particularly in urban areas, is for the clinician to help the mother to choose the schedule which compromises most happily the baby's needs with her own. For example, a more compulsive mother may be persuaded to employ comfortably a schedule which has some regularity to it, but which permits some deviation toward somewhat earlier or later feeding according to the infant's state of hunger or wakefulness.

What has been said above applies also to such techniques as rooming-in following delivery[2] and breast feeding.[3, 4] Both these techniques have received much emphasis recently, along with self-demand feeding[5] and natural childbirth,[6, 7] in the framework of a movement which justly lays stress upon the naturalness for the mother and infant of such child-care practices. No complete discussion of any of these techniques can be attempted here, but a brief mention of rooming-in and breast feeding seems appropriate.

If a mother feels comfortable about a rooming-in approach, definite benefits would seem to accrue, in a psychological sense. These may result from the mother's enhanced feeling of intimacy with her baby, the greater possibility of active sharing by the husband in the early approach to the baby's care, the confidence in her capacities which a mother, of a first-born infant in particular, can develop, and other associated phenomena. Rooming-in does not seem to carry a significant danger of cross-infection, from all reports.

Certain mothers, however, do not want this approach or are not emotionally equipped to try it, and they should not have such a program legislated into existence for them. Because of their enhanced emotional needs during pregnancy and immediately following delivery,[8] many mothers need considerable support, aid, and attention during this early phase. In individual instances these needs may be considered more important than the favorable potentialities of the rooming-in arrangement. Some hospitals which have tried rooming-in have come to a flexible, individualized usage of its benefits, permitting the mother to change her mind or to ask for more help if the consequent responsibility weighs heavily, or if fatigue or depression appear. The amount of professional nursing help, however, is not significantly decreased over traditional obstetrical practices, as had been hoped for by some.

Breast feeding is being encouraged today in many hospitals and by many obstetricians and pediatricians, in contrast to the active discouragement of such a technique which was popular not long ago. Although the physiological advantages of breast feeding over bottle feeding have become less impressive in recent years with the improvement of artificial feeding, the psychological advantages may be substantial. These lie in the area of the spontaneous pleasure of many mothers in this type of feeding experience and in the resulting warmth and intimacy for the infant. Some hospitals, however, have employed strong pressure on mothers to undertake breast feeding. The studies of Newton and Newton,[9] among others, have shown the limitations of such an approach, since a significant proportion of mothers who have conflicts about this practice are unable to carry through successfully beyond discharge from the hospital, or may find excuses to stop at a slightly later point. A number of American and European obstetricians, particularly Waller[10] in Britain, have shown a capacity to encourage successful breast feeding in a very high percentage of mothers. This requires the expenditure of a great deal of time during pregnancy in discussion with and preparation of mothers for breast feeding, within the framework of a very close and supportive relationship with the physician or nurse.

No longitudinal studies have as yet had time to examine fully the possibility of conclusive benefit for emotional development accruing to babies who are breast-fed rather than fed by bottle.[11] Again the impression exists that breast feeding can be an immediately positive experience for mother and infant and, under rooming-in circumstances, at least, for the father also. These evident qualitative effects, however, do not call for the strenuous urging of a mother in this direction if her fears or disinclinations are tenacious and deep-seated. At the very least, one can and should reassure a mother who feels guilty over her physical or emotional inability to nurse her infant with the knowledge that a happy feeding experience with a bottle will not emotionally penalize her future son or daughter. On the other hand the advantages of breast feeding are too valuable to be casually discarded, and a gradual approach to the reeducation of women in this direction seems warranted. With the changing status and role of women in Western society, it seems unlikely that an overwhelming majority of educated urban mothers will return to breast feeding. Reassurance regarding the lack of harmful effects on the figure, as well as the use of one night bottle when breast feeding has been established, can free many women from feelings of fear or frustration regarding this experience.

Mother-Infant Unit

The beginning discussion of emotional development has emphasized up to this point certain physiological characteristics of the infant and has also included the emotional attitudes of the parents, particularly the mother. These emphases are not without reason. The need to consider each infant as an individual is a principle which applies to all later stages of development. Wide individual variations can occur within the normal range of sucking behavior, for example. These variations may also be of importance in indicating the infant's general level of maturity or his predominant activity type. Similar individual differences appear to exist in the range of sensitivity to visual, auditory, tactile, or kinesthetic stimuli during the first several months[12] and possibly throughout life, with some modifications arising from later development and experience. More significant, however, may be the way in which these variations from the norm influence the mother's response to the infant's behavior as well as her feelings regarding her own role as a mother in relation to this particular infant. Thus the aforementioned principal factors — the infant's limited emotional behavior, strongly influenced by inborn and current physiological factors at this point, and the parental emotional attributes and behavior, representing the focal point of impingement of the environment upon the infant — interact in a most important and complex fashion.

The importance of this emotional transaction between mother and infant has been recently pointed up by Benedek in particular.[13] Its pertinence for professional workers lies in the recognition of the fact that not only do the mother's feelings about and handling of the infant influence strongly the capacity of the infant to form a relationship with her, and thus to make a beginning contact with the outside world, but also that the nature of the *feedback*, or the emotional responsiveness of the infant to the mother, determines in some measure the quality and nature of the mother's continuing feelings about him and thus to some extent her future handling of him.

The term *symbiotic relationship* has been applied to this mutually reinforcing and reciprocal emotional phenomenon involving both the mother and the very young infant. Both are dependent for emotional supplies upon each other — the infant upon the mother for the warmth and social stimulation which is necessary as an impetus toward later development, and the mother upon the infant for some gratification of her own need to feel "complete" and of supreme importance to her baby, who was so recently a physical part of herself and whom she still regards psychologically as a product of her own. With this concept in mind, it is easier to comprehend the types of challenges to a successful mother-child relationship which may face a mother who is confronted, for example, by the presence of a congenital abnormality in this "part of herself," or who may approach her first-born with intense eagerness only to find an unusually unresponsive baby with a low index of psychomotor activity. The mother is of course the mature component of this psychological unit, with other sources of emotional supplies available to her from her husband and family. Thus her capacity to give emotionally to the baby is a most important feature. It is not the whole story, however, as the above illustrations may indicate.

This observation has some relevance to the feelings which parents in general and mothers in particular have been prone to develop following the barrage of educational mental health material which they have received during the last 15 or 20 years, to the effect that they alone are responsible for any disturbance in the parent-child relationship and, consequently, in the child's infantile or later behavior. This question will be discussed more fully at a later point, in regard to the problem of neurotic behavior. At this juncture it can at least be emphasized that, although parental conflicts about certain aspects of child-rearing are important determinants of the child's later behavior, there are always multiple factors involved in such behavior. Such additional factors include the infant's innate characteristics and the feedback phenomenon, already mentioned, and may also include, as Bowlby[14] and others have suggested, certain highly individual characteristics, largely inborn, of the later patterns of the child's growth and development, together with certain incidental crises over which parents have no control.

The appearance of many books, pamphlets, and magazine articles recently "in defense of parents," in reaction to those of some years ago which criticized parents strongly, emphasizes the need for a balanced professional viewpoint in this area. Preventive mental health work based on scientific principles should be neither "for" nor "against" parents. In its application of scientific knowledge, it should include a complete understanding of the challenges facing parents, together with a certain humility regarding the incomplete state of that knowledge. Fortunately, the environmental pressures, of which parental conflicts form a large part, are those which can be most easily dealt with preventively or therapeutically.

The Feeding Situation

The broad implications, for emotional development, of particular feeding techniques, insofar as these are understood, have already been briefly discussed. It remains to examine more carefully the individual feeding situation as a focus of early contact with the environment, in order to point up those facets which relate specifically to the process of emotional development. The necessity for such a thorough scrutiny of this process arises from the impressions of many observers that profound influences upon the child's later behavior may stem from his experiences during feeding in the first several months of life. Middlemore[4] has made careful investigations into this area, particularly regarding breast feeding, and has developed the concept of the "nursing couple," incidentally underscoring the importance of the feedback aspects mentioned earlier. Escalona[15] has also devoted careful scrutiny to feeding behavior of very young infants. She has pointed out the highly sensitive response of infants to transient changes in the physical vitality or emotional state of the mother.

Certainly the way in which the feeding situation is handled has important implications for further development, at least as an index of the emotional climate in the infant's family. Benedek[16] has discussed the emotional aspects of this situation in a most helpful fashion. She has drawn attention to the fact that the infant's earliest mental representations of the outside world are strongly, though not exclusively, derived from his response to the kinds of feeding satisfaction or lack of satisfaction which may occur, thus giving or lending an "alimentary" quality to his earliest relationships. It seems clear that, in certain instances, a lack of feeding gratification, which may include a lack of emotional warmth as well as inept or inappropriate feeding techniques, does pave the way for the infant to react to other and later experiences in a way which would support the impression that he had incorporated mentally a concept of the mother as a "bad" or frustrating person, in contrast to the healthier situation where feeding satisfaction seems to induce the incorporation of a concept of the mother as a "good" or satisfying mother. Where frustration exists, the infant's responsive disturbance in feeding seems to act reciprocally upon the mother in a detrimental fashion, as described earlier in relation to the transactional concept.

In a healthy mother-infant relationship, it appears that both satisfying and frustrating elements are present, with the satisfying one predominating. The mingling of the qualities of the experience, with the potentiality on the part of the infant of angry feelings appearing at any time because he cannot wait for satisfaction and therefore must inevitably face some frustration, has led Benedek to impute an ambivalent core to the mother-child relationship, involving the kind of reciprocal transaction already discussed. This formulation has some pertinence in relation to the concept of ambivalence of emotions discussed earlier, since it indicates that the source of these normally mingled feelings toward even loved persons may at least receive impetus from the emotional concomitants of the process of feeding. Other aspects of the early contact with the mother are of course important and are frequently overlooked, such as those involved in caressing, rocking, and singing activities by the mother, providing tactile, proprioceptive, and auditory stimulation of significant degree. The need for satisfaction of such "stimulus hunger" has been stressed by Ribble[17] and others. Behind all of these contacts, feeding and otherwise, lies the need for emotional warmth and social stimulation from the mother, involving the gratification of "affect hunger," as Levy[18] termed it.

It cannot be said that our understanding of this early phase of development is complete in any sense. It is most difficult to study preverbal behavior of the infant and to determine the kinds of early mental impressions which occur in relation to either specific or diffuse types of environmental experience. It is equally difficult to determine how lasting any memory traces may be. These seem to begin somewhere between the second and fifth month of life.

In summary, it may be said that although conscious memories of experience during this very early phase do not seem to be retained, patterns of reaction (such as initial refusal of food, the negative attitude continuing unchanged or becoming diffused to later patterns of reaction toward parents or other adults who urge something on the child), often do persist. Such patterns of response may be covered over later by other mechanisms of adaptation, or may be nullified by subsequent experiences of a more positive nature. A pattern of reciprocal struggle between mother and infant, however, may remain. Thus, attempts to help parents handle the feeding situation in a comfortable fashion for the infant and for themselves (as in flexible scheduling of feeding intervals, with the qualifications previously mentioned), do seem to be justified from a preventive point of view.

On the basis of the above considerations many pediatricians have resisted the recent and almost competitive trend to offer soft-solid food at earlier and earlier stages. Such physicians feel that it is wiser to wait until approximately the third month, when the infant is neurophysiologically more likely to be ready to perform easily the complicated act of neuromuscular coordination between tongue and hard palate which is involved in swallowing solid material. This approach includes also the consideration that the infant's nutritive needs can be satisfied exclusively by his milk intake, with added vitamins, until at least the third month of life, at which time his needs for iron and other dietary constituents begin to become important.

Prior to the third or, in some infants, the fourth month, the majority of infants can only suck solid food. If a mother does not understand this fact, and especially if she feels a need to produce a "perfect" child who performs outstandingly, the introduction of soft-solid food into the diet prior to the third month may lead her to urge its acceptance so strongly upon the physiologically unready infant that he may begin a pattern of refusal. In such a situation the mother may misinterpret the infant's refusal of food — the visible substance of her proffered love — as a rejection of her affection. Again the quality of the emotional feedback becomes important. It is recognized that there are instances where an exceptionally active and hungry baby, who may also be somewhat advanced developmentally, accepts soft-solids eagerly and fairly competently at 2 months of age or even earlier. Nevertheless the possibilities of initiating feeding problems from this situation are great enough, and the need for solid food at this stage is small enough, that caution should be the watchword.

Sucking Needs

Mention has already been made of the various instinctual drives of the infant during this early stage, relating principally to the satisfaction of hunger and the needs for warmth, for sensory contact, and for rhythmic and auditory experience, the latter two being often satisfied during rocking and singing by the mother, carried on frequently in relation to the central feeding situation. It remains unclear whether the response of many infants to being held or wrapped firmly while being rocked and caressed has, as some workers have suggested, some relation to the possible similarities to intrauterine experiences. An occasional overactive baby resists these approaches, while some infants seem to respond eagerly and almost exclusively to such handling.

At least two additional drives of the very young infant can be identified at this point. One, relating to social contact, will be discussed in the next section. The other drive, relating to the need for pleasure in sucking, will be briefly discussed at this point. Sucking represents the only method of ingestion of nutritive materials available to the infant at his earliest stage of development. Thus the strength and vigor of the sucking reflex is of key importance, and any definitive weakening of this reflex can be of serious significance. The differences among infants in the quality and intensity of sucking activities have already been pointed out. These differences may have a large part of their roots in the innate characteristics of motor behavior. Middlemore[4] has described changes in the degree and effectiveness of sucking activity during the neonatal period, however, and has recognized the possibility that the character of the early feeding situation may determine how and to what extent these modifications of basic patterns may occur.

It is apparent early in the infant's development that sucking, which overtly seems to serve predominantly a utilitarian function, soon, or perhaps from the first, acquires a significant pleasurable component as well. The mouth and the adjacent skin areas seem to be endowed with tactile sensitivity of higher degree and greater exquisiteness than any other bodily zone at this stage of development. This may perhaps be true even during fetal life, as the experiments of Davenport Hooker would seem to indicate.[19] It is not surprising, then, that sucking gradually becomes a pleasurable experience in itself, even when later separated entirely from the originally associated act of ingestion of food.

Preceding the development of the hand-mouth reflex, as has been indicated, consciously purposive sucking of the fingers or hand does not exist. Nevertheless various observers have pointed out that, even in the early phase, most infants exhibit a need for pleasurable sucking, often carried out by mouthing the nipple without attempt to express milk in the process. It is equally well known that definite differences in the amount of such activity exist among different infants and in individual infants at varying times. In the majority of instances an infant's individual sucking needs can be met by letting him suck simply for pleasure during or after the feeding experience. Some infants, however, and probably all infants at some time, show such needs at other times than during feeding. A nipple or other pacifier may be of help in meeting these needs. In the light of current knowledge, such an approach does not seem to predispose the infant to later dependence upon sucking or upon any other means of unhealthy self-gratification, as so many workers with children felt formerly.

Lack of appropriate sucking gratification may result from mechanical or technical inefficiencies in the feeding process, or in consequence of a physical defect, such as harelip with associated cleft palate. Whether among the later effects may be serious emotional deprivation manifested by abnormally intense thumbsucking, significant insecurity, or distortion in personality development, is a question which is difficult to answer at this point. Sears[20] and Levy[21] have studied this question, but the results are not conclusive. There is some evidence, however, indicating that emotionally deprived infants show greater sucking needs. Suffice it to say that most infants appear happier and more relaxed when sufficient sucking opportunities are available. The quality of the relationship between mother and infant, as expressed through the mother's handling of the infant during the feeding period, with associated feedback phenomena, is probably more important than the number of minutes of sucking time. For these and other reasons, there seems to be no indication for interfering with either the earlier or later manifestations of the sucking need. Dental dangers now seem to be minimal, as regards permanent distortion in the shape of the mandible and the occlusion of the teeth, if, as is usually the case, the child gives up intensive thumbsucking before the eruption of the permanent teeth.[22]

Special Developmental Problems

It is not possible to discuss in detail the types of deviation from the norm of beginning emotional development which may occur in infancy. The principles already elucidated regarding the interaction of inherent characteristics and environmental influences obviously apply. The infant who is premature, for example, may show difficulties in sucking, enhanced motor restlessness, body temperature instability, or other signs of more primitive neurophysiologic or metabolic organization, as well as a more fetal appearance, even after discharge from the hospital. The special meaning of these signs to the parents, in the particular context of the pregnancy, delivery, and early neonatal period, may at times produce unhealthy response in handling the infant. In cases of prematurity, the smallness of the baby may pose a particular challenge to a mother who may, as many such mothers do, express her fear of hurting the baby who is "so fragile I might break him." (Spock[23] has remarked that "the anxiety of the mother may be inversely proportional to the size of the infant.") Here the capacity of the parents, particularly the mother, to tolerate anxiety, and the almost universal parental susceptibility to free-floating guilt feelings, may combine with other individualized circumstances to produce an overapprehensive approach to the premature but otherwise healthy infant. Hence the value of permitting and even encouraging a mother to become familiar with her premature baby by holding, rocking, and feeding it, at least during the week or two prior to its discharge, with due but not elaborate precautions against infection.[24] At other times these factors may enhance a parental need to pressure the child in regard to milk intake, for example, in order to make him "catch up," and thus to deny any implications of failure or inadequacy which the prematurity may carry for the parents. Fortunately this is not the usual case, but such extremes occur frequently enough to be noted. The same general remarks might be made regarding congenital deformities in the infant, which to certain parents may unconsciously represent objectivizations of the "bad part of themselves" or of feared hereditary stigmata, as well as punishment for certain dietary or sexual indiscretions during pregnancy.

A fairly universal problem during this period is that represented by "colic." This constellation of signs of gastrointestinal discomfort in the infant will not be thoroughly discussed here. It may be said that several recent studies[25] would appear to document the earlier impressions of wise and experienced pediatricians and general practitioners that emotional tension does play an important role, along with other factors such as allergy and the physiologic variability of this stage, in the appearance of the discomfort itself, or at least may result at times in the perpetuation of such symptoms beyond the usual 3 month limit. Many workers[26] have had the impression that severely colicky babies tend to be the more active, restless ones, who may have been more active *in utero* and who may now exhibit greater gastrointestinal as well as motor activity. This impression is not fully documented at present. It is apparent, however, that tension in the family or in the mother is commonly present when one sees severe or prolonged colic in an infant. It is also clear that measures involving psychological support may be of value in diminishing the symptoms. Again the interaction of inherent and environmental forces appears to be at work, even though our knowledge of their exact balance in any individual case is not complete. At any rate neither physical nor psychological factors appear to be the sole cause.

For the professional worker it is important to mention Levine's[27] demonstration of the fact that babies with severe and prolonged colic often have enhanced sucking needs, and that the use of a pacifier is markedly effective in many such instances. Such a technique should, of course, wisely be combined with opportunities for the parents to "think out loud" in the presence of a sympathetic professional person about the resolution of superficial tensions, centering around living arrangements, schedules, etc.

The problem of scheduling brings to focus again the feeding situation and infantile sleeping patterns. Flexible approaches to both these areas have produced significant benefits to many babies, letting them find their own rhythms (which undoubtedly vary, not only from infant to infant, but from time to time), and thus preventing long periods of screaming, irritability, and sleeplessness. Nevertheless it should be re-emphasized that certain parents may respond, almost too eagerly, with the offer of a feeding in response to the infant's slightest demonstration of a fussiness which might well be the result, for example, of fatigue rather than hunger. Situations such as these can lead to sleeping problems in babies who become overstimulated and unable to "release into" sleep. Factors of this kind may also contribute to certain clinical pictures resembling colic. Astute clinicians will be aware of these exceptions to the success of a flexible feeding approach, and may gently have to help such a parent impose on herself a more regular scheduling for the sake of the infant.

In very extreme cases, marked incapacity of the mother to give emotionally to the infant may combine with his inherent tendencies toward apathetic responsiveness to produce a picture resembling depression in the infant, with associated feeding refusal, and consequent disturbance in nutrition to the point of serious wasting (marasmus) even in the face of adequate nutritional supplies.[28] In some such instances, as Lourie has demonstrated,[29] the purposive use of a mother-substitute in the hospital, involving the assignment of one nurse or attendant to the painstaking and slow process of feeding such an infant, has produced positive results. Other conditions, with a basically physical source, can of course also produce a marasmic picture. An emotional component of the type described may at times be operative even in these.

Other less sweeping types of pathological response have been encountered during the first several months of life, including vomiting, diarrhea, and other disturbances. Most of these early infantile problems involve some form of negative response to the feeding situation, but may also implicate the gastrointestinal organ system, and occasionally other systems, in the relatively undifferentiated fashion described earlier. The majority of these disturbances have seemed to appear in an emotional climate which includes a mother (and often, indirectly, a father) who has experienced significant conflicts about the handling of this particular infant or who was unprepared emotionally for parenthood at the time of the infant's birth. In a number of such instances the reciprocal or feedback phenomena already mentioned were undoubtedly also at work, at least in relation to the innate characteristics of the infant's feeding behavior. Many of these disturbances can be prevented by anticipatory guidance and support; others, if more severe, can be treated in the way described by Lourie in connection with marasmus, with the combined use of a mother-substitute during hospitalization and special work with the parents.

It can be seen that, in this phase of development, disturbance in the emotional balance of the symbiotic relationship between mother and infant produces a relatively undifferentiated emotional response on the part of the infant, including physiologic as well as primitive behavioral components, with a minimum of subjective elements involved. This set of observations has significance for future development. Many later psychosomatic or psychophysiologic disturbances have seemed to a number of investigators to have had their roots in this undifferentiated phase of emotional behavior. The exact psychophysiologic mechanisms by which later disturbances in adaptation could produce, in certain individuals, a "regression" to this type of infantile participation by various organ systems in an unhealthy emotional response have not yet been elucidated. Nevertheless, this concept in some form or other has become the central one in recent psychosomatic research. Much work is going on to illuminate the factors which may determine the particular organ system which may participate predominantly in such regressively unhealthy adaptive responses as, for instance, those of the rectum and the colon in ulcerative colitis, the stomach in gastric ulcer, etc. Multiple determinants are clearly involved in such disorders, including inherited, constitutional, or emotional ones, of which the last may act as a precipitating and perpetuating factor.

The nature and degree of the still undifferentiated emotional responses during early infancy thus appear to be important for later emotional development and its vicissitudes. Whether specific environmental experiences during this phase exert specific effect upon later psychophysiologic functioning remains a moot point. Some workers believe that, for example, the very young infant who is given suppositories repeatedly by an anxious or compulsive mother may respond to this mingled pleasant and unpleasant stimulation of the anorectal mucous membrane with a heightened predisposition to later bowel or sphincter dysfunction.[30] In our present state of limited knowledge we cannot predict with assurance that such a result will occur, even though this effect has frequently been observed. Moreover, if such a disorder does arise, we can only say that this type of environmental experience is one of several predisposing factors of the types mentioned above. It is known that certain infants have undergone early stimulation of the mucosa of the rectum or lower bowel from this or other causes, sometimes in connection with physical illness, without clear evidence of later bowel dysfunction. In our present state of preliminary understanding it seems wise to help parents avoid *unnecessary* manipulation of various parts of the infant's body, without frightening them into anxious overcaution. Later experiences of this nature, such as those involved in toilet training or in early attempts to "break" thumbsucking, may be viewed from the same standpoint, as important influences upon, but not absolute determinants of, vicissitudes in emotional development.

not wise to frighten a mother who, for needs of her own or because of a particular cultural background, seems to be intent on weaning her child a few months earlier than the recommended time. Sometimes such a mother can be helped to wait at least a short time by the anticipatory knowledge that such an approach will run less chance of difficulties. Better still, if possible, she can be given time to talk a bit, if she can do so easily, about such things as her need, perhaps, to compete with her older sister in the rearing of her children, gaining reassurance from the worker that differences in rate of achievement do not reflect upon her comparative capacities as a mother.

Special Problems

Since the central emphasis in the infant phase has been upon the beginning differentiation of the ego, it will be wise first to consider briefly the vicissitudes of ego formation as the paramount, though not the most frequent or commonly obvious, problem arising at this stage. Studies in this area have been numerous, but the limitations in knowledge are still great. Spitz[44] has shown, for example, in confirmation of the results of the earlier work of Chapin,[45] Bakwin,[28] and others, that infants reared from the very early months in an institutional setting, with limited staff, where virtually no social stimulation was provided and no continuing mother-substitute relationship was available, tended to exhibit striking failure in their later capacities to develop relationships with adults. Such infants were apathetic and unresponsive and were markedly retarded, sometimes permanently, in intellectual, motor, and social development. In addition, they appeared much more susceptible to infections than are infants reared in a healthy family emotional climate, in spite of excellent physical care. These institutionalized infants showed blunting or failure in the development of differentiated ego functions. Other infants, who had enjoyed a close relationship with their own mother for the first few months, developed what Spitz termed serious depression following sudden separation from their mothers, when there was no provision of an adequate mother-substitute.

The implications of these and other studies cannot be fully summarized here. It is apparent, however, that extreme emotional deprivation, involving lack of warmth and social stimulation from a continuing mother figure, can adversely influence intellectual, social, emotional, motor, and even physical facets of personality development. Such adverse influence can also show its effects predominantly in one of the above areas, as, for example, in the type of "environmental" retardation in intellectual development which at times is seen in a severely emotionally-deprived infant.[46] Such a phenomenon may occur in institutionalized infants, but may also appear in an infant living in an intact family where a disturbed mother cannot offer these basic gratifications. The effects of gross maternal deprivation upon social and emotional areas of development have been well described by Bowlby,[47] expanding the earlier work by Goldfarb,[48] in his description of the tendency toward shallow relations with adult figures and consequent impulsive, antisocial behavior, which is often seen in children who have been institutionalized for long periods of time or who have been shunted through a long series of unsuccessful foster-home placements.

The most extreme example of developmental deviation in ego development is seen in certain children described as autistic[49] or atypical in ego development.[50] Such deviation may occur in the presence of an intact family, as opposed to an institutional setting, although the family emotional "climate" is often a deeply disturbed one, and the child may completely fail to undergo successfully the aforementioned process of ego differentiation. In such instances the child either is unable to establish a separate "self," and remains withdrawn and unable to have independent relationships, or he may have begun to take this step but has regressed in the face of some emotional trauma. In these cases the commonly manifest inability of the mother to "give" emotionally to the infant seems also to involve a deficiency in feedback, related to some inherent or constitutional limitation of the child's capacity to respond, with a breakdown of the transactional relationship between mother and infant.

A significant outgrowth of the concepts just summarized has been the trend away from the placement of young infants in large institutions, in favor of their location in foster or adoptive families. On the basis of these and other considerations adoptive practices have been modified in the direction of the encouragement of the very early placement of infants in potential adoptive homes, if possible during the undifferentiated phase — i.e., prior to ego differentiation — or at least during the first half year of life, at a time when the infant can fairly readily accept a mother substitute. When adoption is not possible, foster homes have been considered preferable to institution placements. Foster homes may not be ideal, however, and "masked" emotional deprivation can occur in such settings which may be of equal malignance to that seen in large institutional settings. Careful selection of foster homes then seems vital in order to secure adequate supplies of emotional warmth for such infants. Small institutions, well staffed with trained personnel, may be more effective for such purposes than some foster homes.[51]

Other and milder problems which establish their roots during the first year include certain sleeping problems related to the aforementioned eighth month anxiety. In certain cases, mothers may feel an intense emotional need to return at the infant's every cry. Thus a cycle may arise, involving fatigue and overstimulation for the infant, with consequent hidden resentment toward the mother, with the result that the infant cannot drop off to sleep, and struggle ensues. Help for such mothers is indicated, based on recognizing in advance the developmental quality of this crying and aimed at achieving a sort of gradual weaning of the infant from its night-time dependence on her.[23]

It remains to consider briefly certain manifestations of psychophysiologic or psychosomatic disorders which may appear during the first year of emotional development. The most potentially serious of these relate to gastrointestinal function, and involve prolonged and severe diarrhea or vomiting during the second half of the first year. Chronic disturbances in gastrointestinal function have been seen to correlate with periods of stressful separation from the mother, or at times when she is preoccupied or depressed. The infant often shows an answering depression, associated with emotional and behavioral regression, indicating that the diarrhea or vomiting may help to discharge tensions at such times in a regressive fashion similar to tension releases during the earlier undifferentiated phase. Studies of these and related conditions have been carried out by Lourie[29] and Prugh,[52] as well as others. Knowledge in this area remains sketchy, however. Many of these manifestations respond in non-specific fashion to the mother-substitute approach discussed earlier, combined with measures designed to reverse often severe metabolic consequences of the diarrhea or vomiting. Physical measures alone, however, often do not seem to produce significant improvement. Rumination, or paradoxical pleasure in the mouthing of regurgitated food, may appear in this phase and have similar causative features, as Richmond's[53] studies have indicated. Again certain biologic predispositional factors may be involved, as well as emotional feedback difficulties.

Similar clinical pictures may be seen in infants who suffer from obscure physical abnormalities, such as congenital diaphragmatic hernia. In certain of these infants, similar psychologic components may be present, as the result of tension and discomfort on the part of the infant, the impact of the hospitalization which may be necessary, as well as the tension and/or guilt of the parents over their failure to help the infant feed or develop effectively. Again the observations made earlier apply to the parents' feelings and reactions to the physical component.

As another example, premature infants, if born without associated congenital abnormality, ordinarily remain somewhat behind others in most aspects of development for the first year of life, catching up during the second year, if no other problem intervenes. For the parents the emotional meaning of this retardation, especially if associated with misconceptions regarding the cause of the prematurity, is probably the most important single determinant of their handling of the child. Again anticipatory knowledge and frequent, supportive contacts with professional personnel during the early phase of parental activity can often prevent unhealthy overapprehension and guilty protectiveness, or too vigorous denial of the defect and resultant "pushing" of the infant at this stage.[3]

Other disturbances in behavior deserving mention are repeated and prolonged bouts of head-rolling, head-banging, or body-rocking, patterns which normally appear in a transient fashion during the second half of the first year. These may become so intense or prolonged as to represent a symptom of emotional disturbance, involving unhealthy methods of discharging tensions on the infant's part and producing various desperate attempts of the parents to prevent these troubling manifestations. Adequate rhythmic gratification, as in rocking or singing by the mother, may prevent or minimize such unhealthy behavior, which often is initially related to anxiety at night in an infant who seems to employ this more passive method of response rather than screaming or crying out. Occasionally, however, such a symptomatic trend is so deep-seated and prolonged that referral to a child guidance clinic is necessary.

In summary, then, the infant during the first year remains strongly dependent upon the mother, although interaction with the father begins to occur. From the point of view of emotional development, he has made enormous strides by the end of this phase of differentiation, but with important individual variation. These include occasional regressions, as well as fluctuations in the emphasis laid upon differing areas of development from time to time. An infant who manifests significant deviations from expected emotional progress should not be considered "neurotic," as this concept implies the presence of a more fully developed mental apparatus. It is true, however, that important patterns of ego reaction to particular environmental situations already have been set up, but these are capable of modification within certain limits. Such patterns of reaction may determine, in significant measure, the type of approach to life which will be characteristic of a particular infant in his particular family. They do not necessarily predetermine the over-all success of his adjustment, however, as some workers have implied.[54] Hence the justification, in this discussion, for the much more detailed approach to the first year of emotional life than that which will be employed in the stages to follow.

A word is indicated regarding the concept of separation. Much research is necessary to aid us in our understanding of what factors determine the pathogenicity of a particular separation for a particular infant. Not all separations from the significant mother-figure, and certainly not brief ones, are necessarily pathogenic. It would appear that the context of forces operating at the time of separation is more important than any such single factor as age, level of emotional development, or length of separation, provided an adequate mother-substitute is available. The meaning of the separation to the infant, the mother, and, indirectly, the father, are the prominent features in this context. Here less tangible but still powerful emotional forces, such as guilt or anxiety on the part of the mother, or special apprehension on the part of the infant regarding new situations, are paramount, receiving their impetus from the previous quality of the mother-child symbiosis. Hence prolonged separations, unless unavoidable, are unwise. These considerations should not mean, however, that mothers should be told that they should constantly remain with their infants. If this were the rule in modern society, frustration and guilt for the mother and complete lack of contact with new figures for the infant would result.

THE SECOND YEAR OF LIFE: DEVELOPING MASTERY

The tasks for the infant during the second year, from the point of view of emotional development, are fundamental and extremely important. Perhaps the most obvious is the beginning resolution of the symbiotic mother-infant relationship, leading to enhanced independence and the opportunity to acquire mastery of basic biologic skills. The on-going psychomotor and intellectual development of the infant permits him to take this step, which includes also mastery of his own instinctual impulses, in the interests of becoming a social being. The most important although not the single determinant of the infant's emotional growth during this phase remains the capacity of the parents to permit him enough independence, combined with guidance, to make possible the most constructive utilization of his own inherent and highly individualized biologic and psychologic capacities.

During the second year of life the infant begins to consolidate the motor skills which he acquired during the first year. By 15 to 18 months most infants have become more or less able to walk, to explore their environment actively, to manipulate objects with varying degrees of skill, and to communicate, at least in primitive nonverbal fashion, with their parents. It is of course difficult to study preverbal intellectual functioning. Nevertheless, the impression of many observers is that the infant tends to think in terms of "concrete" images or mental pictures. Again individual variations are quite marked, however, and during the latter part of the second year certain infants are capable of other intellectual performances, which will be described in the next section. Although the first 2 years, arbitrarily designated "infancy," are often thought of as the period of inability to speak, this generalization is of course inaccurate. A number of infants at 18 to 24 months use single words quite effectively; some by 2 years are using short sentences. Girls appear to advance slightly more rapidly in speech development than do boys. Some infants respond to excessive stimulation from their parents with more rapid speech progress.

Perhaps the most outstanding component of the emotional aspects of behavior during the second year is the developing sense of "autonomy," [38] which often appears to parents to be present in alarming amounts. The relentlessly exploratory toddler who seizes tablecloths, sending a flood of dishes crashing to the floor, or who investigates a Ming vase with demolishing ardor, is a familiar phenomenon. He is equipped with maneuverable muscles and extremities and a tremendous need to do things himself, but is relatively inaccessible to reason or restraint. Behind such drives towards independence and autonomy is a definite sense of power in new-found abilities, combined with emotional operation still predominantly on the level of the pleasure principle and an inability to test reality in more than a very primitive fashion. Boys seem to be slightly more active and vigorous than girls in this phase, according to some studies.[54] Very soon the infant begins to discover, at first somewhat unhappily, that there are certain limits to the free expression of his aggressive impulses, including those components relating to basic mastery of the environment as well as those destructive components mentioned earlier.

Much remains to be learned about the instinctual sources of the apparent cruelty and intermittent destructiveness of the 18 month old infant. Here it will be assumed that a good deal of the toddler's destruction is only incidental to exploration and to constructive but frequently unsuccessful attempts at mastery and the development of skills. Hence the oft-repeated advice to parents to remove precious bric-a-brac from his range and to avoid making an issue of every incident which has destructive results. Nevertheless in his second year the child obtains some real pleasure in destruction and in hurting. These manifestations appear to derive both from the fundamental ambivalence toward loved persons, mentioned earlier, and from the compensatory use of destructive or "sadistic" behavior on the part of the infant, who is presumed to feel small and helpless in an unfamiliar giant world. The ambivalent component can be seen clearly in the 18 month old infant who first lovingly hugs, then playfully bites his mother.

Although aggressive drives represent the major instinctual challenge, drives of a more clearly sexual nature also begin to emerge during the second year. Such sexual stirrings still retain, to a large extent, the pregenital and predominantly autoerotic characteristics of the previous phase. Brief and primitive masturbation of a specifically pleasurable sort, without orgasm, is often observed. This behavior may be of considerable concern to parents, who tend to read adult implications into the infant's obvious pleasure, with resultant fears of fostering a "sex maniac." Other sources of pleasurable sensation may include stimulation of the anorectal mucous membrane. Pleasurable stimulation may occur paradoxically from without, as the result of the use of suppositories or enemas, even though often mingled with unpleasant or painful sensations, or from within, as in the withholding or partial extrusion and withdrawal of the stool, from which many infants gain a kind of pleasure. The still poor localization of bodily stimuli frequently permits such stimulation to be confused intrapsychically with genital awareness and sensation.

Such an apparent shift in area of pleasurable excitation from the mouth to the anus, combined with the infant's obvious interest in and initial lack of disgust for his stool and its characteristics as a part of his body, led Freud [34] to term this period the "anal" period of psychosexual development. Clearly, however, oral sensitivity and associated sucking needs still persist during this phase. Thus the term is valid only if one defines sexual pleasure broadly enough, as Freud did, to include any such bodily excitation, recognizing that oral activity, notably kissing, persists in adult sexual behavior, as does anal stimulation in certain sexual perversions. The tendency today is to regard oral, anal, and later phallic or genital interests and preoccupations as if they were tributaries flowing into and mingling with the broad stream of later adult sexuality, rather than as definitive and clear-cut separate stages.

In addition to the heightened independence, augmented psychomotor capacities, and enhanced capacity for expression of instinctual drives which are apparent, the infant in his second year exhibits greatly advanced potentialities and needs for social interaction and for increasingly outgoing emotional attachment to the parents. The father now becomes a less peripheral figure, although the mother's importance is still central. In other words, the infant is by no means completely preoccupied with the handling of internal sensations, instinctual expression, and the mastery of skills. His ego is now more nearly autonomous, and more fully differentiated from the mother's, and he has begun to develop primitive symbols of communication, even though words may still be limited. He can thus, through "games," relate to the mother and the father as other human beings rather than as parts of himself, and has come to possess the rudiments of outgoingness. He imitates his parents in simple ways, as in attempting to push a broom or to pound with a hammer. He can engage in glancing social contacts in play with another child, even though his tendency is still to engage in "parallel" play rather than true interaction. He can even grasp the meaning and importance of "giving" presents to his parents or to strangers. Admittedly, he often shows his limited capacity in this area by taking back the gift, sometimes before it is fully delivered. Such behavior seems to represent a manifestation of basic ambivalence, over and beyond the difficulties in sharing which is characteristic of this period.

In spite of his growing psychological and social potentialities, the infant indicates in many ways his continuing dependence upon his parents, particularly the mother, as well as the fragility of his ego autonomy. When in an unfamiliar place or in the presence of a stranger, he runs to his mother. If she is absent, he may cry anxiously, although later he may show withdrawal for a time. When the mother is departing he may cling frenziedly to her, or may strike out at her or the baby-sitter. Spitz[33] has pointed up the fact that manifest separation anxiety in toddlers often occurs most intensely in those who have the closest relationship with their mothers. Thus this phenomenon may not represent simply the results of overprotection or insecurity, even though these latter are often involved in especially persistent or sweeping instances of separation anxiety.

Struggle for Control

From what has been said it may be seen that the infant during this phase is trying to achieve control or mastery in a number of different directions. He is impelled by his developmental impetus to begin to master his environment through his enhanced motor skills, as in beginning self-feeding and the physical manipulation of objects, and in other ways. He must also begin to master his own impulses. Since he has become a primitively social being, he must begin to face the need for some conformity with the demands of social interaction. Much though not all of the behavior of the infant in the second year of life, and indeed for several years thereafter, can be seen as a kind of testing out of the social, i.e., parental, limits to his expression of his instinctual drives, particularly aggressive ones. Beginning evidence of this struggle to control destructive impulses and hostile feelings can be seen in the 20 month old who reaches for a forbidden object, looks toward his mother, and emphatically says to himself, "No, No!" The fact that he sometimes goes ahead with his investigative or destructive plan, following such apparent lip service to parental limits, indicates only his small capacity for "building in" controls in a steady and unambivalent fashion.

As is well known, this struggle for control works outwardly as well as inwardly. The infant's attempts to control his environment include experiments in the control of his parents. Demands, direct rebellion, and temper tantrums begin to appear. Temper tantrums seem to represent diffuse behavioral discharge of tension arising from frustration and anger, often with apparent turning inward or turning aside of aggressive impulses against the parents in a kind of self-punitive way, related to kicking or pounding the feet, banging the head, etc. Control of the parents, in a more safely rebellious way than by direct acting out, is often accomplished by the infant or at least attempted in a negativistic fashion. The period from approximately 18 to 24 months has been designated by some as the normally negativistic stage. During this time, and later, during the brief regressions so commonly seen as a result of illness or minor emotional crises, the infant frequently employs the word "No" or vigorously resists attempts at control by the parents. This tendency may be carried to such an extreme that at times, "No" may be employed in situations which are obviously pleasurable to the infant. As with other phases, this one ordinarily passes away. Parents are therefore well advised to avoid making an issue of every negativism, and to carry through with reasonable confidence and calm, however difficult this may be. Asking the child if he "wants" to do something which is part of an important routine is doomed to failure, especially if the 18 or 20 month old infant is tired or fussy. Quietly announcing a transition in routine, with positive alternatives offered, works much better with a child of this age, as Spock has perceptively and wittily pointed out in his inimitable *Pocket Book of Baby and Child Care*.[23]

The infant's struggle for control of his impulses, and his attempts at control of his environment, may be puzzling and frustrating to parents. No longer is their baby a soft, cuddly, and responsive creature, full of cooing and playfulness. Difficulties in the parent-child relationship may often be dated from this phase, even with parents who have been highly successful up to this point. Here the feedback has been altered by developmental changes, with consequent alterations in the whole transactional process. Again individual variations in degree of activity and autonomy on the part of the infant may be of great significance in determining the success of future parental child-care efforts.

Adaptive Mechanisms

During the second year the infant acquires new adaptive capacities which are important. In spite of his primitive emotional reactions and his general inability to delay satisfactions, he does begin to acquire, albeit haltingly, the ability to suppress or inhibit, and at times to repress from awareness, certain instinctual tendencies, particularly aggressive ones, rather than to act them out directly. He seems also to deny certain painful stimuli, as, for instance, in the absence of the mother, when he repetitively calls "Mommy" even though he knows she has left. In addition, the infant shows the rudiments of identification by imitating the parent of the same sex, even though his capacity for extended use of fantasy in play is still extremely limited and his attention span quite short. Strange animals and sounds may terrify him. Here the fear seems to be based not only on unfamiliarity, but also upon the infant's tendency to project certain subjective feelings onto outer objects. Witness the 2 year old who calls a frighteningly noisy train a "bad choo-choo."

All of these tentative adaptive steps and others appear in the framework of the developing mental apparatus. By the use of these adaptive devices the infant begins to be able to deal with anxiety or tension in more complicated and effective ways than the simple discharge phenomena available to the young infant.

A word should be said here regarding rates of maturation. The primitive adaptive mechanisms described, since they vary considerably in their effectiveness and time of appearance, point up the wide range of developmental rates. During the second year parents often bcome increasingly aware of the comparative aspects of speech and motor development, as well as differences in height and weight, the possibility of such deviations as flat feet, and the like. Although the possibility of noticing mental retardation is now more definite than during the first year, there are such wide fluctuations in speech and motor development that much caution must be observed. Careful observation over a period of time is necessary for accurate evaluation, even with the use of psychological tests. Although Gesell and his associates[55] have made important contributions to the knowledge of intellectual development, many parents, particularly educated ones, have in their anxiety misinterpreted their pinpointing of stages of development. Such parents may need some time for discussion of these concepts in order to avoid unrealistic fears for the future of their infant, who may vary normally by several months at least from the stated "average."

Definite mental retardation, of course, must be faced. Even here, however, caution in diagnosis is commendable in infants and young children, in view of the wide fluctuations and functional I.Q. which Sontag[26] and others have indicated may occur as the result of environmental influence during childhood. The intelligence quotient is not an absolute figure and its predictive capacities show certain limitations in early childhood.[56] Attempts to diagnose Mongolism at birth or shortly thereafter may founder because of the essentially descriptive nature of the diagnosis, with the possibilities of confusion because of family patterns of physical appearance. Even when gross mental retardation is strikingly apparent to the examiner, parents may require some time to assimilate this fact. Overforceful statements of the diagnosis, combined with sweeping predictions and preventive recommendations regarding institutionalization, are often doomed to failure as parents may defensively deny the seriousness of the problem. Because of these facts as well as the difficulty in arranging early institutionalization, it is wise to proceed gradually and to employ repeated tests, letting the family come gradually to any such decision. It is well to recognize that some parents may be able to keep a severely retarded child at home without serious harm to siblings.

Toilet Training

As an example of the need for control, the infant in Western society during his second year ordinarily comes to grips with the socially dictated need to learn to control his sphincters. A generation ago this social need was brought home to some infants of 6 months or less. With the trend in child care methods towards a more permissive approach, the majority of infants in middle class families now first encounter toilet training during the early part of the second year, or during the last several months of the first.

Toilet training has received intense and at times uncritical scrutiny from all professional quarters during the past 15 or 20 years. Its importance as an area of study stems mainly from Freud's observations regarding the impact of environmental pressures upon the developing personality of the infant and young child. The literature is full of impassioned appeals to parents to delay training because of the dire implications of early or rigid practices. Other equally dedicated workers have maintained, from other theoretical contexts, that the timing and nature of training have no demonstrable effect upon personality development or later bowel or bladder function. Actually, very little balanced and detailed investigation, particularly of a longitudinal nature, has been carried out.

The limited data available includes some studies of the rate of maturation of function of the spinal nerves, supplying the external sphincters of the bowel and bladder. Huschka[57] has summarized the available information in this regard. It appears, for example, that the process of myelination of the spinal nerves involved in bowel control, which is ordinarily achieved before bladder control, does not become completed until sometime between 12 and 20 months of age. There remains some question as to whether myelination is necessary for voluntary control. It is also true that individual variations in rate of neurophysiologic maturation do exist. Watson[58] long ago showed that conditioned control of sphincter action could be achieved with the use of suppositories, at six or eight weeks of age.

The currently prevailing point of view takes note of the above neurophysiologic considerations and the admitted gaps in pertinent knowledge. Since voluntary and not merely conditioned control is the goal of such training, the capacity of the child to sit alone, to communicate his needs by at least nonverbal means, and perhaps to participate by walking to the toilet or pot, are other pertinent considerations. Some observers consider it important for the infant to be old enough to want to please the mother by producing the stool appropriately. Worthy of note also is the observed fact that many, though not all, of the infants "trained" (conditioned) by stringent measures early in the first year, show at least a temporary breakdown in control during the second year at the time when voluntary participation in the act must appear.

With these and other related facts at hand, a number of workers have suggested postponing active bowel-training until the beginning of the second year or perhaps the last month or two of the first. It has been said by Aldrich[59] that before this time it is the mother who is "trained" to catch the stool at the appropriate times. Certain authorities have recommended, with some wisdom, waiting until later, and have pointed out the important fact that it is unwise to begin bowel training at the same time as weaning or some other potential emotional challenge, such as the birth of a sibling, a temporary separation from the mother, etc. The evidence from Fries'[60] studies would indicate that infants achieve bowel control more rapidly when training is undertaken either at the beginning or end of the second year, the hiatus being accounted for by the peak of negative tendencies and the struggle for control of sadistic impulses at around 18 to 20 months of age. Individual variations of course apply to any such considerations. Also, Roberts and Schoelkopf[61] have shown that, in our North American society at least, boys exhibit a more rebellious response to bowel training than do girls, which may be related to more vigorous male aggressive tendencies, possibly interacting with a difference in mothers' feelings about the training of boys and girls.

As in other areas involving complex forces, it is necessary to put the few available facts into whatever perspective is currently attainable. Very early and/or very coercive or punitive training, involving shaming, spanking, or requiring the infant to sit on the pot for long periods of time, does seem unwise in the light of existing knowledge, which includes the fact that children with later bowel dysfunction and certain personality disorders, particularly obsessive-compulsive in nature, frequently have a history of such coercive training experience. Not all children undergoing such training appear to exhibit these disorders, however.[30] To many observers[54, 11] the most important factor has appeared to be the personality structure and attitudes toward bowel training of the responsible parent, usually the mother, though occasionally it is a grandmother or other mother-substitute and, more rarely, the father.

To sum up, it can be said that a sound approach involves the beginning of bowel training around the end of the first year or beginning of the second. In such an approach the use of a "potty chair," if available, rather than a "toidy seat," seems to fit the fact that some infants are frightened of the height of an adult toilet. The flushing of the toilet may also cause some anxiety, as the infant may be confused by the sound and also by the fact that this "precious" object, the stool, which he now recognizes as a part of his own body (and the production of which his mother seems to value highly) is dealt with so finally and irrevocably. It seems wise also to take advantage of the gastrocolic reflex, which operates to empty the colon and to fill the rectum by peristaltic waves after the ingestion of a meal. Seating the infant for a few minutes only at a time, regardless of production, has much to recommend it, since constant activity and resistance to prolonged or enforced restraint are so characteristic of this phase. Avoidance of a pitched battle is of course indicated. For reasons mentioned earlier, the infant is prone to join eagerly in any such struggle and can usually "win" by withholding the stool — and incidentally enjoying the sensation — or by extruding it when and where he will.

With the use of an approach similar to the above, many mothers appear to be able to help their infants to achieve bowel control over a period of a few weeks or several months. Regressive breakdowns in control of course occur, but a mother who has advance knowledge of such possibilities will ordinarily be little troubled. Control of bowel functions by this approach may be expected, on the average, to be consolidated by 24 to 30 months, with an occasional child failing to achieve such control by 3 years of age. Children whose control is delayed much beyond this usually represent special problems, arising from some of the sources mentioned above. Such a conclusion must be modified, however, according to the cultural background and ethnic derivation of the family.

A program of bowel training of this nature, recommended in an unevangelistic manner, fits the needs of many mothers. A certain group of mothers in contemporary Western society will feel the need, however, to train their infants earlier and more stringently. Such mothers may come from middle class socioeconomic brackets, where training for cleanliness still tends to be of more urgent significance, or may represent individuals with more intense preoccupation with bowel function and certain obsessive-compulsive trends, or those with strong needs to control their infants. Certain of these mothers may even incline, intellectually, to the more permissive approach. Thus they may, like other mothers in regard to breast feeding, develop strong feelings of guilt over their conflicting needs to conform at once both to the dictates of the experts and to the urging of their own impulses to "get the nasty business over with." Other mothers may be under pressure from grandparents or relatives in the home, or from other sources, including intrapsychic ones, to compete with siblings or neighbors in the achievement of early and scrupulous cleanliness in their infants.

For another group of mothers, also, the suggested program may be unsatisfying. These are the small group of mothers who intellectually subscribe to permissiveness but who actually are driven, by difficulties in handling their own aggressive drives, to the point where they are unable even to begin training. Their conscious fears of controlling or "harming" the infant (often contrasting with unconscious needs for strong control, of which they are afraid) may lead them to lean over backwards and almost seduce the infants into resisting the attainment of control. Such parents may repetitively find a "crisis," such as the impending birth of a sibling or a move to a new house, which leads them to postpone training longer and longer.

The above two extremes of attitudes among parents are cited in order to point up the need for an individualized approach to bowel training, similar to that for breast feeding or self-demand scheduling, which considers the needs of the parent as well as those of the infant. Mothers with strong needs for early training are frequently made more guilty by exhortations regarding later approaches, while those with overly or compulsively permissive trends may find ready justification for their own conflicts in such appeals.

It is thus wise, in well-baby care, to inquire first about the mother's attitudes and, indirectly at least, about the father's, toward bowel training. With this understanding at hand, certain deviations from what has been cited as the currently rational approach may be worked out in the framework of anticipatory guidance. A mother with intense needs for early training may at least be helped supportively to postpone her onslaught for a few months, even if her final approach is earlier than the recommended one, by the implied assurance that she will still be a good mother if her infant fails to gain control at the earliest possible point. Mothers with overly permissive attitudes may be helped to begin training by being given "permission" to train their infants, in the form of reassurance that some training will not harm their children by exerting some control. Such supportive techniques do not touch the deeper unconscious conflicts of such mothers. Nevertheless, some important preventive results may accrue, with the obviation of some battles over the early attainment of control on the one hand, and the avoidance of marked postponement of control on the other.

All of the above considerations are based on the premises that bowel dysfunction and personality disorder are not solely caused by early or coercive bowel training. A related premise deals with the fact that infants do not "train themselves," although many appear to do so by imitating older children and parents, or by responding to nonverbal cues arising from parental wishes, even if these latter may be unrecognized and strongly denied by the parent. The more flexible approach discussed can be of some preventive significance in this regard. At the same time, with this rationale, mothers will not be forced into a mold for which they are not ready, with the result, as Fries[62] has indicated, that they may continue with their previous patterns or may simply become more guilty, confused, and chaotic in their approach. A small group of parents, of course, will be unable to utilize such a framework in any fashion. In such instances, where serious bowel training problems arise, referral to a child guidance clinic, if acceptable to the parents, may be of preventive help.

Much of what has been said has application to bladder training as well. Bladder control seems to be attained later than bowel control, although the reasons for this are complex and unclear. Therefore, day-time training in this area may be wisely delayed until the later part of the second year or the beginning of the third. At this time the infant ordinarily has a bladder capacity enabling him to contain his urine for at least one to two hours, although there is considerable variation. If he is encouraged to sit for a few minutes on the potty seat every hour-and-a-half or so, the infant usually begins to associate the urge to urinate with the experience of "tinkling," or whatever the family word may be. Day-time control by this approach, exclusive of frequent "accidents" or regressive developments, may ordinarily be achieved by 30 to 36 months. Nighttime control usually appears by 3 years or $3\frac{1}{2}$, but may be delayed until 4 or $4\frac{1}{2}$ years, or according to Bakwin[63] even later in certain children with delayed maturational processes in regard to this function. Such an approximate figure is based on the assumption that strenuous efforts are not made to keep the child dry at night by picking him up several times. It is felt that such measures are not necessary for the ultimate attainment of control, though they may seem to be necessary for a mother's peace of mind and convenience.

It is obvious that the approach mentioned above involves a redefinition of the term enuresis, particularly of the nocturnal type, as it has been employed over the past 25 years. The time schedule mentioned obviously will not meet the needs of certain parents, and appropriate flexibility should wisely apply. As with bowel control, such considerations assume, on the basis of important evidence, that a battle regarding bladder training is less healthy than a more casual approach. Studies from many sources, among them those of Bostwick and Shackleton,[64] indicate that persistent enuresis has, as one of several causal influences, the background of premature or coercive training. It is recognized that many infants and young children will achieve bladder control long before the broad time limits mentioned. Such variations in rate of attainment of control relate to sex difference in some measure, with girls often achieving day- and night-time control before boys. Other individual variations in rate of neurophysiologic maturation and autonomic development are also subsumed under these considerations, as are the influences of differences in the gradient of emotional maturation and incidental physical illness or emotional crisis. Once again the factor of personality structure and training attitudes of the responsible parent enters the picture most importantly, as do certain predispositiona' factors of a more basically biological nature.

Discipline

From the previous remarks much of the proposed discussion of discipline can be anticipated. In this framework, the goal of discipline will be regarded as the ultimate achievement of self-control or "self-discipline" on the part of the older child or adolescent. Numerous swings in the pendulum of popular and professional opinion have occurred during the last 50 or more years, regarding the most effective parental methods of achieving such a goal. After oscillating violently from the "spare the rod and spoil the child" dictum of the Victorian era to the opposite pole of "encourage individual expression" of the progressive schools of 30 years ago, the indicator of current thinking about discipline has steadied itself somewhere between.

In Western society (and we cannot properly equate our complex urban civilization with more primitive societies, past or current), the infant does seem to need some limitations upon the expressions of his instinctual drives in order to become a social being, whether in regard to feeding flexibility or destructive tendencies. The important consideration would seem to be that such limitations be geared to the child's level of emotional and intellectual development, and to the parents' attitudes and inner needs for control.

In regard to the second year of life, such an approach can be spelled out in certain areas. Since the infant appears to be testing out his parents in search of limits within which to resolve his struggle between control of his own impulses and his desire to control his environment, specifically his parents, present day Western parents do need to work out some limits within which they can feel comfortable and confident. Perhaps the parents' confidence is more important than the specific details of such limits or their technical application. Some parents, for instance, cannot set important limits without spanking, while others, for personal and cultural reasons, do not feel comfortable with such a technique of control. Our current knowledge would indicate that for the 2 year old and indeed for children of any age, frequent and sadistic physical punishment may produce more rebellion, or unhealthily passive acquiescence, than temperate behavior on the part of the parent. Conversely, it is apparent that, in urban society at least, no limits at all and therefore no punishment may produce equally unhealthy results, with consequent anxiety, confusion, and guilt, and further testing out on the part of the infant or child who receives no consistent models of behavior from his parents. Certain parents, termed "compulsively permissive" by Senn,[65] may follow this pattern. Fortunately these two extremes, of overrestrictiveness and overpermissiveness, are the exception rather than the rule. Current research by Sears and other workers[66] indicates that different patterns of control may be characteristic of different sets of parents, and often of the same parents under differing circumstances, and thus no universal or absolute pattern of control can presently be achieved. The professional worker must rather help the individual parent come to terms with his or her individual child and with himself, with the help of the recognition that developmental phases do influence the types of results which can be anticipated.

For the infant in the second year, it has already been said that strongly punitive measures of control of aggressive-destructive tendencies may have little effect, except in the case of an exceedingly passive or apathetic child. At the same time some measure of control should wisely be exerted, particularly regarding potentially painful or serious situations, such as are represented by hot stoves, sharp knives, or wildly aggressive attacks on others. Most infants are made only more guilty and anxious, for example, by being permitted to pummel unmercifully an overpermissive parent. Firm removal from such situations, combined with a simple verbal admonition, such as, "We don't do that," or "That's sharp; Mummy doesn't want you to get hurt," usually is sufficient. Long explanations or discussions of complicated codes of honor alike are incomprehensible to the 2 year old. Parents need not be afraid to say "No" or to use sterner measures when indicated, however, in spite of the negativistic phase and its implications. The avoidance of an unprofitable struggle should not mean complete license for the infant nor abject submission on the part of the parent.

More will be said regarding discipline and its goal — self-discipline — as the discussion continues, in regard to specific phases. The point of view expressed here as representative of current professional thought can be summed up by the statement that older infants and young children need to know, and indeed want to know, what is allowed and what is not allowed. They appear to need at times, particularly in later stages, some appropriate punishment or deprivation for unacceptable behavior and some praise for reasonable conformity. Parents who are not confident in this regard can often be helped to clarify in their own minds what limits are important for their children and for themselves, as well as for society, thus achieving something more vital than the mere memorization of techniques of discipline, with which they may feel at odds. Although consistency and firmness should be the goals of such an approach, it should be clear that no parent can succeed in achieving absolute consistency or complete objectivity, nor need he feel that he should, in dealing with his children. Perhaps fortunately, parents can and need be neither scientists nor therapists while being parents.

Special Developmental Problems

During the second year the most prominent problems seem to arise from the impact upon the parents of the toddler's newfound autonomy. Most parents are able, with some effort, to retain their perspective until the appearance of a more secure sort of autonomy, involving less of a defensive struggle for internal and external control, which ordinarily takes place gradually during the third year. For some parents, however, the infant's increased ambivalence and his exhibition at times of naked aggression during this phase, may reawaken earlier problems related to their own control of aggressive drives. The cessation of continuingly positive feedback from the infant, as mentioned earlier, may complicate this situation, particularly for parents who have strong needs to be loved, to succeed, or to be depended upon, and who may interpret the infant's greater independence and negativism as a rejection of or implied reflection upon their capacities as parents. From these several sources one may see budding behavior problems, with greater and greater restrictiveness or, at the opposite pole, increasing permissiveness, or an alternation of the two, on the part of the parents, and an answering and further provoking rebelliousness on the part of the child. The tendency of one or both parents unconsciously to identify him with one of their own siblings, or other key figure, may of course complicate their approach, as may still other factors.

Here again our knowledge of and capacity to predict the eventual outcome of such a transactional struggle between child and parents (one or both, as the case may be) remains unsatisfyingly limited. Obviously the "activity type" of the child enters into the picture, both as a precipitating factor and as one of many determinants of the future course of events. Certain children may show consistent and continuing rebellious or submissive adaptive and behavioral responses to this developmental conflict. Others may change their patterns at 5 or 6 years, from earlier, more direct acting-out of affects related to aggressive drives, to passive, inhibited, and phobic or compulsive conformance, at times to a crippling degree. Although Sears' [66] interesting observations of children in standardized doll-play situations indicate the possibility of more universal responses of children to differing degrees of parental restrictiveness or punitiveness, we must at the present time content ourselves with the simple statement that parent-child and child-parent struggles for control at this stage may be important determinants of later disturbances in adaptation, however these may manifest themselves.

It should be mentioned that such struggles may begin diffusely, in relation to the control of growingly autonomous aggressive drives, or may begin more focally, in the areas of feeding, sleeping, or toilet training, or may spread from one to the others. Insufficient space is available for full discussion of these more localized areas of onset of struggle. As Sears and his associates[66] have indicated, coercive toilet training may be correlated with severe feeding problems, indicating either a spread of the struggle from toilet training to feeding areas of conflict or a rigidity of parental practices in both areas.

Sleeping problems are commonly seen during this phase. The 18 month old infant who leaves his bed 15 or 20 times before going to sleep is a familiar phenomenon. In many instances parents are able to recognize that this developmentally characteristic behavior is a kind of testing out, combined with a wish for social contact and often a fear of being alone, and are able gently, soothingly, but firmly to return the infant to his room. In some instances, however, a struggle for control ensues which continues for years, with the child finding all sorts of reasons not to go to sleep, based on his guilt over controlling the parents, over-stimulation from the parental attempts at control, as well as his need to continue testing them out for limits. Sleeping problems may of course result from true separation anxiety, from the onset of frightening dreams (which begin at times during this phase), or from the influence of physical illness.

Spock[67] and others have well discussed the management of such problems, and have suggested preventive approaches, based principally upon anticipatory guidance. When parents know in advance that sleep disturbances are apt to occur during this phase, they are ordinarily able to employ somewhat greater objectivity in dealing with them once they arise.

Various psychosomatic or psychophysiologic disturbances may have at least a portion of their roots in the second year. Constipation or diarrhea as well as other manifestations which do not become apparent until a later date, such as colitis, fecal soiling, and enuresis, may have had some of their foundations in the phase under discussion. As described earlier, multiple factors play a role in the genesis of these disorders. The developmental conflicts just mentioned, however, may be of significance in relation to points of fixation which may result, supporting later regression to this level.

Mention has been made of certain distortions in personality development which may date from this phase. These include certain obsessive-compulsive disorders, either in gross neurotic form or in the form of enhanced personality traits of meticulousness, overorderliness, overconformity, "stinginess," and others, including the respective opposites of these traits. Again the impact of controlling parental forces, often centering around toilet training, is only part of the picture. Nevertheless enough is known, at least regarding continuing struggle begun in this phase, to underwrite preventive efforts such as those described earlier.

In addition to the possible problems arising from struggles for control, a second set of deviations may result from disturbances in the infant's ego development. Obviously these two clusters of disturbance are inter-related. Although the differentiation of the self has by now proceeded to the point of vigorous autonomy, frequent regressive reactions of the infant's ego may be seen. Many of these appear to arise in response to separation from the mother, as involved in hospitalization of infant or mother, for example. At times, however, a severe depression or other disturbance in the emotional balance of the mother — or an answering response on her part to the father's disturbed adaptation — may produce a psychological rather than a physical separation between herself and the infant. Ordinarily these reversions on the part of the infant to greater dependence or his temporary losses of certain independent functions, such as the capacity for self-feeding, disappear as the separation ends. Much preventive help can be given to parents in understanding this fact. In rare instances, however, with certain infants predisposed by somatic or psychologic factors, this regression may proceed to the point of dis-solution of ego development, with a loss of the differentiation of the self and the capacity to test reality. Such a regression may persist in the form of a disturbed picture of psychotic degree.[68] In addition to other factors, such situations ordinarily involve a previous disturbance in the mother-infant relationship, which has interfered with normal ego differentiation though not completely prevented it.

Too much emphasis should not be placed on the immediately fore-going description of such deviations in ego development. Such cases are fortunately rare. Their occurrence, however, does give us some inkling, in a negative sense at least, of the importance of healthy ego development during this phase for later personality maturation. Anticipatory guidance may be of help, but in more flagrant instances early referral to a child guidance clinic may be of greatest effectiveness in preventing firmly fixed distortions in future personality development.

THE PRESCHOOL CHILD
DANE G. PRUGH

Fact Versus Fantasy

At the outset of the preschool age period, the young child has made tremendous strides toward the crystallization of an independent person-ality capable of considerable autonomous function. He has some capacity for control of his instinctual drives, for beginning communication of thoughts and feelings, and for the development of positive relationships. He has consolidated his basic motor skills to a considerable degree. Large-muscle movements still predominate, however, and fine coordinations of fingers, eyes, and cerebral cortex are just beginning to be possible. During the preschool period the "sense of initiative," as postulated by Erikson,[38] appears in full flower, although the capacity to carry through with projects undertaken is still limited.

By the middle of the third year, the child has ordinarily acquired enough mastery over his instinctual drives to permit a fair degree of control in the interest of obtaining the approval of his parents. Such mastery lies at first principally in the areas of some control of more primitive aggressive and destructive drives. Sphincter control, although in process, may not yet be fully established under the current toilet training approach, particularly in regard to urinary accidents during the day or wetting during the night. Thus, one can say that the child during the third year is taking sturdy steps toward the development of the reality principle, involving beginning capacities for postponement of immediate gratifications in favor of more long-term and socially acceptable goals of behavior. Hence, the relieved and pleased feeling parents often experience in facing the "sunny threes." Much unevenness of course still exists during the whole of the preschool period, with steps forward frequently followed by plateaus or regressions. It is easy for the most comfortable of parents to forget this tendency toward fluctuation in development and to feel puzzled, resentful, or guilty when regressions in particular occur.

As the age of 3 approaches, there is a gradual tendency for the child to conquer his negativism, and to operate in less ambivalent fashion. (Some ambivalence of course persists, in muted measure, for several years.) Thus it would appear that he gains greater freedom to use his energy for the development of intellectual capacities and for beginning creative outlets through play and the use of fantasy. The child's ability to share his possessions or the attention of an adult shows considerable increase through the third and fourth year, as does his interest in and capacity for group participation. Not many children are ready for nursery-school-type experience prior to 3 years, however, and a few may be unready until 4, particularly those who do not show the usual 3 year old's newfound (though still variable) capacity to separate from the mother without more than transient anxiety. This is not to indicate that every child needs nursery school, as some authorities have implied. For many children and parents, however, a nursery school can have important benefits in the direction of education in group participation.

Together with these evidences of augmented and more serenely autonomous ego capacities and functions goes a flowering of speech development. The ability to articulate more effectively and to employ symbolic expression of thought processes in words, and by 3 years in definite sentences, appears to parallel the ongoing myelination of the central nervous system (to be completed by the age of 6 years approximately) as well as the disappearance of primitive neuromuscular reflexes. Piaget's[69] basic studies of the language and thought of the child should be given first place in any discussion. Development of abstract thinking is beginning by the age of 3 or so. This does not ordinarily reach the maturity level necessary for reading word symbols and employing simple mathematical concepts, however, until the age 6 or, in some cases, 7 years. The capacity for learning is of course facilitated by other developmental steps, both in regard to the employment of memory and the acquisition of learning through imitation and play.

One of the most prominent features of the child's intellectual development during the preschool period is the appearance of the capacity for fantasy formation. This species-specific faculty is made possible by the continuous maturation of the central nervous system, particularly the cerebral cortex, with the concurrent appearance of symbolic thought processes. Thus is laid the groundwork for all future creative acts of imagination. Undoubtedly this capacity takes root during the period from 2 to 3 years. It bears fruit, however, in the 3 year old, whose extended flights of fancy are well-known to parents.

"And then I knocked him down, that big bird, and he knocked me up and then he flew up into the air and I kicked him into the sky, and he never came back." This brief excerpt from the associative verbal chains of fantasy of a normal 3 year old indicates, among other things, the limitations in logical processes of thought for this age group, particularly under the circumstances of play or some strong affective stimulus such as fear or anger. Piaget has termed this type of thought process "prelogical." Rational or logical processes, of course, are apparent under certain conditions, and become increasingly prominent and effective as the end of this period approaches.

The excerpt given also gives a hint of several other important characteristics of the mental and emotional life of the child of three or four. One of these has to do with the striking vividness of the fantasy itself. Children during this phase of development ordinarily are aware that they are "pretending" in developing such an imaginative flight. At times, however, this awareness may be lost temporarily. Such failure to distinguish fact from fantasy, or fantasy from reality, may occur at times of weakening of the child's ego, such as under conditions producing strong anxiety or during physical illness, when regression to an earlier level often occurs. At such times the child may react as if the fantasy were a fact. Witness the 3 year old who one day ran around his nursery school room attempting to frighten other children with the statement, "The big bad wolf is going to get you." After a time he became so convinced of the reality of this fantasy that he cowered in the corner, wailing, "The big bad wolf is going to get me."

From the quoted excerpt one also may apprehend another important aspect of the fantasy life of the child in this period. In the fantasy given, the child performs an impossible feat, that of kicking a huge bird into the sky, "and he never came back." The young child feels small and helpless at times in the face of the inevitable contrast between his own powers and those of the adults around him. It is of course true that at other times, during anxious moments, he gains comfort from this same power and strength of his parents. During the moments when he lets his fantasies free, however, he seems to gain a sense of exhilarating control over the forces which puzzle or frighten him, even to the point of imputing to himself a sort of unreal omnipotence. This fantasied omnipotence clearly serves a defensive or adaptive purpose, in the light of the above considerations. At the same time the child, like the little boy and the wolf, may at times become frightened of the consequences of much-longed-for omnipotence, especially when the line between fantasy and reality becomes more than ordinarily thin.

Still another characteristic mental process can be inferred from the above example. This process, embracing all the others so far described, is that of "magical thinking." This is a feature not only of the mental life of children but also, in a quite different framework, of primitive peoples, as in witchcraft, or of psychotic adults whose egos have, along certain planes, regressed to this early childhood level. This type of thought process, later brought under control by rational, judgmental functions of the ego, involves an underlying belief that, for good or ill, wishes will come true. Tied up in this process are the limitations in the time concept of the small child and the tendency to assume that events which follow each other are causally connected. Thus the 3 or 4 year old, under circumstances which further weaken his shaky ego capacities, may fear that his angry wish that a momentarily annoying sibling were dead may actually come true, especially if the sibling falls sick the next day. (The concept of death, until the 9th or 10th year, appears to involve a "going away" or separation, which may be a reversible process.)

One sees the positive side of such thinking, already under some conscious control, in the Santa Claus myth or the half-belief of the older child that fairies will put money under his pillow in place of a newly-lost tooth. The "magical" significance of words to the child (capitalized upon by medieval cabalistic practices) is also of pertinence, with the word standing so concretely for the symbol that the child may be afraid to say the word for fear the thought behind it may come true. In addition, the small child tends to attribute equal omnipotence and magical powers to the parent, and to fear that the parent can read his mind if he has a bad thought. Associated types of animistic thinking in the small child are familiar to adults, who actively pretend to endow animals and objects with life, thought, and words in stories and fables.

Before leaving this topic a word should be said regarding the carry-over into the preschool years of certain aspects of earlier stages of development. In the fantasy life of the preschool child one can see many things, including certain manifestations of thought processes which were discussed earlier. For example, ambivalence can be clearly perceived in the words of the emotionally healthy 3 year old who says to his mother, in time of anger, "I love you and I hate you." Certain apparent derivatives of the incorporative tendencies of the very young infant, discussed in relation to feeding in the undifferentiated phase, can also be identified. For example, the child of 3½ or 4 may often remark to his mother, "I love you so much I could eat you up," an expression which of course may have been used playfully by the mother herself. At times of anger, the expression by the child may rather be, "I hate you, and I hope a big bad wolf eats you up."

Such examples of apparent oral intrapsychic foundations to fantasy formation can be supplemented by instances of seeming anal derivation. These latter are less socially acceptable in Western society. Many are the parents, however, who have been shocked by occasional conversational attempts of the 3 year old, when visitors are present, to the effect that, for example, "I just made a duty as big as a house." Other examples of this continuing interest in anal functions can be found in the "bathroom talk" of many 3 and 4 year olds of both sexes. Again such carry-overs are important principally in regard to later regressive phenomena, since most children repress such thoughts at a later point.

One should not close this discussion of fantasy in the preschool child without reemphasizing its adaptive character, and its importance as the basic stuff of later creative and artistic modes of expression. The child is of course examining all the while, with insatiable curiosity, the phenomena of nature and the world of adults. By giving his fantasy free rein in the process of play and make-believe, he seems to prepare himself for later enjoyment of an artistic nature. Play seems to embrace also the functions of the discharging of certain tensions, the unconscious mastery of anxieties or fears, through activities with special psychological significance. A number of defense mechanisms, to be discussed shortly, appear to be involved in this universal characteristic of child behavior.

Instinctual Drives

During the preschool years important changes take place in the balance of the instinctual impulses with which the child must deal. Individual variations in the strength of instinctual pressures of course occur. These variations, together with the strength of the child's ego, his past experiences and behavior patterns, his specific level of emotional and intellectual development, the degree and nature of current pressures upon his ego from parents and society in the direction of control of the impulses, as well as permission or stimulation in the direction of lack of control, and other factors, determine the success he can achieve in arriving at a comfortable and effective way of dealing with such impulses.

Aggressive drives will be dealt with briefly. The child of $2\frac{1}{2}$ to 3 often shows sadistic, destructive, and negativistic tendencies frustratingly similar to the 2 year old infant's, in the framework of continuingly unrealistic drives toward autonomy and independence. Around 3 years, however, as mentioned earlier, these derivatives of aggressive drives and their associated affects appear to come under greater control. At times, this control is exceedingly shaky, and appears to be reinforced by extremely rigid, sometimes ritualized and rather compulsive patterns of "good" behavior, particularly regarding cleanliness. Some authorities have related this "normal" compulsiveness of the 3 year old to a type of overcompensation for and holding in check of the previously manifest impulses to soil, wet, smear, destroy, and hurt, the impulses which are so prominent during the phase when toilet training and initial conflict with parental discipline are taking place.

During the third and early part of the fourth year, aggressive drives of a more basically constructive nature tend to predominate. Strong outbursts of destructive or sadistic tendencies do tend to occur at times, directed toward "bad" objects, toward other children who possess fascinating objects and fail to relinquish them, or who attack in their turn, or toward loved parents. Gradually, as inner ego controls are consolidated, these outbursts tend to become more isolated and to take the form of temper tantrums, which of course were present earlier also, rather than hostile attack or destruction. During the fourth and early part of the fifth year, "bossiness" or demanding behavior often appears, if it has not earlier in milder degree, indicating a trend toward more socially acceptable attempts to control others. By 6 years aggressive drives of destructive or sadistic nature have ordinarily been handled by other mechanisms, and are most easily channelled into avenues of expression acceptable to the peer group, including pushing, poking, tickling, and verbal methods of provocation. Direct attack by a younger sibling will still of course provoke physical retaliation in the average child.

It should be mentioned that some difference in aggressive behavior between the sexes usually becomes manifest by the fourth or fifth year, and at times earlier. Boys appear to be slightly more active and aggressive than girls from early infancy on, according to some studies.[54] This difference, if valid, is slight, and may not be manifest in individual cases. With the laying down of beginning identifications, roughly between 4 and 6 years, however, boys in Western society frequently develop a tendency to show off their strength and physical prowess, to want to "box with daddy," and to declaim loudly that they are "big and tough." This is ordinarily not yet the self-disciplined and thorough acting out of roles of cowboy, cop, or robber which features the early part of the school age phase. Although these roles are taken, with much bravado, by 4 or 5 year old boys, they give evidence of unevenness and uncertainty behind the "tough" facade, indicating the struggle to overcome the still unmastered feelings of smallness and ineffectualness.

During this period girls ordinarily are quieter, with rapid development of interests along feminine lines, amounting at times to coyness and exaggeration of feminine behavior. This is a relative statement, of course, which frequently does not hold, particularly among groups of girls. Certain girls, for reasons to be discussed, resist beginning feminization and persist in the direction of future tomboy roles. The sex differences in behavior, many of which probably have cultural rather than biological roots, reach a peak after 6 years.

The most prominent change in the balance of instinctual forces has to do with the enhancement of sexual drives during this phase. For a variety of reasons, some biological, some psychological, masturbation begins to appear more frequently and intensely than before in children of 3 and 4 years. This usually occurs about the time finger- or thumbsucking is given up, and appears to represent a self-gratificatory or autoerotic mechanism. These manifestations led Freud to call the period roughly from 3 to 5 the "phallic" phase of psychosexual development. Earlier, in line with his advancing powers of observation, the 2 and 3 year old child ordinarily develops a growing awareness of the anatomical differences between boys and girls. The curiosity in this area often begins to be verbalized at least by 3 or $3\frac{1}{2}$, appearing earlier in some children. The natural question, often asked by both boys and girls regarding the genitals, is, "Why don't girls have a pee-pee too?" Many boys and some girls tend to conclude with preschool pre-logic, that something happened to the girl's genitals to remove a former penis or to place it inside. Girls often openly express a wish for a penis. They are usually comforted by the knowledge that girls can grow up to be mothers and have babies — a knowledge which for a time may make some boys quite jealous.

The origin of babies is of course another topic of interest and often confusion to the younger preschool child. The 3 year old ordinarily is capable of noticing the increase in size of the abdomen of his mother or one of her friends during pregnancy. His natural hypothesis, on learning that the baby is "in there," is to assume that he, or the "seed," got in through something the mother ate and that the baby will get out through the anus or a sort of cloacal opening. He struggles, with the help of his parents, to grasp the meaning of this new concept, just as he struggles with other equally obscure concepts.

Space does not permit any significant discussion of sex education. Spock,[23] Strain,[70] Levine and Seligman,[71] and many others have done so with wisdom and sensitivity. Suffice it to say that this is ordinarily best done within the family by the parents, and is most wisely carried out in response to the spontaneous questions of the child. The timing and the assimilable amount of information are of chief significance. Information is wisely geared to the level of the child's understanding and given in no greater detail and completeness than the child seems to require. An illustrated lecture will often confuse more than it may inform, and it is possible to overeducate a child when he is not actually ready or searching for such help. This latter point is not infrequently left out of discussions of the topic in the literature available to parents. Occasionally, discussion of sexual matters with a child by a professional person may be indicated, depending upon the family's religious beliefs, in the event that parents feel too inhibited or anxious to respond comfortably to their children's question, which of course may be slow to arise under such circumstances.

When Freud [34] pointed out the important role in the development of neuroses played by distortions in psychosexual development, many persons interpreted his remarks, or interpolations of them, to mean that children should be permitted completely uninhibited expression of their sexual drives. Others of course rejected the whole of Freud's work because of their mistaken impression that he felt that adult genital sexuality was the only motivating force available to man. Actually Freud meant to imply neither of these things.

Most professional people today, with varying psychodynamic viewpoints, feel that the child in most segments of North American society needs help in controlling his impulses to "peep" at children or adults, to masturbate openly and at times provocatively, to exhibit his body, and to "experiment" with other children. The current viewpoint simply suggests that limitations upon such natural and inevitable tendencies in small children should not be set in such a punitive or threatening fashion that the child is either drawn irresistibly and rebelliously to this "forbidden" topic, highly charged in our society, or is made overanxious as the result of unsubstantiated threats that masturbation will drive him or her crazy or, in the case of a boy, that the doctor will have to "cut it off" if he persists. It is now recognized that too much "natural" exhibition of the body and the genitals, particularly in regard to parents and children of the opposite sex, may be sexually overstimulating and even seductive in its effects upon the child in our society, although this may not be true in a less highly urbanized and Westernized setting. Letting the child see and handle the parents' genitals in order to foster educational processes, as some sincere but compulsively permissive parents have done, can arouse as much anxiety, guilt, and confusion as would an overly prudish or restrictive approach. If a child of 4 or 5 masturbates at night, it is probably best to ignore this. If he masturbates at times in the living room it may help to let him know, without punishment or perturbation (if this is possible for the parent) that such is not done publicly. Again the challenge is one of providing firm and reasonable limits for the child within the framework of understanding and awareness.

One important development during this phase remains to be discussed in regard to sexual strivings. This has to do with the child's increasing awareness, between the ages of 4 and 6 on the average, of himself or herself with a definite role, that of a boy or a girl, together with the realization that this role has certain connotations in our society. With increasing knowledge of sex differences, the boy begins to understand that he is "made" like his father and that he will become a daddy and marry a woman, the sequence here being not always accurate. One of his first thoughts, frequently expressed, is that he would like to marry mommy, since she is the important woman in his life at this point. This wish is eventually given up in civilized and even in most primitive societies. Nevertheless the relationship with the mother forms the prototype for later relationships with members of the opposite sex. Along with this new feeling comes of course the realistic awareness that he cannot marry his mother because daddy is married to her. The boy may become resentful or jealous toward his father for spending so much time with mother, and may fear, in connection with the magical thinking already described, that his father knows what he is thinking and may punish him. His rich fantasy life may lead him to refer such fantasied punishment to various parts of his body. Since the child already tends to link the genitals with having a baby, the prerogative of married couples, and since the sensations produced in his genitals during masturbation may now evoke vaguely disturbing or exciting fantasies, it is easy for the boy to fear that something may happen to his penis, as might have happened to his sister — that this organ might disappear or perhaps not grow so that he would become a big man like his father. Previous specific threats by the father or mother to harm the penis because of masturbation are much more rare today than a generation ago, but the combination of circumstances described above is usually sufficient to produce a vague fear of damage to the genitals, experienced in the fashion mentioned.

For the girl a fairly converse set of events appears to take place in regard to the mother as the rival for the affections of the father. Obviously fears of damage to the genitals are not involved in the same sense, but the girl may feel that something has happened already to her to make her different from the boy.

The psychological constellation just discussed centers around the Oedipus complex, about which much controversy has raged since the time when it was described by Freud. Over the years, direct observations of children by child analysts, child psychiatrists, psychologists, pediatricians, teachers, and nurses, have confirmed most of the facts set forth. When one hears a well-adjusted though momentarily angry boy of $4\frac{1}{2}$ say to his father, "Just wait until I'm big and you're little and I'll have mommy all to myself," it is difficult to interpret this statement in any other framework. It is equally difficult when a basically happy and outgoing 3 year old says to his father, while comparing the size of his penis to his father's, "Daddies don't let little boys' pee-pees get bigger." In neither of these instances had consciously verbalized threats of any kind been made.

As has been implied, data of this type have been collected from many emotionally healthy children, as well as the disturbed persons from which the original formulations arose. It is true that much further study remains to be carried out, in many directions. It is also true that anthropologists[72] have pointed out that children in other societies may not undergo an exactly similar process, particularly in circumstances where family structure is radically different and where sexual matters are not so highly charged emotionally. Nevertheless, the formulation can be said to be fairly well documented at the present time, as far as Western society is concerned.

The basic point remaining at issue is the significance of this phenomenon. Here perspective must again be employed. Current studies indicate that most children spontaneously resolve the Oedipus complex successfully, with boy and girl identifying positively with father and mother and ultimately seeking love objects in the opposite sex. Only under unhealthy circumstances do the aforementioned fears become pathological. Also, after the fourth or fifth year, the associated fantasies seem to be repressed from awareness and rarely again become conscious. Contrary to many impressions, the child of this age does not experience genital sexual strivings in the same fashion as do adults. In this discussion it is not meant to imply that these emotional developments are the only significant ones during the preschool period. Others, relating to social activities, the development of initiative, and the satisfactions of the learning experience, are of course of vital import.

The significance of these emotional phenomena lies, among other things, in their formative influence upon later relationships with the opposite sex. The boy needs to feel loved and admired by his mother, as does the girl by her father. Both boys and girls frequently, though not invariably, seem to carry over patterns of relationship with members of the opposite sex from the model available to them at this period. Here exceptions of course occur, since later changes in the quality of relationships with parents, in the direction of more positive satisfactions, may well nullify to a great extent the possible effects of unsatisfying or unhealthy ones during this period. Where predisposing factors exist, however, events of a disturbing nature, occurring during this period, may arouse anxiety to the point where emotional decompensation may occur, with the development of pathological results from the conflicts and fears described. More specific examples of such potential influences will be given in the discussion of special problems of this period.

For professional personnel it is important to recognize that the period from 4 to 6 is an influential one, and that deviations in emotional development of a neurotic nature may derive from it. From a preventive point of view it is rarely necessary or wise to discuss the details of this period directly with parents. Parents may be helped, however, by the knowledge that an otherwise well-adjusted boy who is constantly challenging his father is going through a phase where he is trying very hard, in a still uncertain way, to act like a man. The converse may be true for the girl. Similarly, parents can utilize the knowledge that it is in general unwise to let children of this age sleep with the parents, since this experience may be too stimulating. One must remember, with humility, however, that many families in low income brackets, living in large cities, have no alternative to this practice. The constructive handling of overanxious or overpunitive attitudes toward the increased masturbation of this phase, and other approaches, may also be wisely derived from these considerations.

Sibling Relations and the Family

With the trend over the past 50 years toward smaller families, at least in the middle income bracket, many children do not experience the birth of a sibling until at least the age of 2. In families where births can be planned, there is some growing recognition that the impact of a new sibling upon the infant between 1 and 2 years of age, who is still a baby in some respects, may at times, though not invariably, be difficult for the infant and the parents to handle comfortably.

Much has been written and more has been said regarding the young child's reaction to the birth of a sibling. Many observers have commented upon the jealousy and rivalry which characterize this response. Such feelings may be exhibited openly, through direct attacks upon the infant, physical or verbal in nature. They may also be covert and indirect in nature, as in the case of the apparently loving child of $2\frac{1}{2}$ or 3 years who hugs his baby brother too tightly or who accidentally knocks the bottle out of the slightly older baby's mouth while "just looking at him." Regressive phenomena may also occur. The 3 year old who begins to wet the bed again, who sucks his thumb vigorously and frequently, becomes more demanding, and smears his food "like a baby," is well-known, as is the $1\frac{1}{2}$ year old who either openly asks for a bottle again or temporarily refuses to drink from a cup. Jealous or hostile feelings may also be displaced onto other objects, such as animals, and the cat or dog may suffer for a time.

Fortunately, most of the emotional and behavioral responses just mentioned are temporary and transient. The emotionally healthy child can usually take a sibling in stride, unless other circumstances or crises complicate the relationship. It must not be forgotten, in the urge to minimize the impact of such an experience upon the young child, that importantly positive results accrue to the child who has siblings, whom he can grow to love and with whom he can learn to share experiences as well as possessions, and more basically, his parents' affections. This is not to say that only children are sweepingly penalized by the absence of siblings, and therefore will necessarily be "spoiled" or disturbed. Again the relations within the family remain of paramount significance, and the reason for having only one child may be outside the parents' control rather than a reflection of a parental problem. The birth of a sibling may be disturbing, but it also may function as a stimulus toward emotional growth.

Perhaps one could sum up these reflections by saying that the feelings of children toward their siblings are like all other human relations, tinged with ambivalence. One may wisely try to help parents deal constructively with the negative side of this ambivalence on the part of their small children. Thus parents can helpfully prepare the 2 or 3 year old, as much as is possible, for the coming birth of a sibling. They can also feel free to permit the child to express verbally some jealousy and resentment toward the new baby, if their personalities can tolerate this, rather than strongly urging him to inhibit or suppress such affects and run the chance of these affects breaking through in more indirect and less healthy ways. In addition they can recognize regressive manifestations as understandable and temporary phenomena. With such a point of view, they can avoid feeling that these frequently associated changes in their small child's behavior are their "fault" or the child's and can give him some added satisfactions for a time, gradually weaning him back to his previous level of adjustment. Such approaches have been demonstrated to have preventive value, as opposed to more restrictive techniques or simply ignoring the child's behavior and its meaning.

The caution to be expressed here has to do with the danger of over-concentrating upon the negative feelings, and striving too hard to cushion the impact of such an experience for the small child. Some parents, for example, have sincerely but misguidedly tried so hard to protect the emotional security of the older child, by giving him a great deal of attention, many gifts, etc., that the interests of the new baby may be almost neglected. The older child may actually feel guilty in such a situation, or may respond to overpermissiveness and tacit encouragement to express hostile affects toward the new claimant to the parental affections with the development of anxiety and guilt, with resultant effects upon his behavior similar to those which are supposedly being warded off. Certain parents have been known to "prepare" a child, in a burst of preventive enthusiasm, shortly after the mother has missed her first period. Here the limitation in the time concept of the preschool child is a serious obstacle to balanced anticipation over so many months, and tension may build up to peak levels in the interim. Answering the child's questions about enlargement of the abdomen, giving answers only at the pace at which the child is prepared to move, probably represents a sounder approach.

Perhaps the important point, in this context and others, is that parents who are eager to promote their children's emotional as well as physical growth and maturation should not need to feel that they must be therapists as well as parents. Here considerations apply which are similar to those discussed in relation to discipline. Certain parents, for instance, will not feel comfortable with the approach suggested above. They may be comfortable only with the limited knowledge that it is wise to allow the child some feeling of participation in the care of the infant, without giving a very young child a chance to hold and drop the baby, thus producing guilt, but also without so overprotecting the baby that the older child is afraid even to look at him. At any rate, the personality structures of the parents and their approach to child rearing should be considered in regard to the type of anticipatory guidance which may be employed.

One other set of thoughts regarding family relations remains to be developed at this point. The preschool child begins gradually to develop a concept of social differentiation, and to see his parents, his siblings, and himself in particular roles within the family. It has been pointed out previously that the role the individual child will fulfill is to some extent determined by the attitudes and psychological orientation of the parents during the prenatal and early neonatal periods. This refers to the tendency of parents to see the infant and young child as resembling, in appearance or, more importantly, in behavior, some earlier key figure in their lives — a father, a sibling, a mother, etc. This identification of the child with a significant person, who may also be the parent himself as a child, or may represent the "bad" or "good" part of himself, may complicate the parent's own identification with his own parents, thus affecting his role as a parent. The transactional relationship between the child and parents — and between the parents themselves, as well as other siblings — may thus depend upon the current balance of identifications, usually unconscious, in addition to such forces as the activity patterns of the child at different levels of development, and intercurrent forces such as illness or economic crisis. Most parents, fortunately, are gradually able to resolve these early identifications of the child with themselves or someone else, to the point where they are able to perceive him as a separate and unique personality and to meet his individual needs.

The point to be made here is that the balance which a particular family achieves in regard to the multiple interpersonal relations operating within it may change from time to time, at different points in the development of one or another child. Intrapsychic factors, as well as external sociocultural or economic forces, may also play a role in these shifts in dynamic family balance. Thus the child's developing concept of his mother as "the one who takes care of you" and of his father as "the one who earns the money" may be altered in times of family crisis. Although such shifts may not interfere with the child's basic sexual identifications, they may result in fluctuations in the degree of satisfaction of his needs, or in alterations in his role within the family. If the father, through economic dislocation, for example, becomes the "one who takes care of you," while the mother earns the money, the child's concept of roles must necessarily be adapted, at least temporarily, to this shift. If a sibling becomes ill, the balance of gratifications from the mother ordinarily is altered to some degree, as it is if the mother becomes seriously depressed and unable to meet the family's needs. In the latter instance the child's own role may shift, particularly if a harassed father must find substitute gratifications from the child in the face of the wife's inability to give emotionally to husband or child. The child may thus find himself forced to give more gratification than he receives, although naturally of a different sort, at a developmental stage when his needs for support may be particularly intense. He may instead find himself put into the role of a sibling of the father or of the mother, or perhaps may become a scapegoat for displaced tensions. If his behavior changes because of certain types of illness or emotional disturbance, he may, in families of certain ethnic backgrounds, find himself "isolated" from the rest of the family. Thus shifts in parent-child transactional relationships, involving fluctuations in emotional feedback, may result from alteration in family balance. No discussion can be included here regarding the important sociologic concept of the roles of the sick person and those who interact with him in Western society, upon which Parsons[73] has cogently commented.

It is impossible to do more than sketch the outlines of this important area. For one thing, our understanding of those complicated and multi-determined processes is extremely limited at this point. Lindemann[74] and others have contributed important insights into the interpersonal "epidemiologic" forces involved. Much significant research is now going forward, by Caplan[75] and other workers, who have been interested in the positive forces which hold families together in a healthy state of balance, as well as the factors which operate to produce pathological crisis situations. Our grasp of these concepts remains tenuous, particularly as regards the sociocultural forces which play upon the family and their influence upon family balance, as well as upon individual behavior. Social and behavioral scientists have become interested in this area in recent years, often working with representatives of a number of disciplines. Multidisciplinary research of this kind is necessarily a slow and painstaking process, however, and much initial experiment and practice in interdisciplinary communication by such research teams is necessary before fruitful results may accrue, as they are now beginning to do.

For the professional worker the significance of this elusive concept of family balance lies in the resulting awareness of the fluctuating needs of other family members as well as of the child. Caplan[76] and his associates are at present working on the development of preventive techniques which may be employed for such family members in times of crisis, in order to preserve a healthy state of family equilibrium.

Adaptive Mechanisms

At a number of points in the discussion of the preschool child, mention has been made of various mechanisms of an adaptive or defensive nature which have become available to him in the course of developmental strides. These will be only briefly summarized, since a thorough discussion would require the production of a textbook of psychiatry.

By the age of 6 years the child has at his disposal most of the mechanisms employed by the adult. Piecemeal descriptions have already been given of the child's growing capacity for ego functioning in the interests of testing reality, the development of a self-concept, dealing constructively with tensions, controlling inner drives, postponing gratifications in the service of the reality principle, as well as the development of sound autonomy, initiative, beginning intellectual growth and rational judgment, and the acquisition of new skills, and outlets for tensions. It has been pointed out that the child's ego possesses, even before the preschool period, certain primitive defenses such as *acting out* of affects, *denial,* *inhibition,* and *projection,* in addition to such basic ego mechanisms as *regression,* and *depression,* for dealing with anxiety of potentially dis-ruptive nature. Other mechanisms available to the preschool child in-clude *identification,* which has been discussed, *compliance,* the *discharge* of tension through certain bodily functions, *displacement* of affect onto other persons or objects, *overcompensation, withdrawal* of affect (often resulting in the use of fantasy as a substitute gratification), *turning-inward* of hostile affects (particularly those involving a kind of self-punishment, where appropriate, rather than an open expression or acting out of such affects), and a number of others.

All the above mechanisms subserve the socially necessary process of the civilization of the child, as well as the goal of the achievement of the dynamic steady state. Perhaps the central mechanism in this stage is that of *repression.* This has been mentioned before as beginning during the second or third year. The capacity automatically and unconsciously to exclude painful or unacceptable affects or drives from conscious aware-ness, however, gradually increases in strength and effectiveness by the age of 6, to the point where many of the feelings, with associated thoughts or fantasies, which are experienced prior to this point, are more or less permanently lost from awareness. This is the "infantile amnesia" described by Freud.[34] Without repression, assisted and supported by many of the other defenses mentioned, there would be no civilization. Everyone would be completely aware of instinctual impulses of a sexual or aggressive nature and the associated affects, and the acting out of such impulses would take place freely and of course destructively for man and society.

The mechanism of repression involves a related concept, or rather a psychological dimension of the ego. This has to do with the conscious/unconscious dichotomy. The human capacity to keep certain intense, primitive, and often antisocial drives, memories, or affects in a state of exclusion from awareness serves an eminently adaptive goal, in the teleo-logical framework described. Some of these may be less firmly repressed, remaining just below awareness at a "preconscious" level, where they may be available to consciousness at appropriate times. At times of intense conflict or illness, the consequent weakening of the ego and its repressive capacities may permit even more deeply unconscious material to ap-proach consciousness. A normal manifestation of this nature is seen in the fantasies and often distorted but forgotten memories which are found in dreams. In the waking state, the ego attempts first consciously to sup-press and then unconsciously to repress such thoughts, and in the struggle much energy is expended. An increase in the pressure of instinctual drives as a result of developmental changes, as for example in relation to in-creased masturbation, or an unhealthy degree of repression, such as may result from overstrenuous or developmentally inappropriate parental urg-ing for conformity or the control of instinctual drives, may produce somewhat similar results. At such times, other mechanisms such as displacement, denial, or projection may be employed by the ego in an attempt to reinforce its wavering repressive capacities.

One more mechanism bears brief mention. This is the mechanism of *avoidance,* on which phobias are based. The significance of phobias as neurotic symptoms will be discussed in the school age section, along with other advanced neurotic and pathologic states. In this section phobia is mentioned only to point out its relative frequency of occurrence and its generally normative character in the latter part of the preschool phase. The discussion of a phobia is predicated upon the concept of an unconscious dimension to the ego, since the content of phobias is usually unrealistic and superficially inappropriate. Certain childish fears of butterflies, handkerchiefs, clouds, and other such truly harmless objects are understandable only on the assumption that affects from other areas of conflict *are displaced* onto the phobic object. It is true that Jersild [77] has reported that fears of all kinds, including dangerous wild animals (most of which are seen only in picture books) reach their peak of incidence and intensity around the ages of 4 to 6, when children are more aware of potentialities of danger. Nevertheless, other mechanisms appear to be involved, and will be summarized, in relation to the Oedipus complex mentioned earlier.

In the process of struggling with his feelings of rivalry with the parents of the same sex, the 4 and 5 year old child apparently "uses," in a teleological sense, phobic mechanisms. Hostile feelings toward a parent are painful and arouse anxiety. In order to handle these more comfortably, the preschool child tends automatically and unconsciously to displace these feelings onto some other object, dealing with them "at arm's length," as it were. Fear of a horse, bear, or dog is more acceptable to a boy than fear of his father, with his fantasied omnipotence and possible retaliation. With the displacement, the mechanism of projection results in the child's attributing the unacceptable feeling of anger to the animal, who "may be angry" and thus may bite or hurt. Through consequent "avoidance" of the animal, and the unconscious feelings stirred up thereby, the child's ego appears to be less in danger of disruption or decompensation by anxiety than would be the case if the original affect were experienced directly and consciously.

Phobias of this nature have been reported as early as the second year. Occurrence in mild and transient form, involving a few weeks or several months, is so common during the latter preschool period that Freud termed it the "normal neurosis" of childhood. Not all phobias are based on the process described, and not all involve animals. Some have to do with fears of death, of being left alone, of the ending of the world, or of rain or lightning. Sometimes the phobic avoidance itself is not seen, but a type of counter-phobic behavior is apparent. This involves attempts by the child to overcome unconscious fears by, for example, climbing to high places, or frequently seeking out animals and daring them to bite or injure him.

It should be reemphasized that all the defense mechanisms or ego reactions discussed appear to have a basically adaptive character and goal. Some counter-phobic behavior is an important ingredient of emotional health, for example, just as the phobic pattern indicates a constructive working through toward a successful solution of a developmental conflict. Most of these mechanisms may be employed too strenuously at times, however, and when this is so in marked degree may come to represent symptoms of impending or actual emotional decompensation.

One last aspect of ego functioning remains to be considered in connection with the topic just presented. During the latter part of the preschool phase, conscience or superego formation is proceeding slowly but effectively. This development completes the structure of the somewhat metaphorically-termed mental apparatus. With his greater capacities for reality testing, for postponement of gratification, for control of instinctual impulses, and for learning, the 5 and 6 year old child is better able to internalize the standards of his parents, their admonitions as well as prohibitions. He does this with the help of identification and other mechanisms, more or less incorporating certain facets of the parents' personalities into his own set of mental representations, tied up with his image of himself. He also seems to develop more fully the concept of an ideal model, initially the parent of the same sex, although later other figures are taken over. With this intrapsychic equipment, largely unconscious, the child can grow emotionally in a positive sense, based on the identifications and ego ideals available to him, rather than on the basis of the negative affects of guilt or shame in the face of punishment or loss of love, which have largely guided him up to this point.

Some of the immediately foregoing discussion leaps ahead of the preschool phase. It is not meant to imply that the child of even 5 years has consolidated his internal standards of behavior. An inner struggle in the direction of such consolidation, reflected by other fluctuations in behavior, goes on through at least the first half of the school age period, reinforced but at times opposed by the standards of the child's peer group. The beginning development of such internal standards and identifications, however, represent the principal way in which the child resolves some of the aforementioned rivalry with the parent of the same sex. Such positive consolidations of standards reinforce negative, increasingly internalized prohibitions and the forces of repression in gaining control of current impulses and affects and in later molding of ethical concepts and relationships toward the opposite sex.

Special Developmental Problems

A number of deviations in emotional development have been indicated, explicitly or implicitly, throughout this presentation of the preschool phase. Mention has been made of failures in the resolution of the symbiotic equilibrium between parent and child within the broader framework of the family dynamic balance. These may produce various repercussions, ranging from interference with autonomous ego development to a tendency on the part of the parent to infantilize the child. In the latter instance various manifestations of delayed emotional and behavioral development may be seen, from infantile speech to overdependence and passivity. Certain psychosomatic disorders seem to have at least some of their roots in the early part of this process. These disorders include soiling, certain types of colitis, enuresis, asthma, and other conditions in which a psychophysiologic component may be operative. Obviously, somatic predisposing forces are involved in most of these disorders, and regression, in the sense employed earlier, usually appears implicated. Fixation in emotional development at earlier levels is often a part of the picture, with regression taking place, at times of conflict, to the point of fixation, derived either from periods of insufficient emotional satisfaction or of over-gratification.

During the third and fourth years separation anxiety still is apparent. The possibility of emotionally traumatic experience centering around separation has been mentioned as only one of a number of determinants of later disturbed behavior. Illness and hospitalization represent one such potentially disturbing experience. As Levy,[78] Jessner and Kaplan,[79] Prugh and his associates[80] and Robertson,[81] among others, have pointed out, the child of three years and under seems most susceptible to the effects of separation from his parents, as does the previously disturbed child. During or following hospitalization the young child often shows regressive manifestations. These may include loss of bowel and bladder control, enhanced need for the oral autoerotic gratification of thumb- or finger-sucking, increasing demands, negativism, and other phenomena already described under this heading. Manifestations of anxiety may also be seen, particularly over subsequent separation from the mother, but also involved in nightmares, fears (of physicians, white beds, etc.), or more straightforwardly phobic responses. The child of 2 through 3 is less able to test the reality of the separation or the necessary treatment, and his capacity for fantasy may lead to the fear that the mother has deserted him, or has left him in the hospital because he was "bad." Here magical thinking and other mechanisms are involved.

For the child from 4 to 6 separation anxiety may also be involved, and regressive phenomena may be present. More prominent, however, are fears of bodily mutilation, of "having my leg cut off" when an operation for removal of a bony tumor of the leg is scheduled for a boy of 4 for example. Again magical thinking and fears of retaliation for guilt-producing past transgressions are prominent. A boy who feared his leg would be cut off later revealed his related feeling that this would occur in punishment for his having kicked his smaller brother with the leg in question. The relationship to the conflicts of the Oedipus period, with fears of punishment for unacceptable thoughts or feelings, is also clear.

More important than unhealthy reactions in the hospital are the post-hospitalization continuations of regressive or anxiety phenomena. Robertson,[81] Prugh,[82] and others have pointed out the frequency with which such changes in the behavior of the child alter the parent-child relationship. The tendency of many parents to personalize the responsibility for the child's illness is also involved. As is well known, parents often blame themselves, or, if guilt is too strong, project this blame onto the doctors or the child himself, often in most unrealistic fashion. As a result, changes in the child's behavior may be seen by them to be a result of either the hospitalization experience or the illness itself, or both, and they may try to make it up to the child in an anxious, overprotective fashion or may feel the need to push the child back to his previous behavior in a restrictive fashion, in order to lessen their own anxiety and guilt. Consequently, neurotic illness or behavior disorders may be precipitated in this setting, with all the evident reverberations in the family homeostatic equilibrium.

In this discussion little more can be said regarding the deviations in emotional development which may result from acute or chronic illness and hospitalization. Barker, Gonick, and Wright,[83] together with others, have well summarized this area. It should be stated emphatically, however, that not all experience with illness, hospitalization, or operation, is inevitably emotionally traumatic for the child or parents. The same is true for other instances of separation, or for such potentially disturbing experience as the death of a parent. These experiences certainly pose rigorous challenges for the child and family, and it is very meet and right that preventive efforts be expended. These may include, if possible, preparation of the child for the coming experience, the provision of regular visiting opportunities by the parents, the assignment, where possible, of one nurse and/or one physician to develop a continuing and supportive parent-substitute relationship for a very young or very anxious child, the provision on the ward of adequate play outlets and group experience for the release of tensions, and the opportunity to verbalize, with nurses or physicians, fears or misconceptions regarding treatment, and other measures. Among these may be the important help which parents may derive from the anticipatory awareness of the frequency of regressive phenomena of a temporary nature following discharge, and the positive effect of permitting the child greater regressive satisfactions for a time, followed by gradual weaning back to previous levels of adjustment. The preventive value of such approaches has been demonstrated by several studies.[84, 80] Other workers have indicated the preventive significance of special measures for children undergoing operations, including the use of preoperative basal anesthesia to minimize fears and wild struggling, with the child being permitted to go to sleep with the mother present.

Again, however, certain cautions and perspectives apply. It is possible to overdo preparation of a child for hospitalization, or to prepare too far in advance, just as it is with the child facing the birth of a new sibling. Overpermissiveness and too prolonged overgratification of a child's needs following discharge from hospital have their dangers, just as does overrestrictiveness or overpunitiveness. Also, it is unwise for hospital personnel to become too over-concerned about psychological reactions to treatment procedures, to the point where important procedures might be postponed too long or carried through with uncertainty rather than confidence. In addition, frequent or prolonged visiting may have limitations in value, if the parents are so anxious as to be unable to permit the child to make independently satisfying relationships with hospital personnel. Here it may be wise to help the parents cut down their visiting time to short periods on a daily or frequent basis, rather than to restrict or forbid visiting, as is the natural tendency of busy hospital personnel with irritatingly anxious or controlling parents. The value of frequent visiting, if feasible and comfortable for the hospital staff, has been clearly demonstrated [80, 81] in spite of the more frequent crying of children at the time of parental departure in the early days of hospitalization. Such crying, as Bowlby and Robertson[85] and others have indicated, may constructively release tensions which might otherwise be unhealthily repressed.

As regards prevention of potential emotional trauma in general, the principles discussed earlier regarding breast feeding, rooming-in, and self-demand feeding would appear to be pertinent. Preventive efforts are important, but, as has been said, traumatization is not inevitable as a result of separation, hospitalization, illness, or death of a family member. Other predisposing factors are necessary if the experience is to prove deeply disturbing. One must steer a course between the Scylla of unawareness and the Charybdis of overconcern. Some successful grappling with anxiety and conflict are probably necessary for emotional growth, and preventive efforts should wisely not shield a child from all such experiences nor produce crippling anxiety in parents.

A word is in order regarding the challenge presented by foster home placement, in regard to the concept of separation anxiety. As mentioned earlier, the trend has been toward the use of foster homes rather than institutional settings for placement of children from broken homes or other backgrounds. This trend is generally sound. Nevertheless, certain limitations to its effective implementation do exist and should be mentioned. The basic consideration, as Bowlby[47] has pointed out, remains the fact that a child is better off, within broad limits, in his own home, even if disturbed child-parent relationships exist. We now recognize that a child should not too readily be placed in even a good foster home in the face of such problems. He may suffer emotionally from the separation from even disturbed parents, and may more wisely be handled in a child guidance clinic, in tandem therapy with his parents. Moreover the parents, if unready to accept the placement in more than a nominal fashion, may experience so much guilt that they may interfere to the point of blocking successful placement. Every social agency knows this, but physicians, nurses, and other medical personnel have had less opportunity to encounter the actual limitations of placement. For example, temporary placement in foster homes, or convalescent units, of children with medical illnesses, such as rheumatic fever, was carried out fairly widely for a number of years. Recently, however, medical personnel have come to realize that the emotional advantages of leaving the child in his own home, with perhaps some housekeeping or home-making help for the mother, usually outweigh the disadvantages of separation of the child from his parents and familiar environment, even if the home is not a good one in terms of economic support and easy facilities for home care. There are some illnesses, of course, which can be cared for only in a hospital or convalescent setting with medical and nursing facilities. The decrease in numbers of children with chronic illness requiring hospital-type care, as a result of antibiotic and other current therapies, has paved the way for the gradual demise of the old-style large convalescent home. A recent trend, still embryonic, has involved the setting up of small scale institutions, involving cottage-type group living arrangements, with medical and nursing facilities.

It has become apparent also that there are instances where placement in a foster home runs into difficulties because of personality problems of the foster-home parents, rivalry with the foster child or children by the foster parents' own children, if they exist, the reaction of the foster parents to the child's particular symptoms, such as soiling, or other problems. Warm, comfortable, and confident foster parents are not easy to find. It is not at all easy to take such a role for monetary reasons alone; some more basic dedication must be present. Some authorities are beginning to face the possible need for small institutions, or group cottage-type foster arrangements, with substitute parents who are professionally trained, or at least supervised, and small groups of children of varying ages. This is not meant to invalidate the basic premise regarding the greater value of foster homes over institutions for young children, but simply to provide one way of dealing with the shortage of ideal foster homes at the present time. If a child is seriously disturbed emotionally, placement in a long-term residential treatment center may be indicated, sometimes after a trial of therapy in a child guidance clinic, if the home situation is too difficult or chaotic.

It remains to review briefly other types of deviations in emotional development which may be seen during the preschool phase. Mention has been made of phobias, which, like other "normal" psychological manifestations of developmental origin, may, if other forces intervene, increase in intensity to the point of crippling the child's adjustment or restricting unhealthily his range of activity. If a child fears cats, admittedly for unconscious reasons, to the point of avoiding departure from the house for fear he might see a cat, his activities are obviously seriously interfered with, and therapy for child and parents should be undertaken if possible. Fears of the dark or of being alone are also seen. Nightmares, and night terrors, dissociated states in which the child is in a state between waking and sleeping and may be inconsolably frightened, are also manifestations of emotional disturbances if present more than occasionally.

In addition to direct and overt manifestations of anxiety or fear, certain symptoms may appear which seem to serve the adaptive or defensive function of solving, albeit in an unhealthy fashion, important conflicts which might otherwise produce enough anxiety to threaten the homeostatic equilibrium of the ego. In other words, psychological symptom-formation begins to become available to the child's ego by the age of 4 or 5 as an adaptive mechanism. This mechanism is somewhat different from the production of symptoms merely by the intensification of certain normal defense mechanisms, such as projection, turning-inward, etc. However, one does not yet see hysterical neurotic symptoms in any frequency.

The symptoms seen in the late preschool phase have to do more predominantly with interferences in normal bodily function. One of these is stammering, which may begin in the third year, when talking ordinarily becomes fluent. At this earlier stage stammering may simply represent a repetition of confusing words or a difficulty in articulating more complex concepts which are experienced for the first time. Later, however, the stammering may acquire a more symbolic significance and thus achieve the character of a symptom of the type referred to.

In such instances the child may stammer on words which are associated with particular fantasies, usually unconscious, such as those connected with aggressive, i.e., destructive or sadistic, drives. The child may have fears of losing control of his own aggressive impulses, which may lead him to stammer on the word "fight," for example, and finally with all words beginning with *f*, which might call up into awareness the tabooed thoughts.

This situation illustrates the type of "concrete" and magical thinking mentioned earlier, where the word or thought is almost equated with the deed, in this instance, fighting, and the child fears that saying the word symbol or having the thought may make it come true. Thus, through the difficulty in saying the word, the child's ego keeps the thought out of consciousness by repressing it, and more or less denies that it exists. At the same time the anguish of stammering seems to serve as punishment for having the thought or fantasy. Such a symptom appears to represent a kind of adaptive compromise, where the unconscious impulse and the defense against it neutralize each other, albeit with resultant crippling of function. Such a compromise seems to be the best one which the child is capable of making in his present circumstances.

A full discussion of speech disorders is not intended. This would have to include certain types of infantile speech, which often accompany an infantile personality, as well as the consideration of possible somatic predisposing forces.

Other symptoms of comparable type include fecal soiling and enuresis, which can be classified as manifestations of emotional disturbance if they continue into the latter part of the preschool period. Limitations of space do not permit a full discussion of these symptoms. It can be said, however, that in certain cases of soiling and enuresis, the appropriate sphincter acts as if it were paralyzed, releasing the feces or the flow of urine. Enuresis mainly occurs at night, during sleep, and only occasionally during the day. In both disorders, however, unconscious and unacceptable wishes to express anger through soiling or wetting find their symbolic expression through their symptom, even though the child consciously abhors these thoughts and is certainly "punished" by the anguish caused to himself and his parents by his symptom.

Both of these unhealthy mechanisms appear either on a regressive basis, in the face of some acute conflict or intensified anxiety, or as failures to gain control from the training period on. The latter type of symptom is in general the more deeply ingrained, representing the result of fixation at an earlier level, with a less positive response to symptomatic or supportive treatment. One should be careful to look at the total personality of the child, however, including his physical equipment. Some cases, particularly those of regressive nature, such as nocturnal enuresis appearing at 5 years upon the birth of a sibling, may either disappear rapidly or continue as an "encapsulated" symptom, without deep disturbance of the ego. Others may represent only one of a number of symptoms of failure in adaptation. Gerard [86] and Richmond,[87] among others, have well discussed enuresis and soiling, respectively, including the occasional somatic abnormalities which may be involved.

During the preschool phase multiple predisposing forces usually act as determinants, as is true in cases of colitis, mild diarrhea, and constipation which may appear. The latter are more accurately called psychophysiologic or vegetative disorders, in contrast to such pictures as soiling or enuresis. They involve disturbance in autonomically innervated functions of bodily organs, rather than external sphincter muscles, and appear to operate on a more basically regressive basis, with discharge of tension or anxiety being principally involved. In these disorders the symptom does not appear to represent a basic symbolism as in the others described. No specific personality structure or family constellations can be said to be associated with any of these disorders, although certain conflict situations may be more characteristic of children with colitis than with soiling, for example. Predisposing forces, such as inherited potentialities, toilet training experience, incidental local disease, and the attitudes of the parents toward organ function, are all involved in this problem of the "choice" of organ, which is still poorly understood.

Deviations in psychosexual development will only be mentioned at this point, as they will be more fully treated in the next section. Pronounced or compulsive masturbation may often be a symptom of anxiety in the area of handling sexual impulses, or of tensions in the area of aggression, which may be drained off in this way. In addition certain neurotic disturbances can arise because the Oedipal conflicts are not resolved successfully. Unconsciously overpunitive or overseductive handling by parents may be one factor in disturbance in sexual identifications, although these may not show themselves until later. Thus, if, because of his own conflicts, the father is too punitive toward the boy, the child may then be afraid of the father and of becoming a man like the father, with consequent later difficulties in masculine identification and in developing satisfying relations with the opposite sex. More rarely, serious difficulties may result in later homosexuality, and certain later neuroses of hysterical and other types may have their roots in the unsuccessful negotiation of the preschool phase, with later events of course playing contributory, precipitating or perpetuating roles.

THE SCHOOL AGE CHILD

DANE G. PRUGH

Consolidation and Constructiveness

Growth and development during infancy and the preschool period take place with giant strides, albeit somewhat uneven ones. The transition in five short years from a helpless infant to a sturdy and complicated being, capable of communication, conceptualization, and complex social and motor behavior, is a remarkable phenomenon. The parallel increment in height and weight is equally rapid and striking. In contrast, the period between 6 years of age and the onset of the prepubertal growth spurt, is a phase of gradual, at times almost imperceptible, growth and development, steadier and more even in both its physical and emotional aspects. Spock has referred to the child at this stage as the "middle-aged child." Psychoanalytic writers have used the term "latency period" to indicate that certain facets of emotional development are slowed, paralleling the much less rapid increase in physical size and strength. Since the beginning of the phase corresponds roughly with the child's entrance into formal education, the term "school age child" is widely employed, and because of its general acceptance will be used in this discussion of emotional development, regardless of its patent descriptive limitations.

In spite of the obvious difference in the gradients of growth in comparison with the preceding phases and with the succeeding period of adolescence, it is easily apparent that the child in the school age period does not stand still in his development. By the age of 6, most children have become able to undertake the use of abstract concepts, permitting beginning contact with the subjects of reading, writing, and arithmetic. Some children of 6 have not reached this developmental point, a factor which is significant in the face of the arbitrary school entrance required at this time. Fortunately, contemporary educators now recognize this fact and try, where necessary, to individualize early academic programs to allow for individual maturational lags. The beginnings of academic education, however, are also made possible by the child's progress in the emotional aspects of development. By the age of 6, most children are able to operate more independently of the mother and the family than before. This "independence" is, of course, only relative. Nevertheless some degree of independence is present, at least for periods of time sufficient to permit a full-day school program, which involves sharing the affection and attention of a parent-substitute figure — the teacher — with a relatively large group of other children. Significant individual variations in degree of emotional maturation, of course, occur as with intellectual development. As a result, certain children are unready, or less ready than their peers, for such independence. The wise teacher takes account of these differences.

Beginning with this new base line of intellectual and emotional powers, the school age child shows gradual but significant growth in both areas. His intellectual grasp of abstract concepts shows remarkable increase during this phase. His growing independence gradually permits him to explore, in numerous directions, the community outside the family, including his own peer group. In this respect, he is assisted by the steady and relatively consistent consolidation of his own basic skills, particularly those involving motor performance. Although the child has already acquired basic mastery of his motor equipment by the beginning of the school age period, he now becomes able to refine his skills, especially those dealing with neuromuscular coordination and most particularly those involving fine coordination of the hands, eyes, and cerebral cortex. Thus, for example, boys can begin to build complicated structures and can follow directions such as those for games and the assembling of model airplanes. Girls can dress dolls skillfully, and girls and boys can begin to play musical instruments. Hobbies of all kinds begin to develop. These interests are fitful and shifting at first, but as they consolidate, the child becomes able to follow out more effectively his interests in learning, in exploring the community, and in investigating and trying out in play the roles of various adults with whom he now comes into contact.

Together with this gradual consolidation of skills and interests comes a new type of constructiveness in work and play. The child of this period likes to make things. This need was present in earlier phases, in a desultory way. Now, with exceptions, the child is more fully able to carry through successfully with his intent. It is pertinent that Erikson has identified the "sense of industry" as an outstanding characteristic of this phase.[38] Concepts of duty and pride in accomplishment begin to appear and to mature.

In the face of these subtle but important changes, parents ordinarily feel an understandably growing sense of pride and accomplishment in their children. It should be mentioned, however, that even during this steadier period of development, unevenness appears. As Bornstein[88] has pointed out, during the phase from 6 to 8 or 9 years, bits of exceedingly mature behavior often alternate with babyish mannerisms or demanding behavior, especially in regard to situations involving competition with younger siblings. By the age of 8 or 9, the more mature trends described seem to become firmer and more fully consolidated. Thus parents are often led to expect behavior more characteristic of the second or more "consolidated" phase during the first or "swinging" phase. Anticipatory understanding of the ups and downs of the child from 6 through 8 years can be most helpful to parents, puzzled and concerned as they well may be by signs of consolidation and constructiveness which seem to dissolve, temporarily, overnight. Regression still can occur throughout this whole period, of course. In significant degree, however, it is much more characteristic of the early, rather than later, subperiod.

One of the possible complications arising from this new display of skills and accomplishments has to do with the tendency of many children to overschedule themselves. The bursting enthusiasm of girls and boys may lead to demands to enter a number of group activities; for example, ballet dancing or Little League baseball. Parents may be pleased at these developments, but may also be puzzled at the evanescent quality of some of the child's announced interests. The temptation is for parents to take all these interests at face value and to feel worried about the child's lack of responsibility if he abandons the trumpet 3 weeks after its demanded, and perhaps painful, purchase. Certain parents also may find themselves trapped by their own unrealized wishes for achievement along certain lines, or by their desires to give their children what they themselves could not have. As a result, their unconscious encouragement of a school age child's multitudinous interests may lead to such a tightly scheduled set of activities that the child becomes over-tense, fatigued, or loses interest in one or many activities.

The school age child, in spite of his long step forward, is not a "little man." He still needs understanding and firm guidance.

Adaptive Mechanisms

From what has been said, it is apparent that psychologically the most prominent change during this period takes place in regard to the strengthening and consolidation, as well as further organization and integration of the child's ego. This increase in ego capacities, and expanded power of independent operation, is supported developmentally by enhanced intellectual development, more numerous and complex motor skills, and other maturing personality functions. A need for almost ceaseless activity often accompanies these enlarged capacities. These activities are frequently misinterpreted as unhealthy restlessness or tension, which of course may be the case in extreme instances. Normally, however, such activity serves to discharge certain milder tensions arising from the successful struggle for greater control of instinctual drives. This healthy ability to deal with the tensions of everyday life through constructive activity of a socially acceptable nature embodies one of the outstanding adaptive mechanisms now newly available to the child in significant degree. This adaptive mechanism is *sublimation.* Examples of its usefulness may be found in the manner in which aggressive drives can now be handled more successfully through competitive group games, and may be channelled into the activity of acquiring knowledge in school. Sexual impulses, related to curiosity toward the opposite sex, including the parents, can now be dealt with more healthily by *displacing* the involved curiosity onto the exploration of books and ideas as well as the larger community, as a partial replacement for the preschool peeping and experimentation. Impulses to soil or to mess, deriving from the late infantile or preschool period, can find release in constructive creative activities, including drawing, coloring, painting, or work with clay. Energies previously predominantly tied up in the control of sexual and aggressive impulses are thus freed for purposes of learning and experimentation.

This does not imply that creative and competitive activities, and the drive to gain knowledge and skills, are nothing but sublimations for earlier, socially unacceptable, impulses or drives, with displacement of such impulses into other channels now available. Creative activities and the desire to learn *are* utilized by some children and adults for these and other adaptive purposes, including, as Adler has indicated,[89] compensation for feelings of inferiority or anxiety. Nevertheless the controversy which has raged around the question of "art *versus* neurosis" now seems an artificial one, as certain psychoanalysts[90, 91] and at least one literary critic (Lionel Trilling[92]) have indicated. Creative capacities, up to and including genius, have deeper roots than simply psychological and adaptive ones. Inherited capacities, family and social influences, and various other forces are involved. The school age period permits developmentally the flowering of such budding capacities. The child's adaptive need for handling instinctual impulses simply takes advantage of these capacities and the associated social and competitive opportunities.

Perhaps the other most important adaptive or defense mechanism of this period, assisting sublimation and displacement, is that of *repression*. Children during the school age period are much more readily able to push out of conscious awareness thoughts or fantasies deriving from aggressive or sexual impulses than was previously the case. For example, hostile impulses to strike and hurt, or the desire to masturbate for immediate pleasure, can be more successfully inhibited and repressed from consciousness. This increased capacity for repression enhances the impression of a "latent" period, with reemergence of aggressive and sexual impulses and the need for the development of a new, more independently operating adaptive equilibrium in the next period of adolescence. Social anthropologists have pointed out that such latency may also be the result of cultural influences in Western society since the phenomenon does not seem so marked in certain other societies.[72]

Associated with this augmented capacity for repression is a more exact utilization of the "reality principle," leading to postponement of immediate satisfactions for the more delayed and more subtle approval of parents and society, including that of the peer group. Thus the capacity to share and to build up ethical concepts of behavior is promoted, assisted by development of the child's superego (conscience), and his developing ego-ideal.

A number of additional adaptive mechanisms become fully available to the school age child. Most of these have been mentioned before, however, and simply undergo consolidation and more successful employment during this phase. Such mechanisms principally assist, more or less in clusters, the mechanisms of repression and sublimation, as well as the development of the reality principle, and the internalization of the parents' and society's prohibitions and, more importantly, ideals.

Two of these mechanisms are worthy of mention. One is the mechanism of *identification,* which finds its peak in this period. Identifications make their outward appearance during the preschool period, although their roots go even further back. During the school age period, identifications reach out from the parents to representatives of society, in a much more constructive and realistic way than those of the preschool child, who experiments principally with the roles of those individuals with whom he comes into daily contact. The 5 or 6 year old boy already is toying with the more remote and more exciting concept of being a cowboy, in contrast to the 3 year old who tends to choose policeman, fireman, or delivery man. Television has, of course, superficially altered some of these tendencies for younger children. By 8 or 9, many children have expanded their identifications to include teachers, mechanics, doctors, nurses, businessmen, scientists, and other categories, depending upon their economic and social circumstances, the scope of their education, and the interests and occupational choices of members of the family.

Identifications of this nature of course involve the more basic concept of the role of the child as a potential man or woman. This has already been laid down to an important extent by the beginning of this phase. The occupation of the parent of the same sex is of important interest to school age children. In modern urban society, however, various forces during this phase expand children's interests beyond the home circle, no matter what their ultimate choice may be. The point is not that these shifting superficial identifications lead to solid choices of occupational role, based on deeper heterosexual identifications, but that they reflect the child's growing constructive orientation, the quality of his current relationships to family and other figures, and his expanding ego capacities. Identifications show themselves in work and in play. The child's previously developed powers of fantasy are afforded rich outlets in play. Girls, for example, dramatize their roles as housewives, nurses, or ballet dancers. Boys, who struggle more with control of aggressive impulses, shift in games from "goody" to "baddy," from cop to robber, from cowboy to outlaw, or from space pilot to space bandit, indicating that they are thus working out, in play, conflicting forces within themselves. Fortunately the "good" forces usually prevail in such games, at least with emotionally healthy children with reasonably satisfying family and environmental backgrounds. Identification is thus used adaptively by children at different levels of development, and in different ways. It is used consciously and unconsciously, in work and in play. The more important identifications, such as those involving sexual roles, are usually the less conscious ones.

A word should be said regarding the person who now represents the major source of more basic identification outside the family figures. This is the teacher, who acts as a kind of substitute parent, but who, more importantly, enlarges children's horizons and helps to channel their expanding curiosity constructively. Often the teacher does not long remain the object of direct identification. Nevertheless the teacher's personality characteristics are frequently unconsciously adopted by children, and the interest of the teacher in the child is a most influential positive factor in his continued emotional growth. Parents recognize this phenomenon and wisely can support and reinforce it. Certain less secure parents, however, may feel threatened by the fact that the child shows, for the first time, such enthusiasm for a person outside the family. Their fears about the child's growing away from them, combined at times with a fear of criticism by the teacher of their efforts as parents, may lead them to misinterpret and mistrust the quality and extent of the teacher's influence upon their child. More disturbed parents may project onto the teacher their own feelings of guilt about themselves as ineffectual parents, blaming the teacher for the child's difficulties in adjustment. It is, of course, not infrequent that teachers may unconsciously engage in a kind of competition with parents for the child's affections. Individual teachers who may feel uncertain of themselves may likewise need to see the child's problems as the fault of the parents. Ordinarily, the child's problems are no one's "fault," in the sense of conscious wish or design. Nevertheless, these other forces too frequently lead to a certain distance, and to a kind of rivalry, between parents and teachers, which may be reinforced by lack of contact. This discussion cannot include consideration of the ways in which such barriers to collaboration may be removed. It can simply be noted, as Frank[93] and others have indicated, that mutual respect, close contact, and effective cooperation between parents and teachers can and should exert a most constructive influence upon the course of the child's emotional development.

Mention was made of a second type of adaptive mechanism of importance to children of this age period, the mechanism involved in the control of instinctual drives. The term *reaction formation* has been employed for this mechanism. The concept involves "turning into the opposite," described earlier, in which the child unconsciously transforms the expressions of affects into their opposite qualities. Unacceptable feelings of anger or hate toward a particular person, for example, may be repressed from consciousness and only feelings of positive nature outwardly expressed. To a certain extent, this mechanism is employed by many healthy adults, who find themselves showing exaggerated politeness to someone whom privately they dislike. By the mechanism of reaction formation, assisted by denial, the intensely strong and socially unacceptable hostile affects frequently experienced by the child are kept under control. This is accomplished under certain socially prescribed circumstances by a more or less permanent maintenance of the opposite affect. Such a process usually operates unconsciously. Thus the formation of certain character traits is made possible, involving the capacities for forming relationships which are pleasant, warm, steady, and drained of most of the explosiveness and turbulence of affect which mark relationships in preschool children. Such reaction formations, assisted by repression and other mechanisms, are necessary to a constructive degree for the maintenance of civilization. In this manner they assist positive identifications with tolerant and kindly adults, building up important character traits involving consideration for others, kindliness, and other more broadly ethical considerations which are deemed important in our society.

It is possible, however, for these reaction formations to be carried to the pathological point where the child can only express positive feelings and must repress and deny the existence of any negative feelings, even when these become necessary for the maintenance of some kind of emotional homeostatic balance. The child who can never permit himself to become angry or irritated, even in defense of others, for fear of losing control of his affects, finds himself building up tensions which are difficult to drain off in the socially acceptable channels of sublimation. Such overrigidity may lead the child to withdraw from healthily competitive activities and to reinforce his reaction formations with crippling inhibitions. A healthier type of control in our society appears to involve the recognition of, and coming to grips with, the universally present negative affects.

For the school age child this struggle to control instinctual impulses is an important and newly effective one. The tendency toward conformance and certain compulsive mechanisms are also involved, in which children not only conform to outer societal regulations but to inner controls as well. In spite of its frequent breakdowns in effectiveness, the conscience or superego is often harsh and uncompromising, during the early part of the school age period in particular. In a sense a compulsive, rather rigid type of behavior is often seen in school age children. The tendency for these children to hold parents to their own rules is embarrassing for parents, who hear their partly civilized child requiring their observance of certain rules of politeness, often overlooked by the adults despite their natural zeal for their children's social welfare. Particularly during the second phase other overtones of independence appear at home and in school, regardless of more widespread conformance. The inner compulsions often make themselves apparent in the child's games, where rigid, ritualized, often apparently illogical rules are enforced in the peer group. "Step on a crack and break your mother's (or grandmother's) back" gives the key to such compulsions, which assist repression, sublimation, reaction formation, and other defenses, and conform with the demand of the superego by holding in check particularly hostile or rebellious feelings toward parents.

The school age child thus almost overshoots the mark at times in his attempts at conformance and ritual. For the average child this more rigid, pseudocompulsive trend continues with notable punctuations and regressions only up to puberty. There is later a "loosening up," with associated change towards better thought-out and maturely flexible ethical and moral codes of behavior, which are less brittle and no longer so vulnerable to possible exception.

No attempt to describe a child at this or any other phase can do justice to the individual charm, sense of humor, pride in accomplishment, buoyancy, and other positive and attractive qualities which children manifest to parents and other adults. Although this stage may justifiably be described as a relatively more stable period of constructiveness and consolidation, no child is completely static. Each child has his moments of exultation, of superficially unaccountable timidity, of exceedingly mature and praiseworthy behavior, and of infantile temper outbursts or dependent clinging. Sudden advances, surprising regressions, and unexpected plateaus still ripple the surface of the waters of progress in this phase, but with it all there emerges the individual emotional characteristics and personality traits of the child. These are not fully fixed, even though their basic outlines do seem to be sketched in by the early phases of the school age. Emotional growth and personality change can still occur, especially with the help of parents.

Social Relationships and Group Behavior

As has been mentioned, the child during this phase is for the first time able to join in group activities with unreserved fervor and steady participation. Up to this point, the dependence upon the mother, and later upon both parents and the familiar family group, has limited such group endeavors to short periods involving considerable adult supervision. As the child becomes able to share — persons as well as objects — and as his skills increase, he ordinarily becomes involved in one or several peer groups. These groups overlap considerably, and may shift surprisingly as Redl [94] has indicated. The most stable is the classroom group, where the child can gain important status as a respected member as he becomes able to learn and increasingly to contribute to the welfare of the group as a whole. Activity groups, including Cub Scouts or Brownies, church groups, and neighborhood groups, may shift at a rate alarming to parents and often involve a "pecking order," with one or two children suffering as scapegoats for the rest. The same tendency can be seen, though less clearly, in more fixed and supervised groups.

Space does not allow description of the interesting subtleties of group behavior in school age children. Suffice to say that their groups reproduce with surprising accuracy certain features of adult groups, including discrimination and other less desirable qualities. "Bullies" and "sissies" appear among the boys, though the individuals involved may shift as they gain control of their needs respectively to demonstrate their uncertain and shaky strength, or to hold back from any aggressive contact. As Josselyn has pointed out,[95] leaders at this stage are at times "pseudoleaders," dominating the group for needs of their own and are not always the leaders of the future. Considerable supervision is still necessary during this phase, particularly in larger group activities. It should be remembered that, regardless of their initial eagerness and apparent maturity, few children are ready constructively for the enforced independence of overnight camping experience prior to 8 or 9 years of age, and some are not emotionally prepared until later.

During this phase, as children's interests and identifications solidify, groups spontaneously tend to separate into those composed of the two sexes. The original awareness of the apparent indifference of boys to girls, and vice versa, during the school age period was one of the observations contributing to the term "latent" in regard to interest in the opposite sex. It is true that boys in our society are often loudly preoccupied with "masculine" activities, such as crafts and athletics, while girls frequently though not always work more quietly with doll clothes and "feminine" activities. Some girls transiently undergo a phase of "tom-boy" behavior, representing often a certain envy of the boy's freer role in our society, as well as mild conflicts over the acceptance of their own femininity. Girls in general do tend to deride boys as rough and loud, while boys vociferously proclaim their disgust with girls and their sissy activities. Nevertheless, behind the facade of a studied disinterest still smolders considerable interest in the opposite sex. The activities ending in the game of "boys chasing the girls" (or pulling their pigtails) which are so popular around schoolyards with boys — and with girls (who often provoke, with mock protests, even more vigorous chasings) — indicate the presence of such interest, distorted by the unfamiliarity of the new heterosexual role and the lack of social techniques, among other factors. The latency phase is latent only in a relative sense, in contrast to the open sexual curiosities of the preschool phase, now repressed and sublimated, and to the resurgence of heterosexual interest, twisted temporarily by the shyness and confusion which characterize early adolescence.

Discipline

A word is indicated regarding the concept of discipline as it applies to the school age period. In general, the earlier discussion of discipline is of pertinence. It is worthwhile to note, however, that the child at this time poses certain unfamiliar challenges to the parents in their approach to this aspect of child-rearing. The newfound conformance and growing maturity often lead parents to permit the child to make certain decisions for which he is not prepared emotionally. Decisions regarding the type and number of group activities represent examples of such problems. Here the parent may wisely give the child a choice between two different activities, but may run into difficulty in permitting the child to move into a number of tempting activities all at once. Punishment still is necessary at times, and the child, with his growing sense of "right" and "wrong" — still admittedly oversimplified and involving only extremes of choice — may at times invite punishment as a support to his still shaky superego.

Although punishment and reproval remain necessary, they may most safely be reserved for the larger misdemeanors at this stage. Many children are extremely sensitive to criticism, especially as they become more self-conscious and self-aware. Wise parents try to control their urge to teach the child manners all at once. Certain standards of social behavior do need to be maintained, of course, but criticism or punishment can safely be reserved for the larger misdemeanors at this stage. Many children already have extremely harsh internal standards, almost cruelly maintained in their effort to achieve instinctual control and social conformance. Others become so intensely preoccupied with their interests and activities that, for example, they literally do not hear the parent's admonition that bedtime is at hand. Respect for the child's growing individuality and for his independent attempts to achieve maturity is not easy for parents to develop. Fortunately, most parents do gradually become aware of these changes and adapt their standards and disciplinary approach accordingly.

One recent concern of parents and educators has involved the related questions of children's consumption of comic books, television programs, etc. It is perfectly true that these media of communication result in a type of emotional and intellectual stimulation which was not available to the child of 30 years ago, particularly in regard to the aggressive and at times sexual implications of certain themes. Many professional personnel feel that certain types of comics and television programs, even those with themes of shooting, bandits, etc., are not in themselves directly harmful to children, nor do they "plant ideas" in the school age child's mind. The war games of children, observed long before modern media of communication, indicate children's spontaneous preoccupation with such themes. Some of the classic fairy tales involved equally violent, though perhaps more charmingly presented, concepts.

It would appear that, as indicated earlier, school age children have a need to act out, in play, certain fantasies and affects which derive from the earlier preschool period. The school age child, however, is less likely to be frightened by the closeness to reality of these fantasies. Furthermore, the school age child seems to be working out his concepts of morality in the process, as well as his identification with the "good" forces or society. The result is that the "goodies" or the "cops" usually win, albeit somewhat narrowly at times.

Certainly a need is present for comic books and television programs which do not make the role of the "bad" individual unduly attractive. Allowing for censorship from within the commercial concerns, much of which has been promoted by disturbed parents and others, the problem seems to resolve itself into the question of setting limits on the child's behavior within the family group. Some limits need to be set on the consumption of these sources of emotional titillation. Preschool children may be confused and frightened by too much material of this kind. School age children, particularly sensitive ones with rather rigid consciences, sometimes develop nightmares after too vivid or prolonged seances with television. Perhaps the most important consideration, however, is the confidence of the parents in deciding what the limits will be, and how they will be applied, just as in the case with other courses of disciplinary action. Establishing a certain number of comic books per month, or of television programs per day, is not too different from setting a certain number of rides on a merry-go-round, or defining a limited number of pieces of candy.

Intellectual parents are often most concerned about these problems. They fear, perhaps justly, that an exclusive diet of passive entertainment, through visual or auditory stimuli, could dull the child's appetite for more active involvement in more creative and participant outlets. Although further studies are needed in this area, the problem seems ordinarily to resolve itself around the family's interests and patterns of activity. If the parents have other interests and outlets, children generally pick these up through identification and sharing of interest.[96] Passionate interests in comic books or television programs, if these are foreign to the parents' tastes, ordinarily are put into perspective over a period of months or years. Thus a complete interdiction of such interests is neither possible nor necessary in most families. The challenge involved in the setting of limits and in the provision of opportunities for sharing family activities and interests still remains the central consideration.

Special Developmental Problems

During this phase a number of problems may arise. Some derive from the vicissitudes of developmental trends discussed earlier. Among these are the regressive tendencies which appear at times, particularly during the earlier or "swinging" phase, prior to more firm ego-consolidation. Illness of the child, necessary hospitalization or operations, the birth of a sibling, or the death of a parent, may promote such regression, with resultant appearance of behavior and misinterpretations of reality more characteristic of the preschool phase. Such regressive trends are ordinarily transient. In disturbed children, or in those with unhealthy or unsatisfying family relationships, these trends may be more pathological and may form the point of departure, or the precipitating influence, for continuing emotional disturbance. Parents may be greatly helped in their handling of such developments by anticipatory understanding.

One specific type of regression may occur during the late school age period. It is seen commonly in boys, but may occur in girls too. Such regressive tendencies arise from the impending onset of puberty, during the prepubertal period. Certain of the behavioral changes so often seen may begin to appear during the later part of the school age period. Briefly, the beginning physiological maturation and onset of secondary sex characteristics are often accompanied by an upsurge of sexual feelings. The response to this may be, in many children, a temporary regression in behavior, with a revival of old preschool and pregenital problems, representing "unfinished business" in the normal process of development. Boys may become louder, less controlled and less conforming, messier and dirtier, with loud complaints about baths and washing behind ears. Tremendous increase in appetite often occurs, reflecting enhanced physiologic needs leading up to the characteristic growth spurt of this phase, but perhaps also indicating regressive use of food as a source of substitute emotional satisfaction in the face of intensified conflict. The central consideration for professional workers is that the children's behavior is puzzling to the parents. The professional workers can help in interpreting to parents the widespread incidence of such behavior and its normally healthy and progressive developmental resolution. Parents may thus be helped to achieve perspective and to broaden their limits in certain respects, in order to deal with this new phase.

Among other deviations in behavior during the school age period may be listed certain extreme manifestations of tension, which involve muscular activity. The need for relatively constant motor discharge has been stressed. A majority of children in this age group show certain involuntary neuromuscular discharges of tension such as tics. Twitching of the nose, mild grimaces of the face, and occasional movements of the neck are seen transiently, usually over a period of a few weeks or months, in many emotionally healthy children. Parents can be helped to overlook these sometimes troubling manifestations and to avoid unrealistic attempts at control, attempts which cannot succeed but which may increase the tension — and thus the movements. At times, in disturbed children with unsatisfying family relationships, tics are more constant and of pathological significance, with the characteristics of a hysterical symptom. A type of extreme motor restlessness, or fidgetiness, is also seen in this age group, as Winnicott[97] has indicated, and is to be distinguished from chorea, in which emotional components may, however, occur. In contrast to chorea, the fidgetiness is characterized by the essentially purposive quality of the involuntary movements — wringing the hands, fingering the clothes, pounding the furniture, etc.

Academic education begins at this age, and so learning difficulties are frequently manifested for the first time. Some children with mild lags in intellectual development may be unready for reading, writing, or other activities involving abstract concepts and logical reasoning. Others may be unready emotionally to participate in group activities, or to operate independently from the family. Children with mild brain damage, or with congenital predisposition toward difficulties in sensory motor functions, may tend to reverse words or to read in mirror image fashion. Certain passive, rather inhibited children, with conflicts over healthy expression of aggressive tendencies, may be unable to compete successfully in learning activities because of their fears of losing control of hostile feelings, or of losing the affection of others if they outdistance them.[98] Still other children, with conflicts over the expression of their curiosity in regard to sex differences, may encounter emotional blocks in reading because of the unhealthy displacement onto reading of their inhibition of impulses to "peep" or to look. (A fuller discussion of learning problems will be found in Chapter VIII.)

During the school age period, the presence of congenital or acquired handicaps or chronic illness may assume importance. Some children with such difficulties may become over-anxious and over-dependent. Others may attempt to deny any implication of illness or weakness by denying illness and acting as though no such limitation were present. The reactions of the parents to such conditions, as in congenital abnormalities of the heart and diabetes, are of course a part of the picture.

The most important deviations during this phase, from a psychological point of view, arise from the appearance for the first time of definitive neurotic illnesses. For a full discussion of psychopathological problems in childhood, the reader is referred to other sources.[99, 100] Briefly, it can be said that four major categories of symptomatic manifestations of disturbance in adaptation can be seen in childhood, beginning with the school age period. These are similar to but not identical with adult disturbances.

The first of these categories is the neurosis, involving an emotional illness arising from an unhealthy and unsuccessful adaptive attempt to solve intense, unresolved, and usually unconscious emotional conflicts which produce extreme anxiety. In neurotic illness, occurring in psychologically predisposed and vulnerable children, predominantly psychological mechanisms of adaptation are used by the ego to deal with the anxiety, albeit unsuccessfully. Symptoms may simply involve the spilling over into awareness of the anxiety, arising from internalized conflict, as in anxiety neurosis. They may also result from the appearance of hysterical paralyses, which seem unconsciously to solve the conflict, unhealthily, in a symbolic fashion, as in the child with a paralyzed arm who no longer can strike the sibling toward whom he is jealous and angry. Children who experience disturbing obsessive thoughts, or who must perform compulsive acts or rituals, unconsciously atone for unacceptable, guilt-provoking hostile thoughts or fantasies, as the price of controlling the associated affects. Others, with phobias, displace their anger or fear of punishment from their disturbed parent onto relatively harmless animals or situations. A special type of phobic reaction — school phobia — involves a conscious fear of the teacher or of competitive school situations rather than the unconscious fear of separation from the mother.[101] Such phobias appear commonly and transiently in children of 6 or 7 years, often during the first full-day experience in school and frequently associated with "stomach-aches" or vomiting in the early morning on school days. Other, more severe types appear during the later school age period or adolescence, and may involve much more deep-seated conflicts and neurotic trends.

Certain other children — more commonly boys than girls in our society — attempt to deal with such conflicts by acting out directly their unacceptable feelings, of hostile nature in particular. These children may exhibit behavior disorders of aggressive type, which if continued to the point of antisocial behavior may be labelled delinquency.[102] For example, they may steal for revenge or in order to obtain a distorted kind of substitute satisfaction for lack of love; they may destroy things in order to invite punishment, or may act out their feelings in other ways. In certain instances, unhealthy wishes or needs of the parents may lead them unconsciously to condone or encourage stealing or other antisocial behavior in the child.[103] Other children in this group may be utterly unable to postpone need for satisfaction or to tolerate any frustration, exhibiting "impulse-ridden" behavior of explosive and violent nature, with shallow and superficial relations with other persons.[47]

Still a third type of emotional disturbance is represented by children with psychosomatic or psychophysiologic problems. At this point it may be said only that various clinical pictures, including ulcerative colitis,[104] peptic ulcer,[105] asthma,[106] obesity,[107] and constipation or soiling,[87] may contain emotional components of varying severity. In such illnesses the tension or anxiety appears to be discharged through bodily processes, producing disturbance in the function of an organ system, with apparent regressive components, as mentioned earlier. The causes of such illness are ordinarily multiply determined and include, among a number of etiologic factors, somatic and inherited types of predisposition, an example being the allergic tendency in asthmatic children.

The fourth and last large category is that of psychotic disturbances. In such conditions the child attempts to deal with his conflict by breaking off contact with reality, and by withdrawing into a world of fantasy, obviously of less satisfying nature than the world of reality. Thus a beginning disturbance in emotional development may become, in such instances, a mental illness, involving disturbance in basic thought processes and reality-testing, as well as in the handling of affects. Predisposition of psychologic and at times somatic or other nature, seem to be involved in these disturbances[108] and they frequently are exceedingly difficult to treat. Such illness may represent intensification of earlier autistic pictures[49] or atypical ego development, or may be the precursors of schizophrenic manifestations.[109]

In all of these categories of disturbed behavior, conflicts unsolved during infancy and preschool periods serve as predisposing forces, together with current emotionally traumatic events, related physical illness or predisposition, inherited factors, and others. The multiple causation of such disturbances remains a central concept.

As has been indicated, all of these types of emotional or, in the case of psychotic disturbances, mental illness, involve the basic mechanism of rigid and intense *repression from awareness of the disturbing affects arising from unsolved conflicts.* In all these disturbances, the child's ego appears to deal with the resultant tension or anxiety through the unhealthy use of other adaptive mechanisms already described. Conversion-hysterical illness and certain other neurotic problems involve a different mechanism, that of symptom-formation, in which a disturbance in neuromuscular innervation is brought about by the cerebral cortex, without apparent physical change. This symptom-formation apparently deals with the conflict in symbolic terms. No overt signs of anxiety may be seen, for the symptom seems to "bind" the anxiety, which may appear in other forms if the symptom disappears.

Illnesses of these types represent unsuccessful attempts at adaptation, just as do predominantly physical illnesses. Here the unsuccessful attempts at adaptation produce breakdown in the ego's homeostatic balance. Adaptive mechanisms themselves may become "symptoms" if employed too strenuously. This is the case in certain personality disorders, such as the inhibited or compulsive child. Much remains to be learned about the actual neurophysiologic mechanisms, as well as the multiple predisposing forces in all these processes and the specific reasons for the development of one particular type of picture, rather than another.

For the professional worker, the recognition of serious emotional disturbance can obviously be of help in early referral for psychiatric treatment. A great deal can be done to help parents accept such illness as a problem which is not their "fault," nor the fault of the child, and as an emotional sickness which can be treated with real possibility of success. The more obvious types of disturbance are easy to recognize, particularly those involving aggressive or antisocial behavior. However, the child who is withdrawn, markedly inhibited, or extremely shy and passive, may conform quite effectively in school or other groups, and may be difficult for the parents, the teacher, or other professional worker to recognize as an actually or potentially disturbed child.

In many instances, early recognition of an impendingly serious emotional problem can lead to constructive discussion with the parents, and to referral for prompt treatment. In some cases, however, parents are unable, because of their own conflicts, to perceive a child's disturbed behavior as a problem, or at least to admit to themselves or to others their own recognition of the seriousness of the disorder. It is important to state that professional workers need not feel that they have failed if they are unable to help parents face a child's problem immediately. Pushing such a parent too rapidly towards such insight may simply cause intensified anxiety and further resistance to awareness of the problem, because of the severity of associated guilt feelings, or other causes of inability to perceive the problem. In a few instances, premature attempts at treatment of a child's problem, before the parents were emotionally ready to participate actively in the treatment process, have resulted in a stirring up of conflicts which could not yet be handled in a healthier way, on the part of the parent or child, with consequent increase in emotional illness for both parties. Parents and child must proceed emotionally at the pace for which they are ready, to the point which they are able to reach, with wise and patient professional support.

Prevention of milder problems presents an important challenge to professional workers in various fields. Aggressive campaigns to "wipe out" mental or emotional illness, such as have been frequently proposed, often do not take into account the complexity or the subtlety of the problems. More basic preventive measures, involving judicious psychological support and anticipatory guidance for the parents, as well as constructive handling of the child in nursery school and elementary school settings, are described elsewhere in this or other chapters. Prevention, in the sense of early detection and treatment of potentially serious problems in incipient stages, may be as important as these more basic measures. Screening programs have been set up experimentally in certain school systems, and pediatric clinics, settlement houses, or children's camps may be other sources of recognition or referral.

No matter how patent the child's problem may be to the worker, if the parents have not previously recognized the difficulty, a great deal of work and time must go into the discussion with them of the need for referral for treatment. Referrals made without such discussion, or without trust and confidence by the parents in the referring worker, frequently fail. Judgment or criticism of parents should be avoided, and the child's difficulty discussed simply as a problem for which help is available. If a professional worker can work patiently with the parent of a disturbed child until referral to a psychiatric facility is possible, he is accomplishing a reasonable goal. Important also is the later contact and collaboration between worker — whether physician, public health nurse, social worker, teacher, or other professional person — and the psychiatric clinic, during active treatment and follow-up phases. If such referral should be unsuccessful, the worker may have to continue fulfilling a supportive role for the parent or child — no easy task to accomplish without feelings of frustration or resentment. In large measure, the way in which referral and collaborative support of treatment are handled determines the degree of success of psychiatric treatment.

ADOLESCENT GIRLS
ELIZABETH S. MAKKAY

A study of the process of adolescence is most fruitful when we consider what the goals of the adolescent years are, where the girl "has been" and "where she is going," and the relationship of the physical changes to the dynamic psychological changes characteristic of this period.

While the goals of adolescence in a girl's psychological development are, in a general sense, the same as those of the boy's, there are important differences, differences in form and content, just as the earlier phases in the girl's psychological development presented important differences in these ways. But before we proceed to examine the total process of adolescence as it appears in the girl, let us first take a brief look at where, in prepuberty, the girl has been and what she has been doing.

The prepubertal girl is a fascinating child, although not always easy to understand. For one thing she is, to an adult, hard to catch in a quiet, confidential mood. She is not only very busy, but a busybody as well; she is full of activities, a "joiner" who cannot resist being a club member. If she hears about two or three other girls who have formed a "secret" club, she will not rest until she has wangled an invitation to join, and will often attempt to enlist the whole family in her endeavors. Her need for many activities, dancing, music, drama, sports, etc., is often a matter of concern to her parents, who cannot see how she can possibly carry such a heavy schedule and complain because they rarely see her at home any more. However, she relies heavily on aid and support from her family in each new venture, whether it is getting into a new club, taking up playing the recorder, or working with a dramatic group. Her enthusiasms wax and wane, often to the bewilderment of her mother, on whom she relies heavily for the implementation of her plans, but who never knows how long they will last. Like the boy, she has in prepuberty a burst of activity in preparation for the onset of adolescence, and seems to be in a constant battle with time. Although she expects the immediate and enthusiastic support of her parents in accomplishing her aims, she is apt to react to offers of help as if they were a sign of parental interference, and is quick to place the blame on mother if her plans do not succeed.

The intense interest she has in other people's affairs, especially those of older siblings, visitors, and relatives, often is the cause of family embarrassment. She is a busybody because of her interest in "secrets," both other people's and her own, often manufacturing a few in order to feel that she can compete with the older girls and women who have secrets, concerning the nature of which she has already formed pretty definite ideas. The sharing of secrets — what one knows about the physiology of the oncoming adolescent years, menstruation, boy-girl relationships, who loves whom, etc. — forms an integral part of the close girl friend relationships of this period. These "best" girl friend pairs are inconstant in comparison to the later relationships between girls in adolescence, and have a playful imitative quality in which much role-playing and impersonation goes on. Furthermore, the relationship is more exclusive, although shorter in duration, and can rarely tolerate the introduction of a third girl, as it generally does by the 14th or 15th year in adolescence.

The onset of menstruation is an extremely important event in a girl's physical and emotional development; there is no single event in the development of the boy which marks the approach of adolescence so dramatically. This is not to say that the onset of menstruation definitely places a girl in the adolescent phase of her emotional development. The physiological change can take place when a girl is still in the prepubertal phase of psychological development, and indeed today, with the accelerated physical maturation of girls, this happens quite frequently. The girl of 10 or 11 who has her first menstrual period will often show little or no overt reaction to it, treating the menstrual flow pretty much as if it were just another elimination function and one for which she has little responsibility. Mothers who try to teach their 10- or 11-year-old daughters proper hygiene may run up against much resistance from the child, who resents the whole business as interfering with her activities, requiring extra cleanliness, something she is averse to in this period anyway, and certainly an unwelcome reminder of her femininity when she has not yet been able fully to accept this role, still preferring tight dungarees and playing touch football with the boys.

Rarely, if ever, is the onset of menstruation a complete surprise to the girl; if so, it is the result of unusually strong repression of an earlier awareness, and an indication of a strong inhibition of the normal processes of gathering sex information during the latency period, an inhibition which may handicap the girl in other areas, both socially and intellectually. The best-informed girl, however, still experiences menstruation to a greater or lesser degree as a trauma or injury to her body. Feelings of guilt stemming from masturbatory activities, along with an increased awareness of sexual feelings and tensions, are often tied up with the idea of self-injury. Old anxieties regarding bedwetting may revive in the fear of an uncontrollable body discharge. Feelings of shame and disgust which may have been originally attached to elimination may reappear, centered on menstruation. While all these and other anxieties may be focused on menstruation, they should not, in the normally developing adolescent girl, become the dominant attitude toward this physiological function.

The anticipation of menstruation has not only its negative features but many positive ones as well. The girl often looks forward to "becoming a woman" not only in a spirit of competition with other girls, but also with many fantasies and expectations that her whole life will change, and by this means she will receive the longed-for respect, admiration, love, and attention belonging to her new status. When the event finally occurs, such fantasies bring a feeling of disappointment and bitterness for a while because the world stays the same, her family continue to treat her in the same manner they did previously. The proud announcement, "Mother, I'm a woman now," often brings only a wise smile from mother, and perhaps a loud laugh from siblings and father.

Signs that all may not be going well in the important process of identification with her sexual role in adolescence are an attitude on the part of the girl of absolute denial, which may take an extreme form when the girl refuses to wear menstrual pads, or shows hypochondriacal reactions such as migraine-like headaches or varying abdominal pains.

This leads us to a consideration of the general process by which a girl achieves identification with her sexual role, one of the important goals of adolescence. So interdependent are the other goals of adolescence that any discussion of identification involves the drive toward independence, the achievement of close relationships with friends of both sexes, and finally, the ability to choose a mate, marry, and fulfill her primary feminine needs in the roles of wife and mother.

The developing process of identification plays an important part in the lessening of the old parental ties. In both boys and girls the liberation from earlier parental ties, necessitated by the need to prepare for an adult role in life, is brought about by a double and concurrent psychological process. Devaluation of the previously overestimated parent, and the concurrent search for new figures with which to identify, begins in preadolescence in both sexes. There are some interesting manifestations of this in the prepuberty girl. The overestimation of a teacher, mother of a girl friend, or camp counselor occurs together with and as part of a process in which her own mother is devaluated. Mothers constantly hear the rhetorical question, "Why can't you be like so-and-so's mother?"

It is understandable that for the girl the need to devaluate her mother in order to form new identifications in her search for her independence is a more trying process than is the case with the boy, whose problem of identification is focused largely upon his father. While the boy can loosen his ties to his father without running into so much danger of losing the source of gratification of his dependency needs in his mother, the girl must run the risk of invoking hostility from the person on whom she still needs to be dependent. An increase in hypochondriacal symptoms during a girl's adolescence is not an unusual occurrence, and seems to serve the purpose of reassuring herself of her mother's continued concern and care for her as a dependent child.

While a change toward being "fresh" and rebellious is often the cause of major concern in the parents of adolescents, this is not serious once the concerns of puberty have been overcome and the child becomes more confident of her own ability to achieve and to establish a separate identity from her mother. However, if a new real motive for hostility toward the parent enters the picture — for example, learning that one is adopted, the divorce or separation of parents, emotional withdrawal of the mother due to depression (menopause frequently may be a cause of depression, irritability, and emotional withdrawal in mothers of adolescent girls), a more serious disturbance in the girl's emotional life may occur and exert an unfavorable influence on her subsequent destiny.

In preadolescence the girl is trying on different roles for herself, play-acting different parts in a quite open fashion. The search for new figures for identification provides in part at least the impetus which makes her so active and busy in preadolescence.

Although there may be a frequent change in the person who wears the title of "best girl friend" or "chum" — an intensely close and possessive relationship between the two girls for a time, followed by sudden quarrels and break-ups — in early adolescence this process is an important one in preparing the girl for longer and more lasting friendships built on more sublimated and altruistic interests in one another's welfare, which is characteristic of the friendships between girls in later adolescence and, indeed, throughout their adult lives.

An important factor serving the purpose of unifying and solidifying the many partial identifications the girl makes in early adolescence, identifications which later merge into an abstract ideal, is the girl's increased self-love which, while it prevents too many identifications and increases self-confidence, can for a time make the adolescent girl a pretty difficult person with whom to live. This self-love has a transient component of megalomania, which manifests itself in increased demands for new clothes and other material benefits from the family, often with what seems to be little regard toward the welfare of other members of the family. She is intolerant of any criticism, moody, and unpredictable. The slightest criticism or disappointment may throw her into despair, or seemingly trivial successes lead her to heights of happiness and renewed self-confidence. Since her fantasy life is very active, she is often preoccupied, negligent of responsibilities, forgetful, and tactless. She is strongly partisan, and to some extent this tendency toward overidentification remains a well-known feminine characteristic in later life, often interfering with her ability to be objective and wise in her judgment of people and situations. At the same time, her use of fantasy, her ability to "tune in" on other people's feelings, as well as a greater awareness of her own inner perceptions, form some of the basic feminine characteristics so important in the successful fulfillment of her role as wife and mother.

This brings us to the process by which, in adolescence, the girl's search for new objects to love, and to be loved by, changes from persons of her own sex to the opposite sex. Interest in boys by no means begins in adolescence. Although her status and intimacy needs are fulfilled primarily through her relationships to other girls, she has been, throughout the preceding school years, formulating definite ideas about boys, what they are like and what kind of boy is the most deserving of her admiration. Although she takes the position that boys are not likable creatures, she admires them and is secretly convinced of their superiority. If, under group pressure and in order to maintain her status with her girl friends, or under the influence of an older girl friend, a girl must have a boy friend in the early adolescent years, she may be quite aggressive in obtaining one, but there is no real emotional need for physical contact with boys at this period. The reason that this is so is not because the girl is unaware of the intensified sexual urges and body tensions associated with the hormonal changes of this period, but because she is capable of using fantasy fulfillments and gratifications rather than the physical contact and activity more characteristic of the male. The dominance of passive characteristics in the feminine personality favors the development and utilization of fantasy in the release of sexual tensions; masturbation activities are utilized also for release of tension to a somewhat less degree than in the boy. It is also probable that the protected, hidden position of the genital and reproductive organs is one of the important determinants of the development of these feminine characteristics of sexuality in the girl. As a result, the girl tends to spiritualize her physical sexual feelings, a tendency which persists in adulthood, but along with the capacity to experience physical sexual gratification as well.

The need to "fall in love" over and over again is stronger in the girl than in the boy, and while she is less aware of the sexual character of these feelings than he is, there is a pattern of progression in heterosexual love relationships similar to that of the boy. A frequently necessary ingredient in the "falling in love" process in early adolescence is that the object of the girl's adoration should appear to her to be unattainable. A movie star or other hero of the day possesses this necessary quality of the love object of the young girl — unattainability — and therefore is a safe object around which her early fantasy can be built. Within a short time, however, someone nearer her, a favorite male teacher or uncle, may become the center of her fantasy life, with intensification of feelings of love, hate, and competition with other girls. The next progression in love object is the older adolescent boy, also unattainable but not quite so hopelessly unattainable.

During this period the girl may receive much attention from other boys, but often quickly rejects and devaluates the "attainable" ones, calling them "jerks," "slobs," and "babies." Thus she protects herself from too early sexual experiences for which she is not emotionally ready.

The following is an illustration of this phase in the "falling in love" process:

A 14-year-old girl writes to her friend: "I was thinking of the problem I had last year and how silly it was. How could I love a teacher: Every time I read last year's diary, I can't help laughing. It's so silly and stupid. It seems like every year I end up falling in love and you know what kind of love that is (hopelessly): Last year I fell in love with one of the boys I sat with down at the beach. I'm right now trying to forget him, but it's so hard. I hope I forget him by next summer. I'm always liking a boy that doesn't like me and hating a boy who does. Do you suppose I'll ever settle down? I hope so."

Although it is a normal process for a girl to fall in love many times before she reaches late adolescence and early adulthood, this does not imply that this is an easy, smooth process for her. The falling in and out of love so frequently is in itself disturbing to the girl, who is puzzled by the intensity of her feelings and their seeming inconstancy. She is plagued by feelings of self-doubt and guilt, and concern lest she turn out to be a woman of "light" fancies and whims. If strong, these feelings, plus such other factors as parental objection to her attachment to a particular boy, may lead her to a too-early selection of a mate and premature engagement or marriage.

By the time the girl has reached the period of late adolescence, which may extend into her early twenties, she has become capable of not only choosing her mate, but of offering him a fully developed capacity for love, encompassing both her rich inner personality and her well-developed capacities for physical sexuality, which reach their final, fullest development through the added experiences of marriage and motherhood.

ADOLESCENT BOYS
LOVICK C. MILLER

Someone has remarked that adolescent boys are exactly like adult men except more so: they dream more, curse more, tell more dirty jokes with more interest, brag more, have a greater sense of prestige-loss over failure and a greater sense of achievement over success, and intellectually they explore more in every area. It might equally be true if someone had said they are like men except less so, since they produce less, are less creative, have less physical sexual experience, and less interest in responsibility, success, money, and the future. The problem for the adolescent boy is to become more like a man in the latter sense and less like one in the former sense.

By the time the boy reaches adolescence he has a fairly consistent idea of *who* he is, of what he *can* and *cannot* do, and what he can *expect* during the next stage of his life. He has a fairly stable set of values and ideals, and a range of basic psychological mechanisms for coping with stress. With the onset of adolescence the integration achieved thus far is subjected to a host of new pressures. These he must synthesize into an integrated psychic system which can deal successfully with the privileges and responsibilities of adult living. We might say, then, that the basic problem faced by the adolescent boy is to integrate past experiences with present physiological and social stresses, and with future expectations, into an ego identity which fulfills his masculine ideal and which is potentially capable of fulfilling the roles of an adult male in society.

The following material on the adolescent male is organized in terms of five primary tension systems which dominate the individual adolescent's life: (1) need for greater independence, (2) pressures for decreased autonomy, (3) sexual tensions, (4) hostile tensions, and (5) increased self-esteem. In describing individual adolescents' attempts to integrate these basic processes it is hoped that a general picture of this life period will be obtained.

Need for greater independence. Adolescence is a transitional period between a dependent and an independent state. Since birth there has been an ever increasing need for independence, but in adolescence the pressure increases. Boys begin to rely more upon their peer group than upon parents for their basic values and style of life. This need takes many forms of expression: one mother was driven to distraction, her 16 year old boy refusing to get a haircut because his best friend was also a "long-hair." Often parents describe their son suddenly becoming acutely self-conscious about his appearance, demanding clothes to keep in style, whereas previously no cajoling could induce him to care about himself. At this period the boy constantly demands that he be allowed to drive, to go to bed when he wishes, and to get up when he likes on nonschool days. This is the period when the fantasy develops of going "down south" or "out west" with the gang of boys in an old jalopy. It is also an argumentative period. Boys wish to assert their ideas, to let parents know that things can be done better. Often, too, boys will form close attachments to adults outside the family, particularly people who have lived differently and think differently from their parents. It is through such attachments, through reading new books and listening to new ideas, that an identity separate from that of parents is achieved.

Usually for the boy, independence from the family unit proceeds with only a modicum of disturbance, particularly when he senses the need and the parents can accept it. Some boys, however, tend to demand more independence than adults judge them capable of accepting. Others tend to assert themselves in such provocative terms that society finds their demands difficult to assimilate or tolerate. One senior, years after graduation from high school, was frequently singled out by his teachers as having been a "bad influence in school," "impossible to get along with." This was a very talented boy, one whom all respected in many ways; but in his need for individual recognition he wanted to destroy. He was a leader of a group of boys in school who were the principal editors and contributors to the school newspapers and magazines, which kept the school in constant revolt against the administration. School spirit was at an all-time low because the leaders of this class were against everything in current existence and in favor of changes impossible to be achieved.

When commenting about his senior year, 4 years later, one member of this "disillusioned" group compared the newspaper which he had edited to one in another section of the country. The editor of the other paper had written a series on American school life, printed several thousand copies of his articles, and sent them to India in hopes of establishing an exchange of points of view with Indian high school students. Later, this series of articles became the basis for obtaining foundation support for a tour of high school editors to India.

Here, then, are two solutions to the independence struggle. In the latter case the editor identified with and participated in the problems of adult society. This participation not only was acceptable, but was rewarded by society, and this identification also helped him to complete his own ego-identity. He is now a full-time journalist of promise. The former editor, rejecting the possibility of identification, fought the existing society and demanded changes. Four years later he was still confused as to what he wanted to do.

Another solution to the independence struggle frequently found in adolescence is a pseudomaturity pattern. One 14 year old boy disassociated himself from his own age-mates to be with seniors. He proudly proclaimed that he was a greater "booze-hound" than most college freshmen. His greatest gratification occurred when people mistook him for an 18 year old. He always falsified his age, dated girls a number of years older than himself, and bragged about being bold and boisterous in their presence. "Big deals," fast and dangerous living, run-ins with the law, "wild" house parties were his principal conversational topics. The most striking feature about this boy during his 4 years of high school was that he changed very little. He mellowed somewhat, wondered at times why he had been in such a hurry to grow up, and was able to take life a little more seriously, but for the most part he remained a "big operator" throughout.

An aspect of the need for independence frequently found in boys who seek it through assertive action is a sense of disillusionment following success, as if the independence so highly esteemed in fantasy was disappointing in reality. One brilliant senior, president of the student council, and generally admired by students and faculty alike, wanted to run away two months before graduation because he could see no purpose in it all. He had won most of the honors for which he competed, and yet he felt let down. Another boy was the principal writer of a highly successful and talented musical, yet he was depressed for days following the production. Another boy put an enormous amount of time and energy into "doing" things and getting elected to offices in various organizations. When it came time to graduate, he too wondered "why?" This is a syndrome limited principally to seniors, and seems to be based in part upon the natural withdrawal of school interest when thoughts turn toward college. But a larger part seems to be due to much of the activity in adolescence serving to conceal underlying tensions — as long as you do something then you do not have time to think about things. When the work is over, and success and independence obtained, these boys are left again to face their inner tensions. Much activity also springs from competitive rivalry with one's peers, the rivalry serving to demonstrate one's own self-worth through external symbols. To be editor of the paper, president of the student council, etc., gives one the sense of being "more" important than the next person. When these props are removed through graduation, or when motivations for independent strivings are based upon the need to *escape internal stress,* disillusionment sets in due to the inability to integrate physiological or social tensions satisfactorily except through action and constant assurance of competence. In contrast, when the motivation is based primarily upon the need to *establish an independent identity*, then the boy looks forward with eagerness to the more complex situations of adult or college life which will provide further opportunity for growth and development.

The dependence-independence struggle is not always resolved through a trend toward increased independence. When humans find themselves in conditions of stress with which they cannot deal successfully, they often long to return to the dependent state in which they were protected by parental figures. This wish to remain dependent is often strongly activated in adolescence when the boy either has not resolved his ties to parental figures, or else when external conditions are overwhelming. As the time for adult responsibilities approaches, as the pressures for an individual identity mount, and as psychological separation from the family begins to take place, the boy becomes aware of the lack of continuing nurturing supplies from parents for which he longs. At such times dependency needs become manifest in such problems as being unable to leave the family to go to school. At boarding school he is the homesick boy, at public school he is "mother's boy" — childish, immature, depending heavily upon teachers to take care of him. In its most pathological state school becomes a place to be feared, and the boy stays home because of this fear. School phobias in adolescence are indicative of more serious disturbances than at earlier ages, and generally require professional aid. In such severe cases there is often an unusual family situation in which the boy is very much involved, and the fear of school is a displacement of his fear of what might be happening at home while he is away at school. One case was a sophisticated-appearing 14 year old who was able to get along very well at school as far as the other boys and faculty were concerned, but would collapse in the infirmary for days at a time. Finally he broke down completely, sobbing for hours on end that he could not stand to be away from his home any longer. This puzzled him, for he felt unwanted at home, his father was unbearable, and his mother had a chronic deteriorating disease. In further talking it became quite obvious that although he had an adequate social facade and a "pseudomaturity," inwardly he felt very much a child, not yet ready to be out on his own. He also was mindful of a family joke, often repeated, that he had been an unexpected and unwanted event in their household, the mother having been told that further pregnancies would produce deafness. This in fact occurred, and it was the operation to correct the condition which led to the mother's current illness. In his mind there was the certain conviction that his birth was responsible for his mother's current illness.

More frequently the problems of dependency are disguised. One boy with peptic ulcer talked constantly about how much he enjoyed the keen competition of a "tough school," how he would prefer the English school system because it demanded even greater discipline and competition. The one thing he feared, though, about his particular school was a general tendency for students letting down, taking it easy, after they had been there awhile. His mother further elucidated his dependency, commenting that he depended on her for the most minor decisions, such as asking her each time they ate at a restaurant if he should remove his coat. This boy constantly had to defend himself against his dependency needs both by active striving and by directly expressing these needs to his mother.

Dependency frequently takes another form in the attitude that no matter what happens everything will come out well in the end. Such boys seem to go blandly through the day, sometimes anxious, often not, but generally taking no effective action to aid themselves. One boy expressed it well when he said he believed in predestination — it didn't make any difference whether he worked or not, because it was already decided what his future would be. Frequently such boys are poor academic performers.

Pressure for decreased autonomy. By the time a boy reaches adolescence society expects him to have given up much of his autonomy and to be capable of being a cooperative member of a group. Ordinarily he has learned to control his eliminative functions, to regulate his sleeping and eating habits according to custom, to regulate his anger, to be able to give and take in interpersonal relations, to share, to limit and postpone his individual demands, and to work with a group for the benefit of all members. But the boy's capacity for cooperation is subjected to severe strain with the onset of adolescence. For one thing, he comes to depend more strongly upon his informal peer groups.

These groups usually demand much greater conformity and cooperation than the original family group, and therefore the adolescent tends to do not what "he wants" but what the group wants. This explains to a large degree the intensity of fads at this period, for doing what others do is proof of group identity.

The capacity to control his autonomous wishes in order to be able to participate in such groups is quite important to the adolescent boy, because not only do such groups serve as a medium for achieving independence, but also much of the socialization process itself takes place within these groups.

Here the adolescent learns the vast store of unwritten knowledge about life which is communicated only between peers. This knowledge might be the intimate details of sex behavior as participated in by both sexes;

the breaking of moral taboos such as in stealing, truancy, etc.; the discussion of the personal characteristics of adults, particularly the side which adults try so hard to keep others and themselves from knowing; and the more personal views on the great problems of mankind, such as religion, politics, morals, etc.

When a boy is unable to participate in group relations he is generally retarded in his emotional development. Avoidance of such relationships is usually a sign that the boy is not successfully coping with social or biological tensions. The group is composed of individuals who come together to share their inner tensions, and in this way draw upon each other for achieving mastery of these new and strong feelings. The mastery process in a group, however, seems to have one special characteristic, namely, the boy uses the group to explore tension, but not to reveal his fear of exploration. Boys discuss almost every phase of life. They tell of petting adventures; of talking down the teacher; of evading the police car; of getting slapped by their girl friends for being too bold; of getting disciplined for being too argumentative; of getting put on the police docket. What they do not discuss is their failure to venture forth in some new area. When the group senses this fear in a boy they frequently use him as a scapegoat, which serves to increase the group members' own self-esteem while covering their own fears. For the scapegoat this results in a major loss of self-esteem and an unusual sense of loneliness.

When a boy has little tolerance within himself for the tensions underlying such group discussions, or when he has little adventure to contribute to the group because of his fear of exploration, or when he has not been able to limit his own autonomy needs, he tends to avoid the group or to be expelled from it. This eliminates the main social avenue used by most of his contemporaries for mastery of these feelings. Such boys have to tolerate not only the anxiety arising from the continuation of the conflict, but also they have to tolerate the increased sense of loneliness and hostility arising from their inability to participate in the group. One boy dramatically expressed the pain associated with such loneliness when he said he craved a friend so much that he found himself just "wanting to crawl inside anyone whom he could trust." This boy found such a friend, as frequently happens in the course of counselling interviews. Also, one friend often is the avenue for finding other friends, tending further to break down the sense of isolation. Finding a friend seems to be one of the sure signs that the repression underlying his isolation is lifting, and that the boy is on his way toward a more integrated and mature solution to the problems of growing up.

Isolation is a dreadful experience in adolescence since there is not yet a sufficient sense of self-identity to master the anxiety aroused by the lack of support of the peer group. It can, however, also be a constructive experience if it does not create sufficient anxiety to cause a general disruption of the integrative capacity of the ego. From time to time adolescent boys like very much to escape from the continued pressure of the group, but they generally like to do so at their own choosing rather than to know it occurs at the hands of others.

Society, too, places considerable pressure upon the boy to give up his autonomous functions. Athletics demand greater cooperation from individuals as team sports replace the sandlot, coaching and systematic training replace the Sunday afternoon get-togethers, and umpires replace the perennial arguments. Other extracurricular activities, such as school papers and magazines, debates, club activities with elected officers, politics, etc., all become sources of interest that demand much sustained effort, necessitating a curtailment of individual autonomy.

But the greatest pressure comes from the school itself. There is a large transition from grammar school to junior high. The boy is faced with demands for more work in less time, for higher abstractive abilities, more individual initiative with less adult support, and more emphasis upon achievement and competition. In addition to this increase in work demand, the adolescent becomes aware that school is his major preparation for adult life, which he will soon be entering, and to do this he must have a trade, a business skill, or a profession. Each thing he does brings with it the realization that it is not only satisfying or frustrating at the moment but also preparation for the future.

Most boys accept the need for greater curtailment of autonomy placed upon them by both society and their peers. Occasionally we find a boy who disguises his unresolved autonomy needs by throwing himself with great gusto into various cooperative activities, such as athletics, politics, or journalism. Such a boy tends to be overconscientious, always demanding things be done "his way," becoming extremely upset if they are not. One boy joined every major activity in school except athletics and constantly tried to become principal leader in each activity. When he succeeded he was frequently at odds with other members as a result of his insistence on domination. Because of his inability to resolve this conflict between wanting to be a part of a group but also wanting the members to go his way, he frequently became depressed following failure and ostracism. In the course of counselling interviews he began to recognize the extent to which his autonomous demands had not been resolved. This led to greater awareness of the needs of others, and then to a reduction of his interpersonal conflicts.

The greatest source of difficulty relating to autonomy occurs in that group of boys who have not acquired the skills necessary to meet society's increased demands at adolescence. These boys frequently lose interest in trying to conform to society's pattern, and "go it alone." In a recent study Peck[110] found that 84 per cent of the 229 children appearing before a juvenile court in New York City in 1951 showed a reading retardation of 2 or more years. Half of this group manifested a disability of 5 or more years retardation. This research team pointed out that the typical pattern followed by these boys was to find themselves hopelessly lost in school as the demands became greater. Frustrated and feeling inadequate, they began to truant to avoid the constant sense of failure. When not attending school they became lonely and fearful of the law, and began to seek companionship. These groups of truants, to ease their tensions, then began to find activities, frequently delinquency. Cohen,[111] enlarging on this concept, points out that delinquents have the same values as do conforming members of society. They are boys who have the values, and at the same time the unconscious recognition that they do not have the skills necessary to achieve what society has outlined as "the successful life." In their delinquency they are trying to reduce their own sense of inadequacy.

Sexual tensions. At adolescence there are accelerated physiological activities which become manifest in a number of ways. There is a new growth spurt described in an earlier chapter, which changes the image that a boy has of his body and requires relearning physical coordination. This change in the body-image is often disturbing. One boy described in detail his embarrassment with his new size and awkwardness, being especially self-conscious about the size of his hands. He went to great lengths to hide his "hams," as he called them, and was sure that other people felt the same way about their size. The adolescent boy has to learn to live, so to speak, with a different body.

In addition to the change in body size the adolescent boy gradually becomes aware of other changes. He notes such things as pubescent hair, nocturnal emissions, dreams which are sexual in content, erotic erections of his penis, and changes in his voice. These body changes symbolize that fundamental changes are taking place within him, and often they become a focal point for anxiety arising from other sources. They signal that he is becoming sexually mature, which means he has acquired a new apparatus for the expression of new sexual energies. It means he must seek out other objects for the expression of his sexual and tender feelings than he has had in the past. Up to adolescence, the mother, or such mother-substitutes as teachers, nursemaids, aunts, and grandmothers, had been the sole recipients of his tender feelings. Girls his own age had been avoided, teased, or considered to be another boy. At adolescence he takes another look at "friend Jane" and begins to recognize qualities hitherto-fore unseen.

The process of seeking out new and acceptable objects for the mutual exchange of sexual and tender feelings is not a simple one in our society. The adolescent learns or already knows that there are certain taboos placed by society against irresponsible expression of these new energies. Society demands that expression with objects of the opposite sex be post-poned until such time as the boy is ready to assume more adult respon-sibilities. Despite its being a highly individualized experience, society sets the rules under which the experience takes place. For the adolescent boy there appears a dilemma: here is a new and exciting experience, but it is forbidden for the time being. Accepting the presence of sexual im-pulses, but at the same time postponing their expression through genital discharges in sexual intercourse, poses one of the principal developmental problems for the boy.

For boys, masturbation becomes the principal means for the manage-ment of sexual impulses while at the same time postponing mature genital expression. Kinsey[112] reports that 99 per cent of males masturbate by the time they are 20. Despite this universal practice, attitudes differ widely. Some boys accept their sexual needs and discuss openly their pleasure associated with masturbation. One 14 year old boy said he masturbated almost every night, that it was a very real source of pleasure to him, and that his fantasies "get really low, down in the ditch, almost anything you want to think about I think about." Other boys tend to be more self-conscious, keeping their activities pretty much to themselves, and fol-lowing a general pattern of self-indulgence with increasing need to con-trol the habit as they get older and find heterosexual objects. At times boys appear so guilty about masturbation that the act becomes a major focus of anxiety. One boy, in the course of counselling interviews, an-ticipated discontinuing interviews when the topic was raised "for fear of having his morals corrupted." This was a very immature 14 year old whose alcoholic father had deserted the family when he was a small boy. His mother abhorred everything pertaining to masculinity or sexuality. When he was able to discuss his feelings about masturbation, he said he had always wanted to know, but he was afraid, for "nobody from good families masturbated." When he went away to boarding school he found it to be a common topic of conversation of even boys from the "best of families." This boy was greatly relieved to learn from an adult, whom he considered to be a trusted authority, that there are no harmful effects from masturbation at this age and that in fact it usually serves a useful purpose in the process of growing up.

Masturbation serves not only to relieve sexual tension. It is during the manipulation of the penis that the adolescent boy prepares himself for an active heterosexual life. His fantasies during this time are usually rich and varied. This fantasy activity serves as a practicing ground for the actual heterosexual activities which are to come later. It is for this reason that one worries when adolescents manifest extreme asceticism, compulsive masturbation, marked repression of sexual feelings, or excessive guilt about sexuality during early adolescence, thus suggesting that the synthesizing work of the ego is not progressing normally and that trouble can be expected when the next stage, active heterosexual activity, is reached.

If growth and development are progressing normally the adolescent boy greets his awareness of sexual maturation with a relatively positive and uncomplicated attitude. There is generally an increased sense of self-esteem and pride, the boy begins to "feel his oats," often to the regret of his elders. He enjoys this new experience, and accepts it as a sign that at last he is "growing up."

When, however, the boy experiences these internal changes as threatening, then any number of reactions may set in. In general there appear to be two differing modes of defensive reactions, nonacceptance and acting-out, which represent two polar extremes of an adjustment continuum. Individuals generally do not use one particular defense to the exclusion of all others, but tend rather to use various defenses at various times. Occasionally, however, they do restrict their defenses to such an extent that they appear to fall close to an extreme of the continuum.

Some boys appear to limit nonacceptance specifically to sexual content. They appear at ease with their contemporaries and generally have social skills adequate to be considered "one of the boys." These are conscientious, hard workers, often interested in athletics to a mild degree, and tend to take themselves quite seriously although they are not without a sense of humor. They enjoy relationships with contemporaries, both male and female, as long as the relationships are not too intimate. When sexual themes are discussed they find themselves embarrassed, and evade bull sessions where such topics are discussed. They feel extremely guilty about masturbation and constantly struggle to control it, but despite themselves they indulge and find themselves obsessed with sexual thoughts. Because of their guilt, masturbation often does not adequately relieve their tension. This leads to further masturbatory activity, and a compulsive cycle is set up.

When the nonacceptance is more pervasive we find these boys often becoming hyperintellectual. This intellectualism seems to enable the boy to be less emotionally involved in his interpersonal relationships. One boy said he was not interested in people unless they liked to argue about esoteric subjects. He decried the lack of such people, particularly among girls. This lack of suitable friends made it almost impossible to make close relationships.

Occasionally we find the repression resembling asceticism, where the boy renounces all interest in sexual or tender feelings. One 14 year old boy denied all interest in such feelings, saying he never thought of girls, he never intended to get married, he never had sexual dreams, he never masturbated, and he thought any show of tenderness was a sign of weakness. He had never had positive feeling for his mother, whom he could not tolerate. He intended to emulate his father, an impressive person with a brilliant career, by rigid self-discipline and the surrendering of personal desires. In interviews this boy was cold, analytical, and challenging, constantly demanding facts and clarification of statements, and maintaining a haughty, contemptuous attitude. As one frequently finds, such rigid self-denial could not be maintained by this boy. His controls would episodically break down. At such times he would get involved in impulsive anti-social acting-out by stealing, destructive dormitory pranks, etc.

If counsellors or therapists are available, the boy using repressive defenses frequently seeks them out, because the conflict between the new sexual tensions demanding expression and the attitudes which make expression unacceptable create considerable anxiety for which they urgently seek relief. They often respond quickly to psychotherapy, one reason being that the incomplete mastery of these tensions is common to all boys of this age, and unlike adults, they use their informal peer groups for purposes of integrating conflicts. In adolescence it is permissible to talk of one's interests and to a certain extent one's concerns and fears about sexuality, for this appears to be society's way of providing a favorable setting for individual mastery to take place. When boys are freed to the point where they can make use of this natural social process, then development continues normally. One has to be careful, however, in not encouraging premature group participation for these boys, for although there is the urge to master the feelings, there is also the recognition of the anxiety which accompanies the lifting of the repression. One boy continuously avoided any discussion of the area, becoming silent or irritated whenever the subject was approached. He was told, in an attempt to ease his self-consciousness, that most boys his age frequently engage in a mutual exchange of sex information through jokes and stories, and also that masturbation was a quite common practice. He later brought out that this information increased his anxiety, for it highlighted another sensitive area, namely, how different he was from the other boys.

The boys who tend to act out their sexual feelings also can be arranged along a continuum. There are those who seem to act directly upon their sexual impulses, and tend to do so with little thought for their female sexual partners, but with a great deal of thought of the effects of their acts upon their male contemporaries. These are the boys who spend hours describing their exploits, making their repressed contemporaries slink away into the shadows. In this way they often displace their anxiety, letting the repressed adolescent carry their guilt as well as his own. Sexuality for them has been divorced from tender feeling, and the problem here is to bring the two into close harmony. Such boys are not likely to find their way to a counselor, for generally they do not feel anxious or concerned.

Another aspect of the sexual problem is that of homosexuality, which disturbs adolescent boys considerably more than girls. In early adolescence it is a common experience for boys to feel sexually attracted to other boys and to engage in mutual masturbation. Kinsey reports that by the 18th year 34 per cent of the male population have engaged in at least 1 homosexual episode. A large number of boys think about it but do not act it out.

Homosexual interests result from numerous factors, but are closely associated with two: (1) in certain socioeconomic groups, the social prohibition placed upon heterosexuality after onset of physiological sexuality forces boys, because of their assertive masculine strivings, to seek other outlets, and (2) if the assertive drives have themselves been unhealthily repressed we find a turning toward the same sex to avoid anxieties in heterosexual relationships.

It is the latter situation which usually results in more serious conflict over homosexuality, for here it is based on fear of women in general. Often when this is the case we find that the boy identifies himself more with a female image than a male. Such cases need professional attention. Although the fear of homosexuality is widespread, and homosexual experiences are not infrequent for adolescent boys, homosexuality is a state generally passed through in adolescence and only in special cases does the concern linger.

Hostile tensions. At adolescence, there is a heightening of *aggressive* tension similar to that for sexuality, but the source is to be found in the increased pressures arising from the sexual and social demands being placed upon the adolescent, rather than upon some central physiological source. The adolescent boy has to integrate these new tensions by means other than the direct expression of the primitive wish to destroy which lies behind the hostile impulse. Most boys find complementary modes for expression which modify the basic wish but do not inhibit their assertive masculine strivings.

There appear to be three general types of boys who have come to accept aggressive and destructive impulses to the point where they cause little concern to themselves or others. The first are the boys who have channeled such impulses into hard competitive sports. Another group are the boys who are known as the "hustlers" — the boys who channel their aggressive drives into more social activities, such as work, management of school newspapers, etc. The third are boys who seem to have no special outlet for their drives, but who at the same time appear comfortable with such feelings, being assertive when the situation demands, accepting other people's aggression without becoming defensive, and generally giving the impression of needing neither to assert themselves nor to avoid aggressive feelings within themselves or in others.

When their own aggressive feelings or those of others are anxiety-provoking, we find defensive reactions developing. Frequently the defensive process is closely associated with both sexual and hostile tensions, making it difficult to know which presents the greater source of difficulty. Quite often an adolescent who represses both assertive and sexual urges says that when he was younger he was quite aggressive. One boy described it as feeling "on top of the pile, as if the world was all mine." Rather suddenly, around 13, the pain of aggressive competition became too intense. He found himself fighting with his contemporaries more and more and coming out on the losing side. Rather than being at odds with his peers and suffering the pain of repetitive defeat and further loss of self-esteem, he gradually withdrew, adopting more indirect ways of asserting himself through the use of words and his keen intellect. Such boys are often intensely aggressive intellectually — slashing, cutting, showing their superiority by flaunting their knowledge. What seems to happen is that in the prepubertal period these boys have sufficient tolerance for anxiety created in nonsexual competitive and aggressive activities, but with the coming of the new sexual tensions, which they are unable to master gracefully, they become overwhelmed to such an extent that even the once satisfying aggressive play becomes a nightmare. They retreat to a more secure position, choosing their tongues and their minds as their weapons.

Often we find, however, boys who have a high degree of tolerance and acceptance of sexual desires, but who develop a reaction formation against their aggressive wishes, turning them into their opposites. They usually appear as nice, polite, cooperative boys who never give anyone any trouble. Their aggression is well concealed, seldom coming out directly. One boy was fascinated with guns. He belonged to the rifle club, was an expert shot, but said he never hunted because he could not bear to hurt an animal. Another boy gave innumerable instances where he would go out of his way to avoid hurting other people's feelings. He told, for example, of working in the kitchen with a number of other boys. A new boy was assigned to an easy job, and when he finished he left. The remaining workers agreed that next time they would give him a hard job, and leave him to do it alone. When the retribution was under way our boy became soft-hearted, and broke his bond with the older kitchen hands to help the new boy. This same boy became extremely uncomfortable when he learned the entire school population planned to riot in chapel in protest of an act by the dean. Any show of aggression, even with the support of all his contemporaries, would have been an extremely unpleasant experience for this boy. Boys that go to such extremes in inhibiting aggression may develop characterological symptoms rather than neurotic ones. The first boy mentioned above was close to failing out of school despite a very bright mind; the second had an extreme stutter. His stuttering was bad whenever he felt tense, but in situations where he attempted to conceal his anger he simply could not speak.

Frequently we find a boy who feels quite uncomfortable with his own aggressive feelings and who is easily hurt by the aggression of others. He generally suffers considerably in a group of boys, for they sense his underlying fear of aggression and take advantage of this weakness. Such boys frequently resort to verbal aggression, which seems safer to them than more forceful assertion. A typical situation for one of these boys occurred one day at the breakfast table. The boy was late and the other boy, who was the waiter for that day, refused to serve him. He did nothing, but raged inwardly, and finally dismissed him as "an insignificant prep," the most devastating safe aggression he was capable of expressing. This same boy remembers, as the two most outstanding events of his four years of prep school, first, the time when he successfully beat a friend for a scholastic prize, the friend being unaware of competition, and second, the time when he was doped up with caffein and "demolished" the opposition in a debate. He felt safe in being competitive and assertive so long as his friend was not aware of the competition, and he felt elated when he was able to win in verbal duels. The fact that these two events stood out in his mind showed the importance to him of being able to be assertive even though for the most part he felt inadequate in this area.

Probably the most prevalent type of aggression in adolescence is the aggression which is acted out. In a mild form this is quite typical of the population in general, seen in such things as practical jokes, horseplay, etc. When it takes on a definite antisocial flavoring it gets into the broad category of delinquency, which cannot be dealt with here. The delinquent adolescent, unlike the repressor, intellectualizer, hustler, manager, athlete, etc., *acts* upon the impulse rather than repressing it or channeling it into constructive forms. Like all those who act out, they tend not to internalize their anxiety but immediately to discharge it and the impulse as well. They also avoid counseling or therapeutic situations, and usually can be reached only at the time of their crisis, when society temporarily substitutes for the individual conscience which appears to be lacking.

Increased self-esteem. Many writers have stressed the increase in self-esteem which characterizes the adolescent period for both boys and girls. We frequently hear such expressions as "He is feeling his oats" or "He thinks he is hot." This increased narcissism occurs when the adolescent feels capable of successfully mastering the social and physiological tensions discussed above. The increase in self-esteem, however, seems to be different for boys than for girls. Girls seem to invest more energy in those aspects of the self which enhance their personal appeal, spending hours before mirrors, getting the proper set to their hair, etc. Boys, too, show considerable self-preoccupation, but interest seems to center around their concerns over assertive masculine activities or interests. If athletic, their energies go into competitive sports and muscle-building, and except in special cases this investment is not for the purpose of passive attraction but for assertive action; if intellectual, into fierce intellectual debates; if social, into school politics or rivalry for the affection of their girl friends. When such outlets are blocked we find these boys obsessed with themselves, not usually in terms of how wonderful they are but how wonderful it would be if they could assert themselves fully, whether it is in sports, in the classroom, or on the dance floor. When the energy is released they report unusual experiences. One boy suddenly found he was scoring an unusual number of goals on the hockey rink, taking examinations with unusual ease and confidence, and speaking in classes where he previously had been unable to express his opinion. Previous to this he had retreated into himself, ruminating for hours each day on self-improvement techniques. Self-improvement previously meant inhibiting all assertive and aggressive feelings. When he was able to have more tolerance for such feelings he found a new confidence in himself and new feelings of self-esteem based more on real accomplishment than on dreams of what he could do if only he were the perfect individual.

Often we find that the energies are neither utilized for constructive purposes nor completely inhibited, but oscillate between the two extremes. One boy expressed this conflict when he became obsessed with having eight eggs for breakfast. He had read that eggs increased virility. His insistence became so obnoxious that he finally had to explain his case to the dean of the school. At the same time that he was in trouble over this affair he wrote a theme on the use of salt-peter as a means for keeping one's sexual urges in check. It seemed that he was in conflict over increasing his virility to the maximum, which in turn might lead to a loss of control.

For boys, increased narcissism usually refers to an increased ability to be assertive and masculine. It means a fuller awareness of the new energy sources at their command which can be utilized for realizing their masculine ideal.

In summary, the development of adolescent boys has been discussed, with use of case material to illustrate the way in which various social and physiological tensions become integrated into a self-image which provides the boy with a stable unity to enter the next stage of his development. Because of successful mastery of earlier developmental problems, most boys seem to greet adolescence with eagerness, as if at last they had reached the promised land. At this time there is an increase in the demand for greater independence and autonomy, and an increase in sexual and aggressive tensions which must be integrated into the self-image obtained prior to adolescence. All adolescent boys use the various defensive procedures against these tensions to some degree, but for certain ones the defensive aspects seem to encompass a large part of their personality structure, impeding natural development. Often boys having difficulties in one area will have difficulties in other areas, but this is not necessarily the case. Finally, increased self-esteem in boys has been discussed from the point of view of its relation to their capacity to integrate the various tensions, and to utilize this new energy to fulfill their masculine ideal through assertive participation in activities and interests.

ADJUSTMENT DIFFICULTIES DURING ADOLESCENCE
GEORGE E. GARDNER

In order to gain an understanding appreciation of the occasional difficulties in adjustment of children in the adolescent years, particularly of boys and girls from 12 through 15 or 16 years, it will be helpful to review one aspect of development — a prerequisite for development and for the assumption of maturity at any level. I refer here to the oft-repeated observations of professionals in the field of education, in mental health, and in child guidance that learning and development take place only when the child feels secure.

The child's sense of security. From the earliest steps in training in infancy to the acquisition of very complex bits of behavior and intellectual functioning, it is an observable fact that the feeling of security in the potential learner is of paramount importance. Rewards, ambitions, and discipline are secondary to this single factor in adequate motivation of the child. It is of course comparatively easy to note the presence or absence of this factor in early infancy, but it is just as easy for parents and educators to overlook it or to minimize its importance in the steps that must be taken toward maturity and adulthood in the adolescent years. Before scrutinizing the somewhat particular and even peculiar implications of this notion when applied to the adolescent's adjustment, let us examine what is involved in this emotional ingredient of the developmental process — the sense of security.

At best this feeling of security is complex and not too easily reducible to descriptive terms. Many times its value and power are more easily recognizable because of its absence. However, we can say that the child feels secure when he realizes that he is loved, wanted, and enjoyed by his parents; when he is certain that he is not to be abandoned or deserted; when his home has the appearance of stability, assuring that his parents are to be there indefinitely; when he is protected by them from external attacks or physical injuries by other people (including parents and siblings) and by inanimate objects, together with protection and help from them against expressing *his own* undesirable internal primitive drives and impulses; when his faith in the completeness and truthfulness of parental teachings has been affirmed by repeated demonstrations of it; and when he is confident that his parents treat him as an individual worth while in and of himself, rather than as a composite picture of the very best and the most highly prized — or of the most undesirable and unwanted — character traits of his parents themselves or of other relatives with whom his parents may attempt to identify him.

To be sure, there may be additional elements also needed in good parental-child relationships up through adolescence, but these would seem to be the most important factors constituting that adequate and necessary "emotional climate" cited by Beata Rank and her co-workers, and which if present will not fail to produce that state of security so necessary for the orderly behavioral growth and maturity of the child. Not only are these types of relations necessary in the earliest years of development, but it is undeniably of equal importance in the relationship of parents to children who are passing through the complicated adolescent developmental processes.

The parents' sense of security. Now when we turn to certain peculiarities in the types of adjustment that must be made by adolescent boys and girls, we note right away that there are inherent in these particular problems certain factors that place an equally heavy strain on the *parents'* own adjustment and the *parents'* own sense of security, a strain or threat which, although perhaps present to some degree when their children were in the younger age groups, was by no means as intense and threatening as when it is reborn in attempts to help their children with the problems of adolescence. What I would emphasize here is that the parent herself or himself too must have this sense of security to enable — or in fact to allow — the child to mature. More specifically, the parent too must have the power to grow and mature step by step with the adolescent child. In short, if we return to our phrases above depicting the essential elements in the sense of security necessary for the development of the adolescent child, we will find that these same elements must be present in the feelings of the parents as they survey and evaluate their own interpersonal relations with others who comprise the family and social setting in which they live, including the adolescent child himself, if they are to handle in a rational and mentally healthy manner the inescapable problems that their adolescent's growth process will concomitantly posit for them. It is just this possible disturbance of security feelings in both the adolescent child and the parent — which in relation to any particular problem may be referable to disturbance in such feelings either in the child or the parent or both — that makes for many of the "problems" and troublesome "deviations" in the adolescent's growth toward adult maturity.

Steps to Maturity

Let us review briefly some of the steps toward maturity that necessarily must be taken by the adolescent and, while doing so, observe the aids to or the blocks to mature behavior that feelings of security or insecurity in both child and parent may constitute. It should be noted too that in each instance cited, in the case of both the parent and the child, there are both the manifest, open, and observable responses, and behavior relating to a particular "maturity drive" either urging its inception or delaying it, and there are also associated with these varying degrees of unexpressed but nonetheless powerful feelings enlisted in bringing about just the opposite result. The very nature of the problems to be solved by children in this age group elicits these contradictory impulses, which are the basis for the disturbance in security feelings noted above.

Expression of the sex instinct. One of the most impelling thrusts toward maturity which creates anxiety in both the child and the parent is the drive to the attainment of normal and controlled expression of the sex instinct. The expected and hoped-for attainment is a definite and undeviating interest in persons of the opposite sex, of the same age group, as love objects. Not only is this drive inherent in the adolescent's biological make-up; it is stimulated, aided, and in fact demanded by the child's associates and immediate seniors, and the colleagues' continuing acceptance of him is conditioned by his growth and success in this area of sociosexual development. Nonetheless, in spite of these pressures toward maturity, the final assumption of a definitive and lasting identification with persons of the same sex, and the acceptance of the mature role expected of him, present a series of anxiety-creating situations to the child and result in transient and temporary, or very prolonged or even permanent deviations from accepted typical behavior. Such deviations may be transitory and disabling only for a short time; but while they are adhered to by the adolescent they do block his steps to the next step in his psychosexual development. And further, such responses to such anxiety and feelings of insecurity in the child rarely fail to elicit like anxieties and feelings of frustration and a sense of failure in the parent. A review of some of these deviations and their background in adolescence may be helpful.

The most general feeling of anxiety aroused in the adolescent by emerging sex drives is that which arises out of previously inculcated notions that sexuality in any of its expressions is evil or sinful, or, more particularly, and of more serious import, that sexuality or the sex act is by nature associated with aggressive and mutilative activities. Such notions of probable mutilation or physical injury may be deemed by the child to be the fate which awaits him as the recipient, or that he by his own acts as a mature individual will of necessity perform such aggressive acts on another. When through parental or extraparental admonitions and misinformation the child is led to believe in the inevitability of the association of sexual and aggressive impulses, it is not difficult to see that at adolescence the boy or girl is terrified at the thought of assuming such a mature level as that of the adult of his own sex, and development therefore is thwarted despite all the pressures inside and outside the home that urge that this step be taken. The child's anxiety and insecurity just will not allow him to embrace such an identification with members of his own sex.

Perhaps it may be inferred that the child psychiatrist notes this unfortunate association in the child's mind of aggressive and sexual expressions only in a certain few children who come to him for help and who are really anxiety-ridden in respect to other problems than that of sexual expression. On the contrary, there is considerable evidence at hand in respect to the normal child to justify the assumption that in the earliest years this association of mutilation and sexual expression is almost a universally accepted fear and, in fact, that the incisive and complete dissociation of the conjoint expression of these two drives comprises one of the expected stages or levels of development and growth in the child's increasingly accurate knowledge of human behavior. It is expected, however, that this dissociation usually will have been made before the adolescent years have been reached. Seemingly it is one of the "tasks" of early childhood to accomplish just such a distinction in respect to the expression of the sexual and aggressive impulses. Actual experiences to which he has been subjected or which he has witnessed and misinterpreted, together with misinformation or the lack of information, may prevent this "task" from being completed.

Retardation in psychosexual growth. In the presence of the anxiety aroused by the continuation of the association of these two instinctual expressions, the adolescent in many instances will refuse to develop, in the psychosexual sense, until understanding help and guidance on the part of the parent, the family physician, or the child guidance specialist enable him, through corrective information, to regain a sense of security and freedom from anxiety. This failure to develop is demonstrated in various ways. The adolescent boy or girl may attempt to perpetuate his or her present stage of development as if to deny that any advancement is necessary. The child assumes a protective "neutral position" in that he denies any strong positive feelings for the persons or interests of either sex. He seems to believe unconsciously that an absolute and unequivocal identification with either sex is dangerous; hence it is better to remain, as it were, "asexual." The girl adolescent will continue into the middle or late teens the "tomboyishness" and "bisexuality" which are so characteristic of the 10 or 11 year old, and will be more interested in success in games, sports, camping, riding, etc., than she is in acquiring attributes at all referable to femininity. She will continue to hold to the little girl notion (in the interests of defense) that boys themselves are uncouth, aggressive, boisterous, and irritating "pests."

The adolescent boy, too, will tend to prolong his more secure childhood with the refusal of development by denying a positive interest in girls, declaring such behavior to be "sissified" and "unmanly." He declares to others, and convinces himself if he can, that girls are interfering "brats" with no particularly attractive or even acceptable characteristics. The prolongation of, or even sudden reversion to, an interest in games and activities of a much lower level of boyhood development is not unusual. In turn, much to the consternation of the parents, there may be an associated regression to earlier childhood standards in relation to personal care and appearance, and partial abandonment of the previously inculcated habits of cleanliness, orderliness, and neatness. When this latter response is resorted to, it is not difficult to surmise that such favorable habits previously adhered to have now become associated unconsciously with possible acceptability by or attractiveness to the opposite sex, and the adolescent boy will have none of it.

In addition to these atypical responses there are others that signify attempts at deceleration or retardation of sexual interests in both adolescent boys and girls and which, although by no means serious or pathological, arouse the anxiety of the parent.

There is sometimes apparent what is best termed an "overreaction" to sexual impulses, in the form that the adolescent feels and declares that all sex is "evil," that all members of the opposite sex are "bad" and "sinful"; and the child turns away resolutely from all contacts or relationships, however innocent and innocuous, with the opposite sex. He withdraws almost completely from attendance in mixed groups — social affairs, parties, dancing, skating, etc. This self-imposed isolation or withdrawal is a temporary protection against any and all permissible stimulation or gratification of his needs. Unless this withdrawal is prolonged into the middle and late teens, it can be looked upon as a "phase" in development; but if continued in as a fixed response, the child may need help to gain insight as to its true meaning, its unrealistic basis, or in fact its harmful effects.

A second protective device used by adolescents to deny the existence of deep anxieties in respect to sexual interests or practices is that device known as an "intellectualization" of the problem. In this response the adolescent covers up and minimizes his or her anxiety in the sexual sphere by concentrating on endless rumination in respect to problems beyond herself or himself in the area of social issues, or in respect to the problems and ills ("anxieties" if you will) in the world at large. This is the time of the fervent, engrossing engagement of the adolescent's attention and activity in the problems of "remaking the world," the concern with utopias — either ultraconservative or ultraradical. What the adolescent is doing here, of course, is projecting into the intellectual world the problems and anxieties that beset him in his own inner personal life. It aids him in an unconscious denial that these nearer problems exist for him, and in the pretense that the only anxieties which trouble him are those relating to the social order at large. As in the case of all the other protective devices of the adolescent, this "intellectualization" of the sexual problem is also a temporary phase, one quite needful at that particular moment, and should not indicate to the parent a serious pathological trend. As a matter of fact, regardless of their origins, such concerns for the eventual betterment of this world are sometimes the beginnings of constructive creative programs and interests of the adult citizen.

As stated above, these may be temporary phases in the development of the particular adolescent, and they usually are just this. On the other hand they may, any one of them, constitute prolonged blocks to development. At any rate they can be of concern to the parents and they create problems of varying degrees of intensity for them. The bases of these parental problems and conflicts are not difficult of analysis. On the one hand the parents naturally wish that their child will progress toward adult development in a sexual sense. Any evidence in the child's behavior of a block in that development is interpreted by the parents as due to possible failure on their part. Their security and acceptability as parents are threatened.

But this is only one side of the parental conflict in respect to this stage in development. Almost equally strong as their desire and need for the child to identify with the adult role of the same sex, and to show a readiness to act in regard to the opposite sex — as do the children of relatives and neighbors — there is the associated opposite drive that their children should not, "at least not yet," evidence fixed attitudes exemplifying progress in this direction. The parents may, owing to their own education, training, and experience, have an abnormal or exaggerated and unrealistic fear of sexuality in general, or they may be able to see only the possible risks and dangers that confront the adolescent child. Hence, because of this, they may wish unconsciously that the child shall *not* grow up — may feel that their own freedom from anxiety and their own continued feelings of security, as well as those of the child, are definitely dependent on the child's *not* developing adult sex interests and expressions.

Thus the parents, in the face of these conflicts, must do their best to examine critically the possible motivations marshalled for and against the assumption of maturity by the child, with the hope that such insights will give them more tolerance, or at least more inner security, in formulating their responses to the forward or backward steps that the child seems to be taking. It may be that guidance from more objective sources than the parents themselves is indicated, and as can be seen from the above outline of the factors involved, guidance for the child demands an associated guidance of the parents, with a detailed review and evaluation of their attitudes, needs, and fears. It is just this sort of review and reevaluation, self-conducted or aided by another, that I emphasized above as the necessary steps in growth and behavior that the parent must make, *pari passu*, with the maturing, adolescent child. It too is a "learning process" or perhaps in some instances a "relearning" or reeducative process; and it too, if it is to be successful, can only be accomplished in a milieu of security and freedom from anxiety.

The Acceleration of Development

I would like now to consider for a moment a second major though somewhat different problem in normal adolescent development, one that arouses anxieties and insecurity feelings in both the child and the parent. This refers to the possibly undesirable (to the parent) *acceler-*

ation rather than retardation of development of the adolescent in a social, educational, vocational, and psychosexual sense. In this instance, as contrasted to the developmental blocks commented on above, the child is seen to attempt to assume adult modes of living in these various areas long before one might reasonably expect him to do so when one considers his actual age. In this situation the child seems to be trying to take two or three steps in development during a time span where one step alone would be enough. Such a child strives for — and strenuously cites his intention to gain — an independence in actions, in ideas, and in ideals that has little or no reference to those held desirable by the parent or indeed previously adhered to by the child himself. He is, in short, "overreacting" to the notion that he is to continue longer dependent upon the largesse or even the love of his parents. His internal impulses, plus the accepted and voiced standards of his colleagues, urge a renunciation of this dependency. Feelings of security relative to colleagues, rather than in relation to parent figures, are now in the ascendancy in his range of needs.

Needless to say, such an acceleration in development is not assumed by the child without continual misgivings, and in fact it is assumed often with intense anxiety. Detailed analyses by child psychiatrists have exposed these underlying fears and worries. The child, in short, is conflicted. He wishes to attain an adult position, but he fears it because he fears his own competence to deal with his internal drives and to deal with the external reality of an adult level as well. His needs for the security of parents and parental love — in short, his need for a dependency position — are still operative and repeatedly assert themselves.

On the other hand the parents too, faced with such attempts or demonstrations of acceleration in maturing, or drives for independence, are beset by the anxieties aroused by two conflicting drives; and these anxieties too are frequently recognized when we deal with the parents of children in this age group. There are, first of all, the anxiety and insecurity that may arise out of the feeling that they are no longer loved by the child, no longer needed by the child, and this is easily interpretable that *they the parents* are now to be "abandoned" or deserted by the child. In addition, however, there is the natural wish and desire on their part that their child, like all other children, grow up and act like an adult. Only such a culmination is acceptable to them if they are to be considered by themselves, as well as by others, to be competent parents who have successfully fulfilled their duties. Needless to say such conflicts and threats in reference to their notions of themselves as parents can be very acute, and call for considerable self-appraisal undertaken in as objective a way as possible.

The devaluation of the parent. There is one aspect of this acceleration, and in fact it is an aspect of quite orderly, gradual adolescent development, that is particularly difficult for the parent to accept. I refer here to the bludgeonings of *devaluation* that are heaped upon the parental head by adolescents during this stage of growth. It would seem to be an absolute necessity for children to take their first steps towards independence and away from dependency on their parents by means of a wholesale denial of any worth in the parents themselves, or of any value in the ideas, notions, plans, and hopes that the parents may voice.

There is a devaluation of the parents seen in the criticism of the parents' home, the homemaking qualities of the mother, or even the clothes and jewelry worn by either or both parents. The adolescents become extremely critical of the social and political ideas of their parents, and in fact take great delight in puncturing, if they can, the most idealistic notions, and even the religious tenets, which previously were held as a sacred part of their culture.

Nowhere is the attempted repudiation or devaluation of the parents or the parents' ideas and values seen more clearly in this age group than in relation to the carefully made school plans and vocational choices that parents have determined upon for the child since his or her earliest infancy. If the school as a whole is temporarily accepted by the child, it is certain that the type of course that he has assumed at his parents' direction is probably, according to the youngster, the worst possible course, or too hard, and surely will, he insists, never be of any use to him in later life. There is a suspicion on his part, of course, that the principal and the teachers are in league with the parents to see that such silly school plans are carried out effectively. Vocational choices and preferences for a lifework change from week to week. They change with new schoolmasters, or they change with the advent of new children in the vicinity.

To return again to problems typical of adolescence, there is the secretive phase of adolescence, in which the child now looks for confirmation or denial of his ideas and opinions to someone — almost anyone — beyond the home, anyone else except the parent. It is the age of the girl chum or the boy pal whose knowledge of facts and values and estimates of worth are inevitably truer than the parents'. This is the stage of short answers or no answers to questions that have to do with the plans of the evening or with plans for the weekend. Disdainful looks or looks of resigned tolerance greet the parents' genuine concern in what the boy or girl may be doing. This is the stage also — just to give you a useful hint — when the boy wishes that once and for all his father would give up following that much overstressed idea that the textbooks on child guidance have told him is the best procedure for bringing up an adolescent boy, that it is necessary to be a pal to junior. Junior at this stage wants pals, all right, but he does not necessarily want a parental pal, particularly when he senses that his father is as self-conscious as he himself is in his resigned dutifulness. Rather he wants pals of his own age who can share with him his concern and curiosity regarding certain very important problems of growing up, and the parent-pal is certainly of little or no use to him at such engrossing times. At this stage of his son's adolescence the wise father will begin to fish and to golf alone again — or with pals of his own age.

Again, finally, there is the strong resistance to early, healthful hours, and even stronger resistance to early, cooperative rising in the morning. The former is, of course, a determination to accelerate the move toward maturity, and unfortunately, if acquiesced in, results in a pseudoacceleration or a pseudomaturity on all fronts which none of us care to see in our own or in others' children.

I think we can see in these various phases of the adolescent drive for maturity and independence the alternating phases of a need for independence and a need for dependence. Children of this age do not quite dare give up their childhood *in toto,* nor do they quite dare to refuse to grow up. The parents' role in all this, it seems to me, is to recognize that there are such conflicts inherent in this bizarre, constantly changing type of behavior, and beneath the indifference and devaluation there is a strong inner need for parental aid and parental guidance. Children in the teens do not actually believe they are capable of controlling all of their inner wishes and demands, nor do they really wish to be asked or allowed to do so completely, because they are not quite sure to what lengths they might allow themselves to go. In addition to the recognition of the presence of this fear when the adolescent, in his bravest moments, expresses even the opposite, and the assumption of an air of tolerance toward the child in his conflicts, the parents must be very, very careful not to answer the adolescent's aggressive repudiation with parental aggression toward him or her. If this response is elicited from the parents, a vicious cycle immediately is set up — the "either/or" proposition is established — from which unfortunately neither the adolescent nor the parent can withdraw without severe loss of face.

Helene Deutsch, in her chapter on puberty and adolescence,[113] stresses this expected and in fact necessary stage in development. She states that the means of liberation from an emotional tie to and identification with the parent "is sought in devaluation of previous objects, regardless of earlier relations . . . an increasingly critical attitude and a greater adaptation to reality gradually brings about an abandonment of the infantile overestimation of the parents and the pendulum begins to swing in the opposite direction: the parents are now underestimated. . . ." But Dr. Deutsch does offer the hope and solace that we too would emphasize for the benefit of the parents so afflicted by the repeated and ingenious thrusts of devaluation at the hands of their adolescent children, when she states: "An interesting feature of this devaluation tendency, which deserves some emphasis, is that actually it is not quite as serious as it seems to be, for once the dangers of puberty are overcome, adolescents often resume loving the objects previously rejected and may even be proud of their own similarity to them."

In summary, then, I have selected for analysis responses of adolescent boys and girls which may be cited as "faults" or "blocks" to that orderly step-by-step maturation of children in this age group which parents hope will terminate in a secure self-identification of the child with the future adult role and the functions of the adult of his or her own sex. In the one instance we have noted a possible retardation in development; in the other, the possibilities for a spurious acceleration in it. A point for reemphasis is that these steps in development are models of the learning process in general, and that they can be taken, just as in the case of all learning, only when the child feels secure in his relationships, particularly in his relationships with his parents. The "blocks" and "faults" are then seen to be deviations generated by insecurity and anxiety. Of equal importance, it is to be noted that the parents themselves "grow" and can do so, too, only if they themselves are secure and anxiety-free in the presence of demonstrated maturation in their adolescent child.

VIII

THE MODERN FAMILY
AND THE SOCIAL DEVELOPMENT
OF THE CHILD

THE FAMILY AND CHILD DEVELOPMENT:
A SOCIOCULTURAL VIEWPOINT
KATHERINE SPENCER

The first social unit that the child comes to know is that of the family into which he is born and within which he grows up. In the light of modern psychology we have become increasingly aware of the importance of these early social experiences for the development of the child's personality. In their clinical approach, focusing on the individual child and the effect on him of his family relationships, psychiatrists and psychologists have arrived at some general notions about the personality consequences of particular kinds of early family experience. Social scientists, too, have been interested in the effects of different family situations on the growing child, but they have approached these problems from a broader sociocultural viewpoint. They have taken as a point of departure the family as a group rather than the individual child within it. Impressed with the variety of forms that the family group has assumed in other times and places in human history, they have tried to analyze the functioning of these different family types and their significance for the roles of family members. There has been increasing recognition that a full understanding of family influences in child development requires a combination of these psychological and sociocultural viewpoints.[1, 2] In what follows we shall illustrate one of the ways in which social scientists have approached the analysis of American family types and look at its psychological implications for understanding the child's family experience.[3] This will entail, first, a brief reference to the structure of family relationships in cultures other than our own as a background for comparison.

In social science perspective the contemporary American family appears as merely one among a wide variety of possible family types.[4, 5, 6] Because of its familiarity in our own experience, because it is the kind of family in which most of us have grown up and in which we have an emotional stake, it may be more difficult to view the modern American family objectively, to see its salient characteristics and to analyze the way in which it functions. This is where the comparative cultural approach of the anthropologist becomes helpful. When seen against the background of other family forms, the characteristics of our own family type and their significance for child development are easier to identify.

In their inventory of cultures around the world anthropologists have found a great variety of kinship structures and family forms all of which meet the basic physical and emotional needs of the growing child, albeit in somewhat different ways and perhaps to different degrees. At one dramatic extreme is the extended matrilineal family composed of the women and men belonging to the mother's descent line, a family type that, for example, was until recently a flourishing institution among the Hindu caste of Nayars of the southwest coast of India. Here a child lived in a large, extended family group which was composed of his mother with her sisters and brothers, his maternal grandmother with her sisters and brothers. A child's father did not become a member of this household. He remained an outsider whom the child hardly knew, who visited only at night, and who maintained his residence in and allegiance to the matrilineal household of his own birth. Under such an arrangement many of the economic, educational, and emotional obligations to the child that we think of as belonging properly to a father were assumed by the child's uncle, his mother's brother.

The patrilineal counterpart of such a large, extended family unit is more familiar to us because historically it is from a type similar to this that our Western European family has developed. One of the clearest examples is found in the traditional Chinese family, composed of relatives in the father's descent line — that is, the paternal grandfather, the father, and the father's brothers. A woman left her home at marriage to go and live in the household of her husband, and in this new home she was to some extent a stranger until, with time, and particularly with the birth of her own sons she became emotionally identified with her husband's patrilineal lineage. Under this arrangement a child again grew up in a large household whose members were linked by blood and emotional ties, but in this case his family group was made up of his father's people — his own father and mother, his paternal grandfather and grandmother, his father's brothers with their wives — and as he and his brothers grew to adulthood they too would bring in their own wives and children. In Chinese culture this patrilineal family form was closely linked with the value placed on filial piety and the religious reverence due to the paternal ancestors.

In each of these types of family structure only one of the two possible blood-descent lines, matrilineal or patrilineal, is used to form the nucleus of the kinship system. They are unilineal in structure. As we shall see, the American family does not make an exclusive choice in either of these directions. The fact that it is possible to recruit and organize a family group on a matrilineal or patrilineal principle is linked with other aspects of the total culture of which the family system is only one part. For example, the patrilineal Chinese family operated in a rural culture where land and property were owned jointly and inherited in the father's line and where religious beliefs and customs centered on the paternal ancestors. There is a compatibility, or as some social scientists term it a "functional relationship," between this family form and the economic and religious customs of the culture.

For our present purposes we are more interested in another type of functioning, that is, the influence and impact that the family structure has on the child who grows up within it. In very broad terms, we can say that these extended families offer the child a kind of emotional and practical security that is difficult to achieve in our own family organization. By its very size the household unit presents the child with a number of adults — aunts, uncles, and grandparents — to whom he can turn for affection and guidance. While his earliest and closest ties are with his own mother, the intensity of the parent-child relationship may be attenuated by being spread over a number of adults, the aunts and uncles who act toward him as second mothers or second fathers. Continuity over time is guaranteed in such an extended family. If his mother or father dies, this does not mean for the child a total disruption of his home; the family unit and his place in it continue.

The structure of the typical American urban middle-class family contrasts quite sharply with these large, stable kinship units, which throughout most of human history, and even today in folk and rural cultures, have provided the circumstances and setting in which children have grown up. In the United States today the family group tends to be a much smaller one, usually limited to the mother and father with their children. This group may number as few as 3, and when it reaches 6 or 7 we already begin to think of it as a large family. Not only is the family itself small, but it is usually separated spatially from other kin. The family lives by itself in an apartment or separate house. If there are other relatives in the household, this tends to be considered a problem or even a misfortune rather than an asset.

Unlike the Nayar or Chinese, we do not use extended blood ties on either the maternal or paternal side as the basis for selecting the group that lives together. Although we use the patrilineal line for naming, we consider the kinship bonds on the mother's and father's sides as equally important; we do not feel closer to either side except by the chance of proximity or personal preference. Instead of blood ties, our family system makes primary use of another kinship relation, that of the marriage bond uniting husband and wife, and it is this bond that has been called the "structural keystone" of our family system.[6] Marriage is entered into by the free choice of the young husband and wife, whereas in the extended patrilineal or matrilineal systems this choice is often dominated by the judgment of parents or the welfare of the larger blood-related family group. Where young people are free to make their own choice of a marriage partner, individual personality factors inevitably influence the nature of the mutual choice. In addition to this freedom of contract in the marriage bond, there is a tendency toward complementary equality in the roles of husband and wife, and in these respects our family system reflects the values of democratic individualism current in our culture. While our conception of the family and of the sex roles within it has been moving rapidly toward the American equalitarian model, in many individual cases, and particularly in certain ethnic groups that have maintained traditions from their rural heritage, there are still prominent traces of a patrilineal or patriarchal orientation.

Not only is the American family unit precariously small in numbers and separated from parental kin, it is also expected to be self-dependent economically. When a new family is established, we expect the young couple to set up a separate household. In fact we are disturbed when circumstances make this difficult, as in the housing shortage following the Second World War. The burden of expense in establishing and furnishing a home, and in providing for the birth of children, is a heavy financial responsibility. The recent trend toward earlier marriage, in many cases while the young couple continues in college or professional school, may intensify these problems of economic support and of emotional independence from parents. By contrast, in the matrilineal or patrilineal extended family, the young married couple may be absorbed into an already-functioning household; or the custom of contributing property at marriage, as in the dowry familiar from Southern European cultures, may ease the economic burden. As already noted, our young independent household may be at a considerable distance from the parents of both husband and wife. Usually it is the demands of the husband's occupation that determine where the family will live, and as he moves up in the occupational hierarchy there may be demands to move to a new neighborhood or to another town or another part of the country.

This urban middle-class family begins thus as a small, relatively isolated and self-dependent unit of husband and wife, a unit instituted by the free choice of the marriage partners. It consists typically of two parents and two, three, or perhaps four children. This family lives in a separate household. It may have a greater or lesser number of neighborhood and community ties, depending on the personalities of its members and on the type of community in which it lives, but it must also be ready to relinquish these community ties if the demands of mobility require this in the interests of the father's career and the family's economic welfare.

Although there tends to be equality in the husband-wife relations, the orientation of their respective roles is quite different. In our economic and occupational system the father is usually away from home all day, working at some specialized job, and the time he can spend with his children may be brief indeed. While the children are small, the mother's time and energy are absorbed in their care. The father's daily activities are oriented outside the family, the mother's within it. If the mother needs or wants to work outside the home, or to participate in community activities, she finds a major problem in providing for the children's care in her absence, by nursery school, day-care arrangements, baby sitters, or reciprocal arrangements with neighbors. The absence of "extra" relatives in the home and the substitution of labor-saving devices for full or part-time domestic help have narrowed the availability of others who can fill in occasionally for the mother in her constant care of the home and small children.

The ways in which our small, mobile family unit is related to the technology, economy, and social and value systems of our contemporary culture have been analyzed in considerable detail by social scientists.[5, 6, 7] Here we are primarily interested in the significance of this type of family structure for the experience of the children born into it. In it the child's emotional ties are concentrated on relatively few persons. The responsibility for meeting his physical and emotional needs rests with the mother, father, and perhaps an older sibling, although when there are only two or three children, close together in age, there is less opportunity for the older children to act as caretakers. This places heavy demands upon the mother and means for the child that the channels for his emotional expression are narrow rather than diffuse. If he feels frustrated or hurt by his mother's lack of attention because she is engaged in some household task that cannot be interrupted, there is no substitute mother-figure readily available, such as the grandmother or aunt in a Chinese home, to whom he can turn for temporary comfort or for the opportunity to express his anger and resentment where it doesn't matter too much. In such a situation he has to turn inward to himself, or vent his feelings in bickering and quarreling with a brother or sister.

Not only does this small family offer the child few targets for his emotional expression, but their cultural values place a premium on love and harmony in family relations, and tend to deny the natural needs for expression of aggression. The slender family unit creates a situation where the child is more exclusively dependent on the two adults in his environment, and more vulnerable to the feelings of anger that such dependence will arouse. Parents may become disturbed and even frightened when they recognize the child's aggression directed toward themselves. The question has been raised whether in the long run our family system is not overly conducive of aggression in the child and at the same time overly restrictive of its manifestation.[8]

There is another area in which our cultural values foster the expression of the child's aggression. This is in competition with his peers.[9] In our individualistic competitive culture parents feel, and with justification, that the child must learn to be independent and able to stand up for his rights in the world outside. They know that he will soon have to make his own way in school, and later in his occupation, and that they cannot follow him out into these worlds. He is not going through life, as the Chinese peasant could, with the external support that comes from being integrated in a large cooperative family undertaking. Again we may ask whether our cultural demands for early training in independence and self-assertion do not place a greater burden of insecurity on the child than we realize.

Part of the child's task in growing up is to learn, and to incorporate as his own, the standards and behavior that will be appropriate to an adult young man or woman in his culture. The child's most significant role models for this are his own parents; in them he sees embodied the patterns for adult behavior. To the average young girl in our family system the role model of her mother's activities is readily available; she sees her household activities and plays at or helps with these grown-up tasks herself. At some point, however, this experience is interrupted and her interests are diverted to other kinds of learning and activity in school. Before she herself becomes a housewife and mother, she goes through a period in which her interests are centered outside the home, in school work and perhaps a job in the industrial or business world. In childhood the young boy does not have so readily accessible his adult role model. While he stays at home with his mother, his father goes away each day to a job that is remote from home and that may be technically too specialized for the child to understand. He does not have the same opportunity that he would in a peasant or farm household, to see and gradually participate in the work of grown-up men. Psychologists have pointed out the difficulty that the boy may have in these circumstances in developing a firm masculine identification, and parents seem to take more seriously their fears that a boy will develop into a sissy than that a young girl will continue to be a tomboy. Thus, in our family system the child's problems of adult role identification are complicated by the relative inaccessibility of role models and by the discontinuities in the child's interests at different periods of development, and both of these factors are related to the specialized roles demanded by our technological civilization. In our fast-changing culture we may expect a tendency for balancing cultural mechanisms to develop, and perhaps one of these is already evident in the increasing participation of fathers in early child-care.

At adolescence the child in American culture is confronted with two major problems. On the one hand he is concerned with establishing his emotional independence from the family in which he grew up, and he is looking forward to finding new emotional bonds in marriage and a family of his own. At the same time he faces the practical problem of work and self-support. Our demand for independence in both of these spheres at the same time places a heavy burden on the adolescent, and a greater one than is required of him in many other cultures. We have seen the greater continuity between childhood and adult work-roles that is possible in peasant cultures, and the security afforded by cooperative work within the extended family. Our marriage system also requires a sharper break in emotional continuity. The young people take upon themselves the responsibility for their marriage choice, and both husband and wife leave their parental families to set up their new household. In the extended kinship families that we have considered, the demands for emotional independence are not so extreme; one of the marriage partners remains in his own parental family, and the choice of a mate is supported, if not dominated, by the interests of the whole family unit.

Again, social scientists have asked whether the intensification of problems at adolescence, as we see it in American culture, may not be due to a combination of forces and pressures inherent in a family system that places such heavy demands for independence at this time.[2, 10] The manifestations of adolescence with which we are familiar — the defiance of adult standards and the special symbols, understandings, and conformity within the close-knit peer group — may be viewed as a special "youth culture" that has developed in response to these pressures. The extreme, and often uneven, attempts at independence from adult control are then explainable as a reaction against the overprotection of childhood. This reaction occurs at a time when the child knows he will be required to give up this dependence and protection, and at the same time the peer group affords a substitute to which he can temporarily transfer his dependence.

Adolescence is everywhere a transitional period between childhood and adult life. In some cultures this fact is emphasized by puberty ceremonies which give community recognition and support to the child at the time of this important step into the adult world. Our culture does not afford such a clear-cut point of transition, and the period of adolescent adjustment tends to be prolonged. The "youth culture" can offer a temporary haven, an opportunity to maintain this in-between status and ease the transition during this period when the adolescent is concerned with the fears and responsibilities and privileges of his future independence.

The role of parents in relation to their adolescent children also has its own problems in our family system. In a fast-changing culture parents may actually not know the future reality for which their children are being trained.[7] It is easy for them to feel old-fashioned with the realization that things are not done as they were in their own youth, and they may need to reach outside of their own experience for help and guidance, to neighbors to learn what is happening with other children, or to teachers and guidance experts.

If we look at the total family unit at this point in the family cycle, it is evident that the adolescent is not the only one who must make adjustments: this is also a period of readjustment for the parents. If there are few children, close together in age, the parents will be faced with the prospect of losing not just one member from a large and on-going family, but of losing all of their children within a brief period. This change seems to present more problems for the mother, and understandably so. Up to this time she has devoted her major energies and time to the children, and this change in her family role may coincide with a difficult emotional period for her, that of the menopause. The role readjustments for the father come more gradually, and a break in his work role will not occur until considerably later, with his retirement.

In this brief survey we have presented a sociocultural approach to understanding the family and relations within it. We have focused on the modern family type that is perhaps best known to us, the family that is typical of American urban or suburban middle-class life. In contemporary America there are many variations of this type, for example, toward a father-centered family in ethnic groups that are still close to Southern European cultural backgrounds, or toward a mother-centered family that tends to develop under conditions of social and economic disorganization if the husband and father is absent or has become a shifting figure who cannot be depended on for economic and emotional support. Recent English studies of urban working-class communities have shown the close ties that the young mother tends to maintain with her own maternal kin in the local neighborhood,[11] and such kinship networks may also be more important in American urban working-class communities than this middle-class picture suggests. In any case, a sociocultural analysis cannot in itself tell the whole story; it is but one part of a total framework that includes understanding of the processes of physical and emotional development, as well as of the social setting in which this development takes place.

SOCIAL AND ECONOMIC FACTORS INFLUENCING FAMILY LIFE
ELIZABETH P. RICE

The child and his parents live in an ever changing environment, both within the family and within society in general. These changes are even more conspicuous in families from countries rapidly becoming more industrialized. Over several centuries, the American family gradually changed in its format and roles; but in the less developed countries, these same modifications have come about in a much shorter period of time. The trend in industrialized countries towards urbanization, and now suburbanization, has meant that most of our families today live in urban or suburban areas. Families have migrated away from the farms to centers of industrial development. In early industrialization one often sees the father as the breadwinner, leaving the family in the village or small town to go where work opportunities seem greater with the hope that the family will join him later. As families crowd into cities, living accommodations become smaller, more compact and frequently the family has less privacy. Play space for children may be limited to restricted playgrounds and frequently to the streets. Life becomes more organized and less spontaneous and the opportunities for discovery and exploration, so easily available in the country, are limited for the city child. Thus the adventurous child may quite naturally be tempted to go beyond the behavioral limitations established by his community in the search for adventure.

As families become more urbanized there is a tendency for the young family to leave behind the older parents as the young father seeks employment often at considerable distance from his parents. Families in the United States have a high rate of mobility. Twelve million children were estimated by the Children's Bureau in 1958 to have changed their homes within 12 preceding months. This family mobility usually has the result that grandparents are no longer members of households, and the former close tie between grandchild and grandparent becomes more formalized. Further, also, the young family loses the help which the grandparents, especially the grandmother, gave in the care of the children. Thus one of the former resources for substitute mother care has practically disappeared. In addition, in the present generation there seems to be a desire on the part of both the grandparents and the young families to live apart, to carry out their lives in their own way, and psychologically to be quite separated in interests. These separations have produced both gains and losses to the young family and to the grandparents and, as a result, it has been necessary to develop substitute services to meet the needs filled in the past by relatives. Examples of such are the rapidly developing programs for the aged and the extensive use of baby sitters in young families.

The present-day young mother has come from a generation of small families, the average number of children being until recently only two. Thus she was not accustomed to caring for young siblings in her adolescence and usually had little, if any, direct experience with babies. This has meant that some mothers come to their first pregnancy with little experience in caring for children, and some parents view the approaching addition of a baby to the family with considerable concern. The young mother today tends to be an avid reader of the numerous books on child rearing. These often present to her conflicting points of view about which she may need clarification. Young parents today generally take their role of parenthood seriously and are eager to help towards the optimum development of their children. They usually take pleasure in their children's progress and consciously plan for opportunities which will develop the children's initiative, satisfy their curiosity and provide the experiences required for sound social development.

In their eagerness to be successful parents, there is fostered competition among parents. This reaches a height in the frequent experience of Baby Shows where mothers compete to win the award for the best baby, the judgment often being awarded to the largest and fattest, not necessarily the healthiest. This tendency to compete is shown also in the exactness with which many mothers will follow rigid standards of growth and development and will show concern if, by chance, the baby falls under the average weight and height curves or other developmental criteria. Later this tendency to compare one's child with those of friends is shown in comparison of school records and other social successes. When babies, either because of physical, mental, or social variations are different, parents have difficulty in accepting the difference and in feeling comfortable with parents of more normal children. They sense a spirit of social criticism that stems from the need of parents, especially mothers, to feel they have been adequate in the role of parenthood. Deviations from the usual pattern of growth and development of their children makes them question their own failure, and usually the question is voiced, "What did I do wrong?" Various situations will arouse this self-blaming attitude, such as a congenitally deformed child, a child with school failure, children with behavioral difficulties, or the juvenile delinquent. Later when the marriage may be shaken or broken, the same question is raised, followed by, "How could I have done differently?" However, this desire of parents to fulfill their roles of parenthood with satisfaction to themselves, their child, and the society which eventually makes the final test of the child, has many points of merit, since a responsibility taken seriously, if not overdone, is usually a task well done.

Contrary to the previous generation young families today are more often together. Babies at a very young age are taken visiting, whether this be for the evening or longer. The young child early becomes accustomed to meeting others and of seeing new and different faces and places. This will undoubtedly affect the child's readiness to meet new experiences with greater comfort and security. However, at a later age period when the child is in school and already closely related to his peer group, the frequent moving of families from one school district to another or from one city to a more distant point, is upsetting to children who have already made close friends among their playmates and schoolmates. In one family under study, the children had been moved six times in three years and each time to a different section of the city. It is not surprising that the mother complained of problems with her children who began to show the strain of adjusting so frequently to new experiences. For many children, especially shy ones, the necessity of fitting into new peer groups may create serious problems in their later social adjustment.

Movement of families away from relatives and former friends also results in frequent use of mother substitutes, since generally neither relatives nor household help are present in the home. Thus, unless the child goes with the parent, the common method of child care in the home for assistance during parts of the day or evening are young baby sitters, usually of school age. Under adequate protection, adolescent girls and boys can benefit from such experiences as they learn how to care for children. However, all too frequently such responsibilities may interfere with their school studies or shorten the hours of rest. Without safeguards, too, young people have been on the streets unaccompanied at unsafe hours and exposed to other hazards during their work. Also there may be serious dangers to children if the baby sitters are not properly instructed or if their responsibilities are greater than their age and experience warrant. Many communities now have set certain standards for such care and have regulated hours of work, pay schedules, and extent of responsibilities. In some college communities such experiences have been related to academic courses such as those which discuss the modern family as a social institution.

The family today is a younger family than in the past generation. Brides are now about twenty and bridegrooms twenty-two, whereas a few decades ago they were twenty-four and twenty-six, and in the past even older. This has brought major changes to the young family. With the present need for advanced education for many occupations, it is more and more essential that the husband pursue his education even beyond his age of marriage. In order to do this and also to be married, if he has no other financial resources, his wife usually plans to continue to work to support herself and often her husband until his education is completed and he is established in a job. Working wives, therefore, are a necessary corollary of early marriage. Many such couples establish themselves in only temporary living quarters, sometimes with relatives or friends, in rooming houses or small apartments, until the time when they can afford more adequate quarters. These young husbands and wives, contrary to those of a generation ago, are willing to start in a simple way if such is necessary and take pride and pleasure in working things out together. Their main desire is to be together and to work out their future by helping each other. They are imaginative and planful in their management and are proud of their home, however meagre. For the future happiness of the family this seems a much more promising beginning than in the recent past where young couples delayed marriage in order to start out about where their parents had arrived. Unless circumstances are too meagre, this experience of working together towards a desired goal for the family may result in stronger family bonds and more unified goals.

Earlier marriages have meant, for many couples, the postponement of pregnancy until the time when the husband is at work and the wife then freed from the heavy responsibilities of support. Women will vary markedly in their feelings about work. In a culture which has emphasized occupation as a goal for both men and women, some will wish to carry on a career and prefer this to raising a family. Others will want children but may regret the giving up of the job and associates, while others will happily surrender the job to the satisfactions of a home and motherhood. Most mothers, irrespective of their basic feelings, will go through a period of readjustment when they give up work and will usually refer to the loneliness they experience at home all day and to the separation from their friends at work. The longer the work experience, the harder, probably, is the adjustment for most women. For some women the socially acceptable excuse of work may be given as the reason for delaying pregnancy when the real reason is much more involved and relates to basic feelings towards marriage, pregnancy, or motherhood. Some women may be able to be better wives and mothers if they have the opportunity of interests outside the home including an occupation. Therefore no generalization in regard to the wisdom of working can be drawn for all wives, but individual differences in feelings, desires, experiences, and

goals must be considered. As the importance of these individual variations have been recognized in progressive communities, services have
been established to help women, who wish to work full or part-time, in
the care of their children. Such modern services as day-care centers and
care during all or part of the day in carefully selected foster homes have
been established in some communities. Day-care centers serve also children who need the opportunity to play with other children of the same
age period.

For some mothers work may be seen as a necessity because of financial
need. Financial need is a relative question since what one family sees as
essential may appear to other families as luxuries. However, it should
be remembered that we regard as necessary in the United States a high
standard of living which requires for basic maintenance many facilities
and much equipment which in the past were considered less essential.
These make it possible for mothers to do the chores of the day without
help which in the past was more commonly available. Such equipment
as washing machines, vacuum cleaners, electric refrigerators, television
and radio have now become standard equipment in the average home.
They are the resources which help mothers to carry the burdens of the
day with less drudgery and which indirectly help to build a happier home
life. Since these are considered necessary by young couples, heavy initial
expenses may be incurred in the first years of marriage. This also contributes to the wife's desire to remain at work at least until the debts of
time payments are reduced.

Along with the high standard of living goes also, in this country, the
high cost of living. Many husbands earn an insufficient amount to meet
such a standard. National statistics show that in 1957 the median income was $4971, which was 60 per cent above that for 1947–1949. During
the same period the index of consumer prices rose only 20 per cent: thus,
on the average, families have gained in real income throughout the past
decade.[12] However, there is great variation in family income. Very large
families tend to have smaller incomes than medium sized families. A
family with 3 children under 18 years in 1957 had a larger income than a
family of any other size, averaging $5363. Over 39 million children were
in families with incomes of $4000 or more, a gain of 25 per cent in this
income group between 1954 and 1957. However, more than 13 million
children were still in families with less than $3000 income. Types of
families with average incomes below the median included those headed
by women ($2763), farm families ($2490), and the nonwhite family
($2764).[12] These lower incomes in a country of high costs and high
living standards mean that supplementary sources are often needed
to meet the standards of family living necessary for the optimum
development of the children. It is fortunate that family incomes have

risen in the last ten years for seldom do we now see the poverty of the last century. Furthermore, along with increased income, there has developed a belief that in a country as resourceful as ours no family should go without the basic essentials of life, namely food, shelter, clothing, incidentals, and medical care. To this end the Social Security program, established in 1935 and revised several times since then, provides in most communities for a minimum standard of living for all in certain categories of need. Improved standards of general relief in cities and towns have helped to raise the living standards of recipients in many communities. However, in areas where the economy is poor or where public opinion has not yet supported adequate standards, some families will still be unable to meet their basic requirements. When such exists there is little choice except for all members of the family to earn what they can. This may place undue pressure on children to earn too early, or at unsuitable occupations, or for too long hours. The realistic need for women's work must, therefore, be seen as a problem often quite different from the woman's desire to work. With the constantly increasing number of married women who work, we support the point of view which states that it is now a well known and accepted pattern in the United States that married women will work at least half-time. Again for some women this will mean additional satisfactions and to their families probably shared happiness while for other women this may mean additional burdens too heavy to carry with other family responsibilities.

Many a parent has the sole or major responsibility for family support because of death, desertion, divorce, separation or chronic illness of the other parent. In 1958, 11 per cent of United States children were not living with both parents. One cause was divorce, the rates for which rose rapidly during the war years but in 1948 began to decline slowly. In 1940 the divorce rate per 1000 married women fifteen years of age or over was 8.2 per cent; shortly after World War II it reached a peak of 17.8, but by 1957 it was back to 9.2 per cent. In 1957 the lowest divorce rate was for women with four or more years of college education while the highest rate was for women with one to three years of high school training. In general the marriages of women under 21 years are more often broken than is the case of marriages over 21 years. In 1956 one half of the divorces were granted to couples who had at least one child under 18 years of age. Of these couples, one in nine had as many as three children. These facts are important for those working in maternal and child health programs to consider since early symptoms of family friction and disintegration could be recognized in prenatal and well-child clinics and guidance provided for young parents aimed towards preventing later separations.

Our Social Security program aims to provide, under Aid to Dependent Children, an allowance usually sufficient to maintain an adequate standard of living and hence is a program focused on encouraging mothers to stay at home with their children especially when the children are young. Extension of this program in some states for mothers with children born out of wedlock has made it possible in many instances for such mothers to keep their babies and to have opportunity of bringing them up, thus providing for the child the strengths which come from belonging to a family. These programs have been aimed at the primary purpose of strengthening family life, and when the familiy is broken, of maintaining the rest of the family intact. However, helpful as such programs are, they cannot make up for the loss experienced by the child in a broken family or one without both parents for it is in the home that the child finds his security, develops his feelings of being wanted and accepted, and is supported by a strong feeling of identification. For children who must, for various reasons, be deprived of this opportunity, substitute parents who may be relatives, friends, or foster parents, preferably carefully selected through a child welfare agency, will need to provide for the child the warmth, love, and acceptance the child misses from his own parents. In order to ensure this, some communities now have organized child welfare services to make sure that the child not only receives physical care but that he also has an opportunity for social and emotional development as nearly favorable as possible with experiences he might have received from his own family. For many children substitute parents can only approximate what the child has lost from his own parents, but it is possible with the proper placement to approximate this frequently. Ordinarily, the younger the child when he needs substitute parents the more readily will he be able to accept the substitution.[13]

Not only do we have deprived children but also parents deprived of having children for various reasons. Many of this group will seek children available for adoption with whom to share their home and affection. Not all parents seeking children to adopt necessarily have the capacities and resources of physical, emotional, or economic nature to provide the kind of experiences the child needs. For this reason many communities have tightened their regulations in regard to adoptions in order to safeguard the rights of the natural parents, the child, and the adopting parents. In spite of these efforts, many children are being adopted without the adequate safeguards provided by preadoption studies carried out by social and health agencies. In 1958, 39 per cent of all babies adopted were adopted without such study.[14] Since the shortage of babies available for adoption is so acute, many parents have sought babies in other parts of the world. These are frequently parents who for one reason or another have been denied the privilege of adoption in this country. Efforts are now underway through the International Social Services and the United Nations, in cooperation with children's agencies in this country, to provide for these children, often severely traumatized emotionally by war, maternal deprivation, or starvation, the same safeguards as are provided for our own children, namely, adequate evaluation of the needs of the child, the capacities and motivations of the prospective foster parents and a period of supervision before legal adoption. A home may appear, to many people who do not know the internal situation intimately, to be ideal for a child, but this can only be determined by a skillful and expert evaluation by a child welfare worker.

Separation of families from relatives and close friends, as often happens in a highly mobile population such as the United States, has created additional needs for service from the community. When a mother is ill or needs to be away for a shorter or longer period, there are frequently no resources readily available to help with the care of the children. To meet such needs child care agencies have expanded their programs in many communities to provide foster day care, or full-time foster care to children until such time as the mother can again take over the responsibility. Other community services, frequently under the direction of the local family agency or public welfare department, have arranged for the help of mature, well qualified women to assume the role of the homemaker for all or part of the day when the mother is away. Such service has lessened the number of children who were separated from their homes, siblings, parents, and schools at crucial times when the mother was ill or otherwise out of the home. Further extension of homemaker services, with variations to meet new needs, is seen as essential to meet the needs of families of the future.[15]

In addition to organized community services to assist families, there has developed a very natural mutual sharing between members of the same social group who, in the absence of relatives or paid help, frequently meet the needs of their friends. In this way several young families who are friends will often "baby sit" for each other, do the shopping, have car pools to drive the children to school or recreational opportunities, or even have meals together or share facilities, such as washing machines. This cooperative movement among young families meets not only realistic needs but provides many opportunities for recreation and the pursuit of common interests. Such an arrangement may provide an added strength when the children are adolescent, since the group of families tend to establish the same standards of behavior for their children and to set the same limits. It is an important substitute for the more closely knit family of older days in that it also helps the child to relate to adults other than his parents in a comfortable and accepting way and encourages the parents to share their children with other parents.

Many parents find it hard not only to share children with others but to give them up when the children are ready to leave the home for school, work or marriage. This may be more difficult in these days than formerly, since the number of children are less, though now increasing to an average of 3+ per family, and since the children tend to be nearer of an age. Thus the children are ready to leave the home within the space of a few years and the home seems deserted without them. Recently a daily press reported that six out of eight children in an unusually large family were married at the same ceremony. Successive separations of children often cause major rearrangement of the household, frequently resulting in a move to smaller quarters and sometimes family disintegration. These separations usually come at about the time of the mother's menopause when she may be less able to cope with additional emotional stresses. This separation may be further exaggerated if the child leaves the home to live at some distance away, thus making ready communication difficult. This helps to emphasize the fluidity of the family, its constant changes, and its inevitable transiency. However, with strong emotional attachments, family bonds may be held tightly and distance may be readily cemented when opportunities arise.

Statistics seem to show that there are in the United States more marriages and more babies being born. Fertility rates have increased considerably according to figures from the Bureau of the Census. Whereas in 1940 there were 281 babies born per 1,000 women of child bearing age, in 1956 this rate had increased to 466. Farm women continued to have the highest rate. The figures indicate that half of the children are now in families of three or more children. Mothers with the most schooling showed the greatest increase in fertility between 1940 and 1947. The greatest increase in rate (77 per cent) occurred among women graduated from college; for high school graduates the increase was 48 per cent; and for grade school graduates, 25 per cent. Since World War II the number of babies born has been increasing after a decrease during the depression of the 1930's. The increase is at such a rate that the present high birth rate is often referred to as "population explosion."

New services are being developed or old services expanded to help to strengthen families in their efforts to provide the milieu in which to live happily and to rear children successfully. In addition to those already mentioned should be noted the programs which emphasize prevention of difficulties from arising within families. Such services involve programs of family and marriage counselling, health information, parents' classes, housing programs, leisure time activities, and expanded services of fraternal and church groups. With increased knowledge of problems which need to be prevented and skill in treating these problems, both through help to the individual or family and through community action, family life of the future can be strengthened.[16]

The family is the keystone of our society, for in it children are born and reared to become the adults of the future who will themselves become parents. They will make the critical decisions of the next generation.[17]

SOCIAL DEVELOPMENT OF CHILDREN
ELIZABETH P. RICE

Social development through the various age periods can be recognized as basically orderly, purposeful in its unfolding, but with many individual variations which are dependent on the child himself and upon his experiences. Thus, although there are in a child's social development the usual steps through which he goes from one age period to another, there will be great individual differences according to his social and emotional situation, the opportunities which are available to him, and his mechanisms of response. Of major importance will be the relationship which he has established with his parents and siblings, the atmosphere of the home in which he spends most of his time, the constancy of his relationships especially with the mother, and the regularity and consistency in the child's general relationships and opportunities for development. The importance of the milieu in which the child is reared is central. If the atmosphere provides a milieu of happiness, the establishment of confidence in his parents is reflected later in the child's relationships with others. Conversely, a milieu creating strains and tensions in the child produces feelings of insecurity, and these bring into play those compensatory mechanisms which are the picture of maladjustment, asocial behavior, and unhappiness.

During each of the several periods of social development, parents, too, experience problems of maturing, and learn through the child's behavior some of the adaptations which they themselves must make to the maturing child. New demands are made on the father as well as on the mother during this period. In modern American culture, with limited or no home help, the father has come to be the mother's assistant in taking over some responsibilities for the baby, and in carrying out some of the household chores. When the baby comes into the family, therefore, a considerable change takes place in the familial home as well as changes in the roles played by the husband and wife. The degree of stress which this new responsibility creates for the parent will be determined by the security of the relationship between husband and wife, and their readiness and desire for the baby.

In infancy, responsibility for care is, in our culture usually placed on the mother, who realizes her responsibilities and is aware that she will be evaluated as a mother by her husband, family, and friends. Thus a new mother has to prove not only to herself but to others, that she has the capacity to provide for the infant's needs. Many mothers are unduly fearful of doing the wrong thing for the baby, or doing something at the wrong time. Some support and guidance during this period, to build up their confidence in themselves as mothers, is usually needed.

In addition to these factors, there are also some reality problems to be faced when a new baby comes into the family. For example, the housing situation may be too limited to provide adequate space for another member. Since many young people are not immediately established in the kind of living arrangements which they hope eventually to have, and since some pregnancies come earlier than anticipated, the housing problem may be difficult during the period of infancy. Another realistic problem is the additional expense entailed by bottle-feeding and other necessities, which may well strain some family budgets.

The new baby, especially the first child, may cause the mother to give up some of her interests outside the home with friends and associates. This often gives the mother a feeling of deprivation and denial. With the 24 hour care required by a baby, mothers often feel homebound and isolated, and often need some practical help in order to gain a little leisure so that they can perceive themselves as persons apart from their babies. One result of this is that the baby, in its first year of life, may become exposed to several different persons, more or less indifferent to the child, who substitute for the mother with the effect of confusing the baby in regard to the mother-figure. Some babies, of necessity, may have to be cared for outside the home, at least part of the time, when their mothers for economic, social, or emotional reasons feel that they must return to work, or when mothers are ill or homes are broken. Thus although babies ideally need the care of one mother-person, they may be shifted from person to person.

The new baby will also affect the relationships of parents with the baby's siblings. If the mother has shared with the siblings the fact that a new baby is coming, they will be better prepared to welcome the new infant into the home. However, in spite of preparation, there usually will be some signs of resentment on the part of the formerly youngest child to the stranger who has replaced him. Mothers will need some help in recognizing the potential problems of jealousy and in working these through with the older child.

In the *preschool years* the child becomes more active, independent, and adventurous. He loves to explore but his interest is fleeting and he needs variety for the release of his energy within safe limits. Some differences may arise between parents as to the child's expression of his explorative nature. Frequently the father urges his young son to discover things for himself and at some risk encourages him to experiment, while the mother has a greater tendency to restrain the child and to limit the scope of his activities. This parental inconsistency may confuse the child who is not sure of what is permitted.

In these early years the child shows negativism and his reaction to almost every request made by his parents is "no." Parents often become exasperated, not realizing that it is through this negativism that the child gets a sense of himself as a separate individual and gains a feeling of independence. A child of this age asks many questions, and wants and needs serious and truthful answers. Such answers help him to rely on his parents and to develop faith in their ability to meet his needs.

Many parents have difficulty in accepting some of the problems in language development. This is the time when the child begins to enjoy using words, and along with ordinary accretions he picks up naughty words. Many parents use punishment to discourage the use of these forbidden words, but this may tend to fix them in the child's mind. If the parent pays little attention to the objectionable words, however, the child soon drops them for something newer and more interesting.

The imaginative child at this period has many phantasies. On the positive side he imagines that he has playmates with him; he makes up stories; he likes to dress up. But on the negative side, often, if he is left alone, he feels in danger because of all the phantasies which are a part of him. This fear of aloneness and abandonment is perhaps in retrospect the most dreadful. In his phantasies he may tell false tales which in the eyes of the family are considered lies. Many parents find it difficult to differentiate between phantasies and actual untruths, and may mistakenly punish children for quite acceptable imaginative projections.

Parents need to know what to expect around this age period in order to know the role they should play. The use of parental authority at this time is particularly difficult. On the one hand they do not want the child to get out of control, but on the other they hesitate to be restrictive. During this period the child urgently needs approval from the parent so that he gets, not the concept of himself as a naughty, bad child, but the concept of being loved. He needs this for his own self-image in the development of his ego. If the child gets constant disapproval, he becomes even more negative and balky. Parents can be helped to use suggestions rather than commands, and to avoid threats, especially threats of punishment. However, the wise use of punishment will help both the child and the parent. Many parents, particularly mothers, find it difficult to recognize and accept the slow development of independence on the part of the child. In order that he can grow in this regard, the child needs to feel some freedom to take the next step; but he also needs to feel the comfort and support of a protecting parent behind him.

During the preschool period the child develops new powers primarily through play. Play is the major business of the child and it is through this that he learns how to relate to children of his age, how to share, and how to distinguish what is his from the property of others. He needs playmates of his own age. If these are much younger the preschool child has a tendency to want to dominate the smaller ones, or if playmates are older he has little opportunity to develop his own interests and will try to follow the lead of the older children. Working at play with his own age group the child has the opportunity to develop leadership qualities. Children who have no playmates of their own age or who need the special skills offered in nursery schools will especially benefit from more supervised play opportunities, thus having help in relating more positively to children of the same age and to the teachers as adults. Nursery schools will also help the child to make the transition from home and mother to school and teacher. This step for both child and mother is one of much concern for both child and parent, for it is the first indication of the child's beginning emancipation from the home to take his place in the wider community.

The preschool child likes to have stories read to him. In the early part of the period he wants to be held during the process, and this feeling of comfort and security in the arms of the mother is as important to the child as the story itself. Children enjoy listening to music, and most children have a natural feeling for rhythm. They like to hear lullabies and to be sung to sleep.

During these years the child may develop a real identification with his family and a strong devotion to his parents. With sympathetic guidance he is easily led, especially by the parents whom he loves, respects, and admires. He wants to be like them. He talks like them, wants to dress like them, mimics their mannerisms, and by the same token, he is very sensitive to their criticism. The child enjoys family celebrations, which help to develop in him a strong sense of family feeling. He likes, towards the end of the period, the opportunity to be included in the family's social activities and to be with visitors who come to the home. This develops his feeling of sociable companionship and helps him to relate to people of various ages and personalities. He begins to develop a real feeling of differences in families, and identifies strongly with his own family as being the best.

The preschool child is intensely active, constantly exploring and discovering, and this may create problems of supervision and control for the parents. Many mothers, burdened with the routine tasks of the home, find it difficult at times to be patient with this inquisitive and active child and to be consistent in their care. On the other hand, the child of this age also provides a stimulating interest for the parents, together with much amusement by his quaint efforts to express his thoughts and ideas. Parents gain real satisfaction in having a child who relates so completely to his own family and who feels his family is all-knowing and all-powerful. A mother perhaps has no greater satisfaction than to have a preschool child who looks to her as the beginning and end of his satisfactions and who with great confidence and joy says, "You and I are pals, aren't we, mother?"

The social development of the child during the preschool years involves tremendous strides. His social adjustment at this time will determine his readiness for school for it is during this period that the basic pattern of social relationships with his peers and with adults are developed.

During the *school age period,* the child begins to show his independence in ways which often disturb parents. He begins to question the knowledge and authorities of parents who, in the past, he considered all-knowing and all-powerful. The teacher begins to take an important place in his esteem. He may often display some impatience with his parents and looks outward for answers to persons in the community whom he now quotes as authorities. Teachers and other adults in close contact with the child, such as group leaders, become his role models and he begins to build his self-image as a potential adult around them. He commences to turn his thoughts away from the family group and toward the outer world. He begins to learn that in his group experience he must conform to what is expected of him, both in the school and in the community. He finds that it is not acceptable to be different, and so he wants to be like his peers in actions and dress. He idolizes the same athletic and entertainment stars, and uses the same slang. In the early part of this school age period girls usually like clothes, but toward the end often turn to being tomboys, disregarding all things that are feminine. Boys during this period want to use their hands to build things, and they utilize whatever is readily available or can be salvaged from the family's cellar or attic. For boys these are the days of making carts, automobiles, airplanes — anything that moves.

Because of the child's need not to be different during this period, it is a very difficult time for the handicapped child or for the child who in some way is so deprived that he is unable to compete. Much self-consciousness is developed for the child who cannot buy his lunches in school, or dress as the other children dress, or have spending money like the other children. Experiences of deprivation are especially hazardous for a child of this age since they create a feeling of restriction and of difference. If he is different, the child is likely to be ridiculed by his playmates. The girl with red hair, or the boy with curly hair, the child who does not dress in the local style, or the child with such handicaps as strabismus or lisping — all are targets for the criticism and ridicule of the peer group.

This age period is one of great activity. The child wants to make use of his body, and exerts his energy ceaselessly, especially in the early part of the period. Girls play hop-scotch, jump rope, jackstones, roller skate, ride bicycles, and display interest in all kinds of sports, while boys want to play ball, "cops and robbers," do handsprings, play hold-up games, simulate Indians and cowboys and frequently wrestle or engage in fist fights even with their good friends. This effort on the part of boys to show their physical superiority is a way of developing their concept of themselves as masculine beings. Children of this age group show great variety in their play interests, more so, in fact, than at any other period of life, but interest in anyone is still not long maintained. They are ready to explore, experiment, or try anything suggested. At home they seem to have a way of being under foot, and are always eager to be kept busy. They are always in a hurry; they have little time to wash or eat, and find it hard to leave their play or playmates. This ceaseless activity is especially true in the early part of this period. Play, therefore, takes on a tremendous meaning to the child of school age.

During the early part of this period there is little difference by sexes in the play experiences of children, but towards the end the differences become more marked. Boys and girls grow more intolerant of each other, especially on the surface. To the girls, boys seem very rough and are considered "pests" because of their constant teasing. Girls begin to talk about their disinterest in boys, while boys think it is "sissy" to have anything to do with girls. The sexes are separated in the games but when they do play together it is usually the boys against the girls. Competition and play begin in the early part of this period, but real team play is not developed until toward the end, as children during this period are not quite ready for the responsibilities of team play and the consistency which it requires.

Group experiences are at their height during the school years. At first there are small groups, and later gangs and clubs. Usually these are rather short-lived. Often one gang is hostile to another, and neighborhood frictions are aroused. In urban areas, gang warfare has become a serious problem in juvenile delinquency. There is an exclusiveness in the selection of individuals who have the privilege of joining these groups. A group seeks a private clubroom or clubhouse, and there is much competition among children for the unused cellar, garage, attic, or other neighborhood facility. At the end of the period secret societies are formed, always exclusively for either boys or girls, and never mixed. These societies have names, secret passwords and gestures, pet phrases, "uniforms," insignia, pledges, and in other ways are surrounded with secrecy and mystery. Many of the phantasies of earlier periods hold sway through these secret societies. Depending on the interests of the group, asocial behavior may take place.

"Best friends" are common during this developmental period. Usually there is one person who is the best friend, but there may be a rapid turnover in persons holding this honored position. There is frequent quarreling between best friends, but the quarrels usually are resolved. Best friends are chosen on the basis of ready availability, usually live nearby, are in the same grade at school, or are members of the same club group. Jealousies frequently occur between best friends especially when a third person becomes involved. These friendships at this age may become a very exclusive affair. Such complete identification is often an indication that a child is having difficulty in relating to several persons or to group experiences. The choice of friends at this period usually has no relationship to similar socioeconomic status, except as the parents bring pressure on the child to conform. A little boy may have his best friend "from the other side of the tracks," despite the disapproval of his parents. Early in the school years the child has little sense of socioeconomic differences, but relates to the other child for the satisfaction gained primarily from playing with him. It is only later that he takes on some of the parental prejudices and begins objective selection of his associates.

Children of 6 or 7 mimic what they see, read, or hear. They play house, the little boy being the father and the little girl the mother. Thus they act out their feelings toward their parents and imitate their parents' expressions and intonations. Later they show their feelings towards their teachers when they play school. Through such play the extent of aggressiveness of certain children and the submissiveness of others can be observed as, for example, when some must always be teachers while others are more comfortable being pupils.

Girls want to do as mothers do, cooking, washing, and caring for babies while boys act as fathers act, building carts and autos. Children naturally show an interest in nature. They love to have cookouts and to build fires. They want to know about birds and stars. This is a natural time to develop their interest in the out-of-doors and to create feelings of pleasure and security in natural experiences. Their imaginations are reflected in their curiosity about the sexes and reproduction and their curiosity rises when questions have not been satisfactorily answered. School age children are observant and curious about all aspects of life.

Children of this age often feel comfortable in expressing their affection toward animals. The child feels the animal's loyalty and responsiveness and gains, thereby, a feeling of security and acceptance. The famous picture of the boy with his dog is characteristic of the child at this age. At this time, too, the child acquires a feeling for property rights. He usually has his own allowance for spending if he comes from a middle-class or well-to-do family, and he gets a sense of the value and use of money. He learns respect for other people's property and the protection of his own.

There is still a strong family loyalty during this period. The child relates strongly to a sibling as *my* brother or *my* sister as illustrated by a child who wept copiously because the other children laughed at her three year old sister who was not able to speak clearly while reciting a poem. Around the age of 9 and 10 siblings are allies, standing up for each other against outsiders. Older siblings have a strong feeling of protection and warmth for the little child in the family. They show loyalty to their own home even though it is inferior to the homes of other children, thus showing that the home has meaning and value to them.

School age children often seem to pay little attention to parental wishes and commands. Parents become concerned because the child is loud-voiced, generally noisy and careless in manners, and they fear that all their teaching has been to no avail. They are often happily surprised when these same children behave much more maturely when visiting or are otherwise on display.

Children at this stage are full of rhymes and riddles and play many guessing games and conundrums. They love to dress up, play charades, and go calling in adult clothes. This is another indication of their desire to take on adult roles and simulate their parents. This is also an age for collecting and hoarding anything that is available. To do this they may send away for samples of interesting or strange things. At this period children often tend to revert to biting, sucking, and chewing and chewing gum is constantly desired. Such behavior may reflect difficult developmental problems which the child is facing.

As the child grows older, increasing emphasis is placed by parents on the child's school performance, and the parents tend to compare the success of their child with that of others in his group. Parents have a need for the child to conform and to succeed at least as well as a neighbor's or friend's child. With failure in school the child experiences a loss of self-esteem and a deep sense of humility, because at this period the school is a very important aspect of the child's life and one in which he strongly desires to do well. His identification with the teacher means that poor school performance is especially hard for him to face, since he is not living up to the teacher's expectations of him either. Too much parental pressure on a child who is not succeeding in school, or the need of certain parents to force the child to attain certain goals may create new difficulties for the child in his ability to face his own self-image. Toward the end of this period the child begins to experience not only the pressures put on him by his parents to meet the hoped-for level in school, but also his own inner drive to be successful at games, in competition, and at parties.

Children have very real worries during these years as they take on more responsibilities and begin to react to them with anxieties and tensions. They may reflect the fears and concerns which other persons have about them or which they see reflected in characters in life, books, or television. They tend, too, to be concerned about the unfamiliar or the unexplained, and seek answers to these. Some children continue to feel fear, often stimulated by adults, of the dark, robbers, certain animals, or storms. Perhaps the greatest concern of the child during this period, however, is about himself, and his ability to do well. Children who have increasing responsibilities in the family, such as care of younger children, or home tasks, may have some apprehension in taking over these adult responsibilities, and may begin to think anxiously of how they will meet such requirements in adulthood.

Many children at this age tell some untruths, oftentimes when the parents force them to tell what they wish to conceal. They try thus to protect themselves against the inevitable punishment which they anticipate, because of the way punishment has been meted out in the past. The degree of such behavior may also reflect the degree of success of the parents in the past in discussing problems with the child. The child at this time may steal. He may use this means to gain popularity or friends or to compete with peers. Often he has little use for what is stolen. The act of stealing useless things, however, provides him with the satisfactions of having things even though he may not have love and security. Stealing, therefore, expresses his insecurity or lack of affection and is usually a way of working out some of his inner conflicts expressed or submerged. If more than occasional, stealing may be an indicator of more serious problems which lie unsolved.

Some children who feel unwanted or unloved, or who believe they do not belong at home, may tend to run away as a means of begging for more attention and display of affection. Sometimes running away is an expression of the child's desire to escape from himself because he may not be living up to his expectations of himself or those of his family. When school is boring or hard and parents are pressing him to meet goals which he is finding difficult, or when school becomes too confining for his teeming imagination, running away may partially meet some of his needs. Obviously the child who runs away is a deprived child who is seeking satisfactions not available in his experience at home, in school, or in the community.

There are also certain socioeconomic changes which make life difficult for the child of school age. Urban living gives the child less chance for activity or adventure than is the case in the country and limits his opportunities for exploration. Leisure time activities are largely outside of the home, different for each age period, more passive than active, and are often commercial, thus requiring the use of money. For this reason alone socially and economically deprived children may not be able to use the recreation opportunities in the community.

A child at this age wants and needs to be taken seriously. He wants others to be interested in his activity and his goals and is very sensitive to ridicule. So great are his needs for physical expression and so keen is his imagination and his desire for discovery that he cannot readily be restricted.

This middle period of childhood is one of marked social development and of clarification of the child's capacity, intellectually and socially. Throughout the school age period the child needs the steady influence and direct guidance of parents and teachers and the security of knowing that they are behind him, supporting him and accepting his limitations. During this period he begins to relate to others outside the family, and to be challenged by the numerous interesting experiences of life beyond his home. If pushed beyond his capacities he will show attitudes of confusion, conflict, and frustration. How he succeeds will depend to a large extent on the soundness of his early development and on the readiness of others to help him make his adaptation to fuller life experiences.

Persons working with children need to have an understanding of the child's experiences in his home, with his parents and siblings, in his school and in his play experiences in the community. Such understanding will indicate in what ways any deficits in the child's experiences need to be filled in and strengths gained. Thus parents, teachers and leaders in leisure-time activities, working together, can round out the child's needs in his efforts to meet the increasing responsibilities of late childhood and the young adult years. During these school years the foundations are laid for the child's ability to support himself and to be ready for the opportunities and obligations of marriage and parenthood.

Adolescents will show some variations in social development according to the social setting in which they live. Farm adolescents will vary from small-town adolescents, or from adolescents in urban areas, in accordance with the opportunities available for social experiences and the way in which the adolescent utilizes his leisure time. There will be variation, too, according to the family's socioeconomic status, and hence the kind of social experiences available to children, such as the use of the family automobile, the size of the child's allowance, the provision of things which cost money, and the kind of home from which the child comes.

Differences in cultural backgrounds affect the ways the child attempts to establish his own independence and to separate from the control and domination of parents. Cultural modes of behavior which tend to increase the opportunity for boys and girls to socialize tend to lessen the evidences of emotional tensions, whereas those which separate and protect the adolescent from free associations with the opposite sex tend to increase the emotional tensions. These cultural restrictions and modes of behavior may actually increase the boy's or girl's pressure to express adolescent drives to a degree greater than the cultural customs will permit. Thus, in understanding a particular adolescent, it is helpful to know the mores of the family and of the subculture in which he lives and how these are coinciding or conflicting with the common mores of the community. Since the adolescent wants to do and to be like his peers, marked differences in parental restrictions of freedoms as compared with those of the community may confuse him in regard to his own social behavior.

The adolescent is always an individual who is caught between wanting his needs fulfilled, and wanting to be accepted as a grown-up, adequate in himself to meet his own needs. At one point the adolescent wants and is ready to accept the same kind of attention, interest, and affection from his parents as in the past, but then seems to want to throw off this dependence. Parents are confused by this duality. In regard to behavior, the adolescent shows in his play with his peers a swing from active, energetic, romping play to quiet, rather sophisticated, inactive interests. Such swings in social feeling and social behavior are unpredictable and, therefore, confusing to parents.

The adolescent is very eager to be accepted as an important member of the family and to be valued as such. He likes to be consulted in regard to family affairs and family planning, and he likes to feel on a par with his parents in regard to many family affairs. He still wants some companionship with his parents, desiring a give-and-take relationship which approaches an adult relationship. He likes to confer with his parents in regard to his own planning, his social life, clothes, schooling, job, and other important concerns, but often feels unable to do so. This will upset all parents at one time or another. Often the adolescent likes to be involved in family thinking and planning and welcomes counsel and advice given when it is asked for, but not when it is volunteered. The kind of companionship the adolescent wants with his parents is a reflection of the relationship with them in the earlier period; it achieves fuller fruition at this period.

One of the major problems of adolescence is the relationship to the opposite sex and to love objects. This is always a changing relationship in adolescence and, oftentimes, a mixed one. In general, the adolescent's first interest during this period is love of self and of those like himself, these aspects complementing and supplementing each other. He has strong friendships. He tends to be fairly selfish, at first, because of his extreme interest in himself. Parents complain that he is not interested in helping others, nor is he considerate of others. The building up of his self-image as that of a satisfactory adult is a prime necessity in his social development.

From this love of self and of those like himself, he then turns to love of a person outside the family, usually a person of the same sex. In adolescence he may carry over the love of teachers, evidenced in his school age period, or of an older person, but this becomes a much more intensified interest in a person of the same sex at this time. Usually between 13 and 15 years the adolescent boy begins to have heroes whom he worships, and the girl often has crushes on older women. The boy tends to idealize heroes such as the baseball player, or a TV star. He pins their pictures on his bedroom walls and often carries on an ardent correspondence with them. This experience, though quite tiresome to his parents, is a safe one for him because it directs his attention to individuals outside his family and to persons far removed from him. It is in a way a transferral of his feelings from his parents, with whom he has been so very close in the past, to another adult idol to whom he can now relate with strong feelings of affection. Such transfer to models not always acceptable to parents is a difficult experience for the parents, because they may see in this behavior a degradation of themselves. These experiences, however, give the child the opportunity to develop love relationships. This is a natural development of the adolescent as he attempts to relate to people outside of his own peer group. It is, however, an important relationship to watch because of the fact that some adolescents never go beyond this stage in their love relationships.

From the love of a hero and hero worship, the adolescent normally turns to love of the opposite sex. The child at puberty shows considerable shyness and some antagonism towards children of the opposite sex. One 12 year old girl, when asked if she liked to go to dancing school, commented, "No, the boys step all over my feet," and when asked if she minded this, said, "Yes, I hate men." Other girls will withdraw when boys are around and will show considerable self-consciousness. In similar ways, boys will ignore the existence of girls in their presence and will find means of escape from them. During this early period of puberty, the child may show changes in feelings and behavior; whereas in the past he may have been industrious, loved school, and been interested in various hobbies, he may now appear to have few interests and becomes quite withdrawn, sometimes very moody. He tends to want to be left alone. This is illustrated by the 12 year old girl who, during an active period at the beach in the summer, commented that she was glad she had a cold because that gave her a day in bed and a chance to be alone. This desire to withdraw in order to have an opportunity to deal with themselves and relax away from the severe social strains and pressures of adolescence, is an important means of escape for these young persons who are always torn in these developmental conflicts. At this period especially, girls may be quite irritable and hypersensitive; they are easily hurt and often emotionally upset by what they consider insults and rebuffs.

Around the age of 15, heterosexual interests are often directed more to older persons of the opposite sex. These relationships often appear to parents to be ridiculous. Criticisms about them by the parents and other adults may greatly disturb the adolescent.

During the latter part of the adolescent period, usually around the last two years of high school, the adolescent arrives at the point of being interested in members of the opposite sex of the same age as himself. He tends to have one relationship at a time. At this time both boys and girls are still shy and awkward; they tend to look at each other with oblique glances, to stray off into corners together, to hold hands, share confidences, plan their lives together, and to be very dependent socially on each other. This involves the beginning of kissing and petting, and of the kind of games which bring them closer together. Real flirtations are carried on. Girls spend much time in improving their appearance, arranging their clothing, having their hair exactly right, and in using cosmetics with great care. This was illustrated by a girl seventeen years old still quite immature in her relationships with boys, who complained that she had spent all her allowance for perfume only to find that the boy she now loved had little sense of smell. In middle or late adolescence boys become particular about their appearance, usually are neat and make demands upon their parents for particular clothes. They begin to use "wisecracks," humor, or simply loudness to gain attention. This somewhat aggressive, rather bold behavior is a way of covering up the self-consciousness of the period. Other children, however, will appear to be quite blasé, not wanting to show their inner feelings. Still others will strive to appear intellectually mature and will try to discuss erudite subjects beyond their knowledge.

Relationships of a boy and girl during middle and late adolescence are often short and intense; they frequently end suddenly with quarreling, as evidenced by some of the poems written by adolescents. In these separations there can be serious emotional strains, and the adolescent may for a period lose his interest and confidence in members of the opposite sex. However, the recovery tends usually to be rapid. Some adolescents will carry on an intense and continuous relationship with one individual and marry that one later. Others will have numerous intense relationships in rapid sequence. Such a variety of experiences with different members of the opposite sex provides opportunities in love relationships which help the adolescent to determine, at a later time, the person he wants to marry. This, then, serves as another developmental experience in social relationships with the opposite sex.

Adolescents who are not ready to relate to the opposite sex may use various means of escaping from this kind of relationship. Some will unconsciously keep themselves unattractive, obese, or unclean in order to be less attractive to the feared opposite sex. Others may turn to physical complaints and use physical limitations, real or imagined, as an excuse for not participating with their peers. A few adolescents will continue to carry on their intense interests in members of the same sex, and thus homosexuality becomes more permanently established and may be the pattern which is carried on throughout life. Some children will tend to overemphasize their school work, and will seek the commendation of their teachers and parents through success at school as a substitute for social success with the opposite sex. These tendencies are symptomatic of the adolescent who is finding the heterosexual adjustment difficult. They are symptoms not easily recognized, but ones which indicate that the adolescent may need help if he is to achieve his next step in social development, his further adjustment to the opposite sex.

During the adolescent period the child's effort to establish his independence is demonstrated in many ways. He tends to renounce the parental standards which have been set up in his family, perhaps finding them more restrictive than the standards of other parents. He feels hemmed in and controlled, and wants to overthrow parental restrictions and disciplines, to set his own limits of behavior, and to make his own decisions. He may even appear defiant in order to show his independence and ability to do differently than his parents suggest. Parents often mention the child's attitude of independence and complain that he will never do what they advise. Clearly, the adolescent has a great need to do things on his own and in his own way. If permitted to do so in certain appropriate areas, he will be able to accept more readily a parental suggestion to do other, more fundamental things somewhat differently. During this period, too, the adolescent wants privacy; he wants to have a room of his own and his own things. He likes secrecy and wants to be able to keep his thoughts and interests to himself and not to be asked questions. He will be more expressive if not pushed too hard to share. He resents being asked for any accounting of himself or of his behavior, even though it is necessary for parents to do this at times. The adolescent is likely to keep a detailed diary, not fully recorded but with points indicating his thoughts and experiences. His diary is very personal to him, and he considers it strictly his private property. It is by writing in his diary that he shares his thoughts with himself.

The adolescent usually feels that his parents cannot possibly understand what he is thinking or doing. He may feel that his parents have not developed to the level of being interested in his interests, or he feels that the parents are old fashioned and that their ideas would not hold weight in the modern age. The adolescent has an idea of the kind of family which he would consider adequate. At the moment his family seems to him to be full of flaws, and much less adequate than the ideal which he has of family life. He tries to improve his family; he wants his parents to appear well groomed, to enter into community activities, to be socially acceptable — in short, to be respected if not leading citizens. Similarly, the adolescent may begin to show some concern for the social order in which he lives. He finds flaws in it; he criticizes the leaders of the past and has an urge to remake and improve society. He becomes interested in various social philosophies, and experiments with these in applying them to his own life situation. He tries to find his own philosophy of life, one that he can live by and one which will hold him to an ideal. The late adolescent is often imbued with great idealism and altruism and his goal is to contribute as much as he can, not only to the family which he hopes to create, but to the society in which he lives. This is the day of exploring and dreaming, of testing ideas and philosophies, and of coming to grip with the whole purpose of life in general.

Adolescents identify themselves thoroughly with their own peer group. They need to feel that they are like the group in such matters as behavior, dress, ideas, and goals. This is a hard period for children who are different because of socioeconomic limitations, or because of physical, or mental handicaps. The adolescent wants to feel that he can do as others in the group do; thus the deprived child is at a great disadvantage. An adolescent who is under much more stringent parental restrictions than the other children in his group will feel different, and will resent the restrictions. The young person, for example, whose parents always require him to be in at a certain hour at night, when this hour is significantly earlier than the hour set by his friends' parents, will feel that his parents are harsh and do not understand his interests, desires, and degree of maturity. There is a strong drive in adolescence for social position, acceptance, and attention from the peer group. The demands of the peer group are heavy; it wants members of the group to be able to be good sports, to have a good sense of humor, to do well in school, to appear attractive, to be good dancers. In a less desirable framework, the peer group may demand stoic acceptance of pain, gang warfare, sex practices, theft, and other such proofs of "belonging."

Belonging to a gang or group has significant effects on the adolescent. If the group is interested in positive experiences such as sports, nature study, or exploration, the membership in the group will absorb the adolescent's interest and time in meaningful ways. However, membership in some groups or gangs may have destructive results on the child's efforts to socialize. Street corner gangs which may develop interests mainly in hold-ups, larceny, or gang warfare obviously create an asocial effect on the child. From these groups, juvenile delinquency frequently develops resulting in arrests, probation, or reformatory experiences. Efforts are being made in many urban areas, especially, to work with these gangs in an effort to meet their needs for adventure and excitement but through socially acceptable channels. Although such gangs exist more often in urban areas and in lower socioeconomic groups, they are not absent in the suburban or rural areas or in higher economic groups. Since the desires of adolescents are the same irrespective of place of residence or social status, these adolescent needs will be met in one way or another, whether socially acceptable or otherwise. Communities and parents, therefore, need to ensure to adolescents the resources for constructive use of leisure time through activities which appeal to this age group.

Pressure from the peer group is felt keenly by the adolescent, and he tries to meet at almost any cost the demands placed upon him. The development of a "youth culture" with its own symbols, standards, and allegiances can help to ease the difficult step from childhood dependence on parents to full adult independence. In growing out of his dependence on parents, the adolescent finds a temporary substitute and support in closer relations with his peers.

In this period parents need help in knowing how to maintain a consistent attitude during the adolescent's progression through these experiences of social development. The adolescent needs to feel that in his family there are firm standards and limits which continue in spite of occasional relaxations, and that these standards of behavior will serve as consistent guides to him throughout the period. He needs to feel too, that his parents will support him in spite of his failures in adjustment. Parents are usually anxious about the child's sexual adjustments, and are fearful of freedoms which might result in sexual delinquency. This seems to be much more acute with parents of girls than of boys, because of the serious consequences of pregnancy. In this period, as before, one of the most stabilizing influences for the adolescent who is making an adjustment to the opposite sex and looking forward to his own happy family life will be the example which he sees of loving parents, a happy home life, and a firm, solid family relationship of give and take.

To live with adolescents is never dull. Every day brings new and different emphases and changes. With an understanding of what the child is experiencing in his social development, the period of adolescence can be a stimulating and enriching one for parents, teachers, and others working with the adolescent, in the support which they can give him in meeting new experiences in life. Looked at in this way, the conflicts of adolescence may be seen more as signs and symptoms of on-going social development than as disturbed behavior.

THE ADOLESCENT IN THE FAMILY
RUTH M. BUTLER

General Considerations

Previous sections have made it clear that the family contributes greatly to the success or failure of the adolescent's social development. This section focuses on those aspects of the family life which a group of mothers have indicated are especially pertinent in considering the social development of their children. During the years 1950 to 1955 inclusive over a hundred mothers of boys and girls between the ages of 17 and 20 years were interviewed by the writer in the course of the Longitudinal Studies of Child Health and Development at the Harvard School of Public Health.[18] These interviews were part of the terminal phase of comprehensive studies of these children who had been followed in this research from birth to their 18th year. However, the children and mothers were unknown to the writer prior to the time of her interview. The families of these children were predominantly of Irish background, although some had originated in Canada, England or Scotland; most of them were Roman Catholic. The families came from the lower middle socioeconomic group. Although most parents had received some education beyond grammar school, only a few had attended college.

The interviews indicate a close relationship between the resources of the family and the child's ability to develop effective social functioning during adolescence. In families where there is a cohesive marital relationship, a regular income, supporting community services, and infrequent stresses or demands, a child has greater opportunity to become better adjusted socially during adolescence and to mature progressively so that he can meet the increasing demands made upon him as a young adult.

In the following discussion, specific environmental factors have been selected as significant in the social experience of adolescents and their parents. This picture should be viewed in the general context of American family life, and of the tensions experienced both by parents and adolescents, reflecting the characteristics of this cultural context. In a culture which is changing as fast as ours, there are inevitable discontinuities between the experience of parents and children, and it is more difficult for parents to bridge the gulf between the generations. At the same time, in the small family unit typical of American culture, the developing independence of the adolescent inevitably brings problems or readjustment within this close social unit.

Housing. Many investigations have been made of the effects of housing as a determinant in child health and development. This discussion, however, is more concerned with the attitudinal changes of the growing child toward the housing unit. In the early adolescent years children usually view their immediate environment critically, in a devaluative manner. Mothers saw this as one of the major evidences of the difficulties they anticipated would occur during adolescence. They recognized that their children were objectively evaluating the materialistic features of the home against the value system of the community. Mothers did not, however, understand some of the positive features of this phase of development. Although they intuitively felt that the children were "growing up," they did not recognize this critical attitude as a steppingstone in their gradual movement toward increased independence. Parents want their children to become adults, but frequently do not identify changes in social behavior as early manifestations of readiness and desire for separation from the family unit. Even the most stable parents were upset by the children's devaluative attitude, and it was not uncommon that the criticisms affected the mothers sufficiently to cause them to become reflective, questioning, and often ill-at-ease. Parents who have cohesiveness in their marital relationship usually can achieve considerable comprehension of the true significance of the children's critical attitude, and thus are able to support one another sufficiently to withstand such discomfort. In these families, although everlasting criticism was a source of annoyance, the family equilibrium was not seriously affected and the children were able to give up some family values and establish new ones. In other families, however, mothers were distressed by this critical attitude, which frequently exaggerated their own disappointment in that the marriage had not fulfilled all their hopes. In a few instances mothers had "put a stop to this," which suggested a serious limitation in permitting the children to express their feelings, so important in adolescent growth.

The generalization that all parents are disappointed, puzzled, and disturbed by these early efforts of the children to separate from the family is a dangerous oversimplification. One must have detailed information of the family to decide whether the child's environment will adversely affect his continued growth toward independence. Similarly, the need for professional services is indicated for families where appropriate independent behavior is discouraged, whether the adverse influence is due to difficulties in family relations, or in the financial situation, or because of unusual stress. It must be emphasized, however, that each helping discipline, whether medicine, nutrition, psychology, or social work, must assume responsibility for comprehensive services; that is, assistance to the family as well as to the child.

Income. Three points about income were frequently referred to in these interviews: (1) the mother's decision to return to work during the child's adolescence; (2) the work and earnings of the adolescent himself; (3) the community's attitude toward the financial responsibilities of the family.

Many mothers return to work during their children's adolescent years. The explanation given is that the increased financial responsibilities of a family with growing children makes this necessary, but some mothers frankly state that they feel a need for outside stimulation and satisfaction. They realize, too, that their children are at a point where they too need to spend more time outside the home. No longer can mothers look for previously obtained gratifications in caring for the children. Mothers described their evaluation of this phase of the children's development as descending on them almost overnight, bringing an acute awareness that mothers as well as children were growing older. This realization sets off a multitude of worries. They find it helpful to be busy, thus taking attention from disturbing thoughts both about themselves and about the inevitable changes in the family. Work makes it possible for many mothers to avoid some of the arguments which the young and middle adolescent sparks off so frequently in the family. The actual physical activity, the preoccupation with the job, is itself a very beneficial diversion. The job does much to strengthen the mother's intuitive wisdom in seeking some way to permit her growing child desirable and necessary increased freedom, independence, and reduced parental direction. It also gives her the opportunity to restore her confidence in her usefulness. Many mothers talk at work with other women about their difficulties, and this frequently results in helping them to put their problems in better perspective. Thus, in our contemporary American culture, working is an acceptable means of enabling mothers of adolescents to achieve the goals of broadening their personal resources in preparation for the middle and later years, while at the same time helping them to relinquish gradually some of the satisfactions previously derived from close relations with their children by offering a sufficiently satisfactory substitute.

In these Growth Study interviews mothers expressed the belief that their husbands had little understanding of the positive values of work for them. Several mothers made great effort to fit their working into a schedule whereby their husbands felt no inconvenience. With other couples there were serious differences of opinion about the mother's working. A small group of mothers described how much they would like outside work, but knew that this would not be accepted by their husbands. Social agencies have a real opportunity to help parents understand their own needs during this period in order that parental attitudes and restrictions will not become obstacles for the adolescent.

Employment of the adolescent. Nearly all the children in the Harvard Longitudinal Studies worked from the early adolescent period on. They secured part-time jobs in their first and second years of high school, and many held full-time jobs during the summer months. The type of work was relatively unimportant to both mother and child, who viewed the job as temporary and to meet specific and limited purposes. Mothers expected their children to use their first earnings for personal expenses, such as carfare, lunch, recreation, clothing, or such special affairs as school proms, and were pleased when their children showed some desire and ability to start saving money. Later, families expected their children to contribute to the cost of their education. Only a few of the families asked their adolescents to contribute to the household costs, which were increasing as a result of the adolescent's use of the telephone, family car, cigarettes, television, and the cost of having clothes cleaned more frequently. If the adolescent had stopped schooling, however, they usually expected the young person to give approximately $10 a week toward the cost of board and room.

Some mothers managed the children's earnings for them, explaining that the child liked to have this kind of help. In these instances one would expect to find other expressions of maternal domination affecting the child's social development.

Community attitude. The families in the Growth Study steadily increased their actual income, the rate and amount of increase being in keeping with the general trend of the past 20 years, and, therefore, the standard of living within this group improved during the study period. Although the amount of available money was greater at the end of the study, most of the women felt that the family continued to feel financial strain because of the increased expenditures of older adolescence. Mothers pointed out that the financial needs of 18 year olds, socially and educationally, were greater than at any other period of development, yet it is at this age that families ceased to be able to claim income tax dependency exemption for their children.

Health. The mothers interviewed were between 40 and 50 years of age, or in the menopausal period. It is, therefore, understandable that they were fearful about their health and were watchful for evidences of their own physical change. Several expressed interest and concern about cancer. They were aware of their own increased nervousness and emotional tension. Often mothers used their physical symptoms to justify their tendency to be either more controlling or more permissive in the management of the adolescent. Others used poor health as the reason for not being able to give the adolescent the guidance needed at this age.

In describing the health of the fathers, it is interesting that several mothers reported their husbands had illnesses of a type which often have a social and emotional component, such as peptic ulcer, tuberculosis, or skin disease. Some fathers were considered problem drinkers by their wives.

In regard to the children, those aspects of health commented on by mothers were closely related to social development during adolescence. Nearly all the adolescents began smoking between their 15th and 16th years. Their mothers wondered if smoking interfered with health, growth, or appetite. None of them raised questions of the significance of smoking in regard to lung cancer. Nearly all mothers themselves smoked, and reported that their husbands smoked also.

From the mothers' point of view, late hours, too, had significance for the child's health. Nearly every mother had found difficulty in controlling the hour when her adolescent returned home. Staying out late was the first major change demanded by the child. Mothers were confused and uncomfortable in responding to this demand. Apparently they found little support from the community, which provided no standard of appropriate behavior in this regard. Families, neighborhoods, and communities differed markedly in their point of view of how late is late. The mother's own decision about time was very important to her, for she felt her decision would be one basis on which the community would judge her adequacy as a mother.

The mother's guidance of her oldest child had family importance, also, in that it evoked the approval or disapproval of the father. The pattern set for the oldest child was expected to be a precedent for the younger children. During this period the mother's adequacy is being tested in a variety of ways. The child participates in activities which result in returning home late, and may become involved in serious social difficulties. It is because of this fear that some mothers emphasized the children's need to have sleep during this adolescent period of rapid growth.

Neighborhood. During the middle adolescent years a large proportion of the adolescent's time is spent in his immediate neighborhood, which is usually made up of families considered by the mother to be "our own kind." Later, the more distant location of schools and of many recreational activities causes adolescents to meet peers in new neighborhoods. This posed new decisions for mothers. Should they call the mothers of these new acquaintances? Should they insist that the new companions be brought home for approval? Mothers were concerned about the possible effect of new neighborhood influences. In discussing this worry, mothers stated it was similar to their concerns in the earlier years, when they tried to overprotect their children physically only to realize that children must learn to protect themselves. Mothers had accepted the fact that the children needed to develop judgment in situations which were physically dangerous. But now the dangers were of a different order; the children were old enough to make mistakes which could affect their social development permanently. Previous social difficulties, such as not getting along with other children, or problems at school, had not worried parents to the same degree as the potential social problems of this age. Illegitimacy and delinquency were the two greatest sources of fear and worry. A parent during this period of the child's growth must accept that the best protection is to allow a child opportunity to manage inner impulses and responses essential in acquiring discrimination in new and complex social situations. A parent must have sufficient inner security to withstand the tension and anxiety inherent to this period of child growth, when the young person needs to explore and experiment in social experiences which present such frightening social hazards.

Closely associated with this extension of the child's participation in the total community are the changes taking place in his recreational interests and activities. Nearly every mother experienced some disappointment when the child first refused to participate with the family in a valued recreational group activity, such as a picnic or a visit to a relative. These refusals seem to the mother to be aimed at disappointing the parents. Such variations in recreation change the parents' relations with the child. With broadened recreational activities, adolescents associate increasingly with those of the opposite sex. Mothers in the Growth Study reported they worried about this. However, they were equally concerned if their adolescents were not developing this interest. Many mothers expressed a need during these years to have more help from their husbands. Even when a mother earlier had preferred to be entirely in charge of the child, now she felt uneasy and longed to share the responsibility with her husband. The new recreational experiences included drive-in theaters, dance halls, and bowling alleys, all of which, in many communities, may contribute to juvenile delinquency. Mothers were acutely aware of the community's judgmental attitudes toward those adolescents who became involved in community problems, and were sensitive to the responsibility placed on the parents by the community. Many mothers reported that they had urged their children to participate in activities in which there was adult supervision, such as school functions, community projects, or church socials, and were appreciative of the community programs which provided such supervised experiences. It helped parents when the school took a stand about the hour when pupils should return from a school dance, or when the church social included plans for escorting the girls home. Mothers felt most worried about recreational activities when their children were in their 12th to 14th years. Most mothers reported that by the 15th year they had come to have confidence in the adolescent's own judgment about behavior at mixed activities.

At this period father and mother begin to realize that once again it would become the pattern for them to spend the major part of their free time together. One mother described how lonely she and her husband felt during the first vacation after their children had grown up. They finally cut short their vacation and returned home, so that they could be with their children. Another mother reported that her husband had commented that they were right back where they had started.

Education. Most of the mothers in the Growth Study had attended high school for a year or two, but only a small number had graduated. A few had gone to vocational schools. A large number of fathers had graduated from high school, and some had gone on to college or technical schools. Mothers had hopes their children would graduate from high school, and were more interested in the fact of their obtaining a high school diploma than in the additional education which the children would gain. Several mothers felt that their children would not be "successful" without a diploma. Having the child complete high school assured the mother that she had met an important parental obligation in the child's preparation for life. Some adolescents had left high school before they graduated, and this was a bitter disappointment to their mothers.

A number of the Growth Study children selected the college preparatory course in high school, but several changed high schools or changed their course during the 4 year period, usually for a lower level one. The first selection suggests that these families held a rather high, unrealistic, educational goal for their children. Although many mothers were hopeful that their children would go on to higher education, few reported that they were financially prepared to meet its cost. Mothers made such statements as, "If it means enough to him, he'll find a way," or they expected the child to obtain scholarships. There was little consideration of the child's own learning capacities in the mothers' pressures for higher education. Mothers seemed to be influenced more by their own wishes to have had more education, and their desires were superimposed on the adolescents.

Many mothers reported that the adolescents' own interests and satisfactions in educational achievements lessened during the high school years. Several said that the children needed more urging to study, made poorer grades, and showed less interest than had been characteristic in early adolescent years. This was acceptable to many mothers in view of the social demands made on the children at this time. Mothers were not disturbed when the children's scholastic achievement was of a lower rating, if the grades were beyond the minimum for continued progress. Parental acceptance of the lower grades was partially explained by the limited value of education to this particular population sample. The factor important to this population as a whole was that high school education includes social behavior as an integral part of the total experience, even though the children's success educationally is based on responses in intellectual tasks.

Religion. The Growth Study mothers thought their adolescents were less interested in religion than during their earlier years, when they had been very conscientious about religious responsibilities. This was interesting, because adolescents are known at times to be rather fanatical about religion. These adolescents, however, needed increased parental urging to fulfill religious obligations. Many of the families were Roman Catholic, and several of the children had attended parochial schools. Most of the parents were very explicit about expecting their children to participate regularly in church activities. By 15 years of age the adolescent began to assume more responsibility for his church attendance.

Parents were very positive about the support and guidance they had secured, during the 20 years of the Growth Study, from their religion and local clergy. Some mothers who had used contraceptives during their earlier child-bearing years now expressed feelings of guilt and regret as they neared the menopausal period. Others stated that they had used the "rhythm" method successfully and satisfactorily. A few in the group had never resolved their conflicts about their responsibilities both to the marital partner and the church, and persistent emotional tensions had resulted.

Ethnic factors. As was previously mentioned, these families were predominantly of Irish background, although some derived from Canada, England, or Scotland. They had assimilated well the customs and cultural values of their community, in which there was a high proportion of Irish-American families. Mothers made little effort to urge adolescents to adhere to the customs and values of their original culture. When the cultural values and customs which guided the mothers' own adolescence differed markedly from those emphasized during the children's development, it was evident that many of the decisions required of mothers during their children's adolescence were especially difficult to make. For example, in this country today, experts in child development place much emphasis on the importance of parents giving sexual information to growing children, in sharp contrast to the point of view familiar to most of the mothers in the Growth Study. Some mothers who had been reared in a conservative religious atmosphere, in fact, were unable to integrate this point of view into their own guidance of children. Although these same mothers were highly motivated toward identifying with the current American cultural value system, some of the difficulties they reported through these years resulted from the shift in cultural values between those held in their earlier life experiences and those held valid during the development of their children. The understanding of cultural values in families is becoming increasingly significant in assessing the adolescent development of children.

Relationships. During the children's adolescent years, many of these parents were called upon to assist their own parents because of health or welfare needs. In some instances it was necessary to take a grandparent into the home. This created problems for the adolescents, who complained that the presence of the grandparent interfered with their social activities. Other adolescents got along very well with the grandparent, but this tended to disturb the relationship between the child and his parent. These mothers complained that the grandparents were spoiling the children, and supporting them against the parents. Grandparents were unhappy when the adolescents entered military service, and their reactions made it harder for mothers to face these separations.

These mothers had been able to separate themselves from their own families since marriage, and were able to react sympathetically and understandingly to the values held by their parents. Frequently they reacted with sadness and other emotions when they discussed their earlier life or some of the disappointments they thought they had caused their parents.

Marital relationship. Adolescence is a period which seems to require some changes in the marital relationship of the parents. Reference has been made to the social activity needs of adolescents as against the readiness of parents to permit these activities. The most important family social factor influencing the adolescent's social development is to be seen in the quality of the marital relationship. Mothers who found satisfaction in their relationship with their husbands were much better able to withstand the strain which the adolescent's new independence created. In some families the mothers had been overly involved with their children in the younger years, and now were unprepared for adolescence and its demands on the mother to allow the child to develop independence. Often these wives felt that their husbands had acquired satisfactions and interests outside the home which were more satisfying to them than the activities they shared with their wives. When the marital relationship was not satisfactory, mothers complained of deep dissatisfaction. In a few instances, divorce or legal separations were obtained during the children's adolescence. Some parents, also, had a high incidence of psychosomatic illnesses. Thus it can be seen that during this period family interrelationships in general are undergoing fundamental changes. Because of this the helping professions have an opportunity to offer important preventive services to families.

The changes which are observed in parent-child relations during adolescence are frequently referred to in popular literature, so that mothers generally are informed of the tensions in a teenager's relations with his parents. In spite of this, mothers are usually unprepared for their subjective reactions to the children's adolescent behavior. They are distressed by the children's devaluation of their families and homes, by the rejection of family values, and by the criticism of the personal traits of the parents. Mothers in the Growth Study described various ways in which the children had "hurt" them, and some were surprised by their intense response to this hurt. They seemed frightened by their lack of control and poise, especially when they recognized within themselves an impulse to react and respond in an equally childish manner. Several mothers described the desperate efforts they made to avoid conflicts with their adolescents. Many mothers found ways to soften the hurt, blaming friends or fatigue for the children's acts and stressing that the children were "not themselves." Able to find no logical explanation for the children's behavior, they intuitively sought rationalizations which helped them to accept their children's attitudes toward them.

A mother's understanding of this aspect of child development will not obliterate all of the distress she experiences at this time. Nonetheless, she should be given greater appreciation that the parental relationship must be essentially so secure that the child may, within limits, safely do what he must do — challenge, ridicule, and devaluate parental traits and values in his own quest for independence. The positive values of this aspect of parent-child relationships were not recognized by most mothers.

It was at this time that some mothers began to realize that there would be some compensations when the child actually left the home. Intellectually, the mothers knew that the children must grow away from them during these years. They thought they wanted this, but it was not until the children caused considerable discomfort that the mothers could emotionally accept this essential step towards independence and want the children to make it.

The most disturbing period in the mother-child relationship appears to be from the 14th to 16th years, but for the most part mothers are able to accept some of the children's individuality by the 18th year. A few of the mothers in the Growth Study could see ways in which the adolescents' independent interests and abilities were adding to the pleasures of the family. There were some, however, who continued to have conflicts with the adolescent through these later years, deciding that there would be no relief for either parent or child until the child left home and was married. Nevertheless, they expected that the relationship would eventually become more favorable.

Siblings. Many changes in sibling relationships occur during adolescence. In the early phase, the adolescent's continuous criticisms of younger siblings, or demands for the same privileges as older siblings, contribute to the general atmosphere of tension and irritation within the family. As the adolescent becomes dominating or controlling of younger brothers and sisters, increasingly mothers are called upon to settle the disputes or soothe the hurt feelings of their children. This adds to the general strain of which many mothers complain during the adolescence of their children. However, toward the end of adolescence, many young people assume quite mature responsibility for younger siblings, a shift in sibling relationships which brings enormous pride and pleasure to mothers.

Friends. During the later adolescent years young people develop their interests beyond their immediate environment and neighborhood. Many of the older adolescents in the Growth Study formed relationships with several peer groups in the neighborhood, school or church. Others gave up interest in neighborhood groups when they joined high school groups. Only a few adolescents had difficulty in their friendships, and this usually indicated that the child had difficulty in other social behavior. When a child left high school prematurely, the mother usually felt it was due to the child's falling in with companions who were a poor influence.

From the 13th year on, these adolescents had friendships with members of the same sex as well as with the opposite sex. They associated with mixed groups; some did occasional dating, others "went steady," a few became engaged, and a few married during later adolescence. The most common pattern of boy-girl relationship was that of "going steady" for a period of 4 to 6 months, after which the relationship ended and a new one was established. This pattern of dating was not disturbing to the mother, because she knew the friend and his interests and felt more security than if the child were "dating" several individuals. Mothers often negated the meaning of these relationships and expressed the hope that the young people would not marry too young, feeling that marriage necessarily resulted in giving up the pleasures of youth. When the children married young, the mothers were regretful. They were fearful of the dangers in adolescent dating, but by the 15th year they felt more at ease. Only a few mothers felt that their adolescents, because of social immaturity, were not yet ready to participate in mixed activities.

In summary, adolescence can be considered a biological developmental phase which involves the entire family unit. Although many families develop greater integration at this period, some family units are weakened or dissolved.

The attributes of families developing greater security are: (1) stable socioeconomic status; (2) cohesive values and goals in the marital relationship; (3) ability of the family members to communicate wishes and needs; (4) an ability within the family to accept individual interests and abilities of one another; and (5) the effective use of community opportunities, such as religious, educational, recreational, health and welfare resources.

The characteristics of families which become weakened or dissolved during the adolescence of a child are: (1) chronic socioeconomic stress; (2) chronic or serious illness; (3) prolonged marital discordance; (4) women dissatisfied with the responsibilities of motherhood; and (5) families unable to use assistance in resolving their problems.

In order to be most effective services for the adolescent should include consideration of family. Traditionally such professions as medicine, education, and social work have centered the volume of their services directly on the child's needs. In these programs work with parents has been motivated from a desire to influence them in ways which will serve the child's needs and without consideration of the needs of the parents themselves. Such community institutions as the court and the church tend to heighten the standards set for parents of adolescents. Frequently these institutions assert that juvenile delinquency results from the inadequacy of the parents; that is, from faulty family life. It is timely, therefore, that all of the professions give greater consideration to those services which strengthen families and thus enhance the child's efforts to achieve increased effectiveness in social functioning and fulfill his potential, a goal to which both parents and professional people are dedicated. If the growing child is to progress in an orderly, sequential pattern throughout his adolescent years, families must have sufficient security to make the necessary adaptations.

IX

THE EDUCATION
AND INTELLECTUAL DEVELOPMENT
OF THE CHILD

THE CHILD IN NURSERY SCHOOL
ROBERT H. ANDERSON

History and Present Development of Nursery Schools

In recent years a great deal of interest has developed in providing pre-school training in group situations for children between the ages of 2 and 6. This movement can be traced to nineteenth century Europe, where the Industrial Revolution created a need for custodial arrangements for the young children of employed women. It had its most significant growth in twentieth century England, where the Fisher Act of 1918 permitted the establishment of nursery schools as a part of the elementary school system. In the United States, nursery schools numbered only 3 in 1920,[1] and the rate of increase was quite slow until the Great Depression and World War II created social and economic conditions which spurred their growth. Herrick and Carroll, in a 1953 review[2] of the nursery school movement, reported that around 20 per cent of all children aged 2 to 5 were then enrolled in school.

For the most part, nursery schools have developed in response to the need for child care, and federal government support has been a major stimulant to their growth. Many have been developed as private business ventures or as cooperative community undertakings; some are operated by philanthropic institutions; others are operated by colleges and universities as centers for research in child development. A few are special schools connected with hospitals and similar institutions and another small number are those in public schools. These public-operated nursery schools tend to be either 4 year old "junior kindergartens" or nurseries operated in connection with child care training as part of home economics courses in high schools and junior colleges.[1]

Many states now permit school districts to use tax funds in support of nursery schools and some have adopted licensing and inspecting procedures. Regrettably, however, all too many nursery schools (especially the commercial and cooperative enterprises) are operated by untrained and incompetent adults whose errors can have significant harmful influence upon the health, welfare, and development of their charges. It is imperative that the high standards for nursery education which have been promulgated by the Association for Childhood Education International, The National Association for Nursery Education and various groups concerned with mental health, should be enforced within each state if nursery education is to achieve its rightful place on the American educational scene.

Characteristics of the Nursery School Child

Although some nursery schools work with children of ages 2 and 5, the majority define their functions in terms of the 3 and 4 year olds. In communities with public kindergartens it is rare to find nursery schools serving the 5 year old; in communities without kindergartens, the preschool arrangement for the 5 year old is more often called "private kindergarten" than nursery school. It seems appropriate, therefore, to limit this section to a rather brief coverage of the child at 2 and to concentrate upon the child of 3 and 4.

The child of 2 is not yet a social being, since his powers of communication are very limited and his social experience has been largely restricted to the home environment in which he has held a central position. His natural reaction to other children is one of pleasure but he is too inept in play and in conversation to establish a satisfactory relationship with them. His legs are short for his body and he tires so easily that a short session of nursery school (2 hours or less) is about all he can take. His teacher must play the role of substitute mother in a more literal way than is necessary later. His demands upon her time and attention make it difficult for her to work with more than a very few children, and generally not more than 6. This makes nursery training for 2 year olds rather expensive.

By the age of 3 the child has become more skillful in communication, in the use of his body, in his responses to social stimuli and controls and in his ability to select and engage in various forms of play. He is less demanding of adult attention, less completely self-centered and more interested in being like others. His expanded interests bring him into more frequent conflict with others (e.g., wanting the same toy) but also enable him to accept compromises (e.g., using a different toy in place of the one Jimmy has). The teacher finds it possible to reason with him more easily but she is also confronted with a more complex behavior pattern in which the child expresses his fears, tensions, and insecurities, as well as his positive feelings, in a greater variety of ways. She helps him to accept his many mistakes and failures as he constantly tries new experiences. She encourages him to "act his own age" through an understanding acceptance of his reactions and deeds. She helps him to adjust to his ups and downs which are associated with his stage of development or with rapid changes in it; i.e. poor coordination, awkwardness in hand and arm movements, speech and language blockages, general discouragement with self become evident to her. She also watches for the signs of tension (nail biting, thumb-sucking, tics, etc.) which are likely to reappear during this period as the child comes to doubt his status within his family and in the world at large.

At 4 the child's physical and intellectual powers have developed to such an extent that he becomes almost literally reckless in his experimentation with them. Ilg and Ames describe this as a period in which he is out of bounds in almost every direction. His tendency to use naughty language is but an aspect of his rapidly developing skill in verbal communication; his air of bravado and defiance of adult regulations is the manifestation of his increasing sense of self-sufficiency; his awakening interest in numbers and the addition to his time-sense of notions like "tomorrow" and "next week" are revelations of his intellectual growth; his eagerness to manipulate and operate toys and gadgets reflects his better muscular control. The child during this period is fanciful and still cannot distinguish between fact and fiction, although toward 5 there is less make-believe and pretending in his play and in his explanation of things.

For the 4 year old the nursery school is analogous to a cafeteria of experiences and "his eyes are bigger than his stomach." He samples everything on the menu, testing his own reactions and abilities. The teacher tries to meet this need by providing new and different toys, equipment and experiences. She helps him to learn what are his limits as well as his strengths; and she rebuilds his self-confidence as often as possible through the acknowledgment of his growth and accomplishments.

Working with the Child

The nursery school teacher, in league with the parents of the child, works toward the positive development of the child's total personality: his mind, his body, his self-concept, his social being. Her task is simpler if she understands his natural behavioral tendencies and is able to anticipate and cope with the various problems his behavior will present. Even before the child appears for his first day in school, she attempts to lay a foundation for his successful orientation by interviewing the parents, meeting and talking with the child, arranging for him to visit the school in advance, and similar preparations. In his first days at school she concentrates on providing information regarding the physical environment, the routines of the school program, the rules and regulations governing social behavior and the privileges he is especially urged to enjoy. She helps the child to resolve his immediate worries about toilet procedures, his physical safety, the teacher's readiness to comfort and help him and the certainty of his eventual return to the home. Once past the orientation period, she next concentrates on his gradual absorption into the pattern of activities in the school.

She realizes that the child is not, and cannot be, perfect and she accepts his occasional "bad" behavior (selfishness, destructiveness, vulgarity, riotousness, excitability) as naturally characteristic of children in the nursery school period. By and large, her success in combating these tendencies and developing "good" behavior (cooperation and sharing, respect for property and rights of others, acceptable manners and speech, self-control, etc.) will depend upon her ability to remain calm and unexcited in the presence of untoward behavior, to divert the child from undesirable activities, to convince the child that her heart is true to him even in his worst moments and to deal with his questions, implied as well as expressed, in a straightforward, honest manner.

When the child hurts another child, for example, the teacher's first concern is to divert the aggressor's attention to something else and prevent further damage. Her next concern is with the hurt child, who may need soothing and comforting and perhaps some advice about "the next time." Finally, she seeks to learn why the incident occurred and to explain the appropriate rule or lesson involved without threatening either child's basic security. Often the teacher discovers through such incidents the aggressor child's needs (e.g., for more experience with "ownership" of things) or his troubles ("she teased me like my sister always does"), and by seeking causes instead of concentrating on punishments she learns to see the child's behavior as a system of action communication.

Destructiveness comes in many sizes and shapes in the nursery school. Because incessant activity is characteristic of the program itself, the teacher must learn to expect a certain amount of accidental breakage, or wear and tear, as the natural consequence of activity. Sturdy and durable equipment should be provided as well as much expendable material which allows the child to "see what happens," and "see what it feels like," and "see what's inside." The teacher helps the child to distinguish between the normal and acceptable uses of equipment and wanton destruction.

When intentional destructiveness occurs, the teacher's tactics again involve the analysis of cause and explanation of the rules or lessons involved rather than punishment. Sometimes she may conclude that she was herself to blame for having ignored certain signs that the child was all wound up and ready to explode: a change in pace or activity might have saved the day. Sometimes she will recognize efforts of the child to overcome certain frustrations or jealousies related in some way to the object or the incident.

Nursery school work, more than any other branch of teaching, involves very close cooperation and association between the teacher and the parents. Often the advice, counsel, and reassurance given to the parents has a more lasting effect upon the child's development than the actual work which is done in the school with the child. This implies that the nursery school teacher's training should include techniques for interviewing and conferring with parents. It implies also that the school should have a suitable lending library (or at least selected reading lists) and a plan for both informal and systematic parent discussion groups.

Criteria for a Good Nursery School

The foregoing comments are illustrative of a point of view which should prevail in a good nursery school. Obviously the most important factor in the nursery school is sympathetic and skillful teaching, and the job of nursery school teacher is only for persons with excellent training and strong personal resources.

A helpful and succinct description of a good nursery school is offered by Gans, Stendler, and Almy,[3] who see it as a place where the young child finds:

> That he can be himself and still receive appreciation, respect, and warm acceptance.
>
> That the world has an order and a routine that he can understand and cope with at his level of development.
>
> That getting along with other people in a friendly way becomes increasingly easier because he is helped, in shared activities, to understand his own rights and feelings as well as those of others.
>
> That there is interest and challenge for his growing powers, but no pushing of them.
>
> That his physical health and well-being are promoted and protected throughout the day.

Since the nursery school movement is relatively new, it has had one advantage over elementary schools in general: it has reaped the fullest benefit of the tremendous advances which have been made recently in the field of school architecture and school equipment design, both in the United States and in Europe. Many schools, of course, are operated in makeshift quarters; yet when blessed with excellent teachers there is no reason that such schools cannot do a good job despite the environmental limitations. The nursery school building[4] is ideally a simple, expandable, and extremely functional unit, equipped with group rooms, work areas, rest or sleeping areas, work sinks, display counters, work benches, specialized storage facilities, and similar features which are in harmony with the varied activities in the program. Its classrooms are far larger in floor space per pupil than one finds in the primary school. It is located on a suitable (safe, attractive, quiet, accessible) site which includes adequate play areas adjoining the classrooms. Usually the play areas for each level will be private, and the entire arrangement is fenced in. For the 2 year olds, who play singly, there need to be such things as large blocks, small wheel toys, boxes, boards, and similar equipment; for the older children there should be runways for larger wheel toys, a fixed climbing frame (preferably of wood), a hillock to run up and down, big (8 ft × 10 ft) sand boxes, barrels, ladders, slides, and similar items. Pet pens, shallow wading pools, garden plots, and digging areas are desirable. The playground ought to be surfaced with appropriate soft materials, such as turf, cork, tanbark, or rubberized pellets, with some of the area hardtopped for accessways and for wet weather use.

In summary, the nursery school is a relative newcomer to the American educational scene. Although its many advantages in the early training of the child are evident, less than 1 child in every 5 has opportunity of nursery school attendance. Even fewer have the privilege of attending a nursery school which would satisfy realistic standards.

The child develops at a spectacular rate and in many directions during the formative years of the nursery school period. He develops his powers of communication, of social interaction, of emotion and intellect, and of physical control, through a rich and varied program. His lack of maturity and his need for experimentation with ways of living require that his teacher be liberally endowed with serenity, adaptability, resourcefulness, and affection. The provision of a suitable physical environment, when combined with the warm and stimulating psychological environment the teacher herself provides, makes it all the more likely that nursery school training can be of inestimable value and benefit to the preschool child.

THE ELEMENTARY SCHOOL PERIOD
ROBERT H. ANDERSON

General Background

The elementary school period in a child's life generally begins with the first grade, which he enters at approximately age 6, and ends when he enters the seventh grade. Sometimes the seventh grade and the eighth grade are regarded as part of the elementary school period, but more often they are designated as junior high school years. Roughly one-third of all American children attend public kindergarten classes for one year prior to first grade entrance. For purposes of this discussion, the kindergarten and the first six grades will be regarded as the elementary school years, which can be divided for convenience into four major periods: (1) kindergarten, or preprimary; (2) first grade, or the initial period of relatively formal schooling; (3) the second and third years of primary education; and (4) the fourth-fifth-sixth, or intermediate-grade, years.

The elementary school in the United States cannot easily be described because it has no universal size, shape, or structure. Despite a nationwide trend toward the consolidation of inefficient and isolated units like the one room "little red schoolhouse" of the past, there remain thousands of such units in operation today. By contrast with these small schools there are many in the large cities where 600, 700, and even 1,000-plus pupils are enrolled in mammoth, congested institutions. In between may be found thousands upon thousands of schools with enrollments between 100 and 500. Research offers little concrete data by which to judge the optimum size of schools for children age 5–12, but it is clear that size alone is rarely a major reason for the vast qualitative discrepancies that may be found from school to school.

Historically, the public schools have been a function of state rather than federal responsibility. The principle of "local control," allowing each community to determine the nature and the quality of its schools, has had the effect of creating regional differences over the country as a whole, and even more remarkable differences between and within states. The financing and management of the schools, always a fairly serious social problem, has reached critical proportions in recent years as local tax resources have strained to meet the needs created by the postwar birthrate, the manpower shortage, new demands for improved school services, and the obsolescence and inadequacy of available plant and equipment. All of these forces have led to even greater discrepancies between the schools in favored and long-sighted communities and the schools in apathetic, declining, rapidly-growing, or short-sighted communities.

While certain aspects of the acknowledged crisis in American public education might be rather easily remedied by more adequate financial support, other problems will be more difficult to resolve. Prominent among these is the unresolved question of the limits of the school's responsibility for meeting the needs of a rapidly-changing society.

By contrast with the relatively simple and circumscribed functions of the school prior to approximately 1920, the modern elementary school has been assigned more tasks than it could possibly accomplish with the available funds, resources, and personnel. The multiplication of "fundamental" subjects, the constant addition of required services, and the increasing tendency of the public to look to the schools for solutions to problems which ordinarily fall within the province of other social institutions, are manifestations of this situation. The elementary school child lives in a world in which change is a watchword and uncertainty is the price of progress. The eminent anthropologist, Margaret Mead, summarizes the situation in these words:

American children are growing up within the most rapidly changing culture of which we have any record in the world, within a culture where for several generations each generation's experience has differed sharply from the last, and in which the experience of the youngest child in a large family will be extraordinarily different from that of the first born. Mothers cannot look back to the experience of their mothers, nor even to that of their older sisters; young husbands and fathers have no guides to the behavior which they are assuming today. So long standing and so rapid have been those processes of change that expectation of change and anxiety about change have been built into our character as a people.[5]

In the face of this problem, the educator is torn between his conscience, which tells him that the child is desperately in need of trained adult help in meeting life's many challenges, and his practical intelligence, which tells him that no man or institution can possibly succeed in being all things to all people. Hence the constant struggle between such writers as Bernard Iddings Bell, counselling the schoolman against his "soft-hearted foolishness" in so willingly assuming duties which belong to the home and other institutions, and persons like Harold Rugg who argue for an expansionist role in the schools. For further treatment of this topic, the reader is referred to Gordon Lee.[6] One need only examine the agenda of any school selected at random to discover that the majority of schoolmen, whether foolish or not, have elected to pit their resources against the total challenge.

Age Characteristics and Educational Needs

Although every child is known to be unique in his own development, studies of child development and behavior, conducted in a variety of settings and for a variety of purposes, have provided valuable help to parents, teachers, and others by documenting the "normal" or typical behavior patterns which are common to all children in each elementary school age period. The following descriptions represent an attempt to summarize certain pertinent data relating to the "typical child" at each of these age periods.

The 5 year old. Few fallacies could be more damaging to the future welfare of children than the common assumption (as reflected in state laws and local policies governing admission to school, for example) that all so-called "5 year olds" are equally ready for school when they enter the kindergarten classroom in September. Even were it not for the great discrepancy in their physical ages, which can vary as much as 20 per cent from the youngest to the oldest in the class, there would still be great variety in home backgrounds, neighborhood influences, play habits, interests, and other factors to be considered. The following description, therefore, is merely suggestive of certain usual patterns and characteristics which might be observed in a "5 year old" group.

Children by this age have usually had few large-group social contacts with peers, so the contrasts of extremes in development become apparent to themselves and to adults for the first time. In general, although the boys tend to be slightly taller and heavier than the girls, the girls are usually ahead of the boys in all-around physiological development. This has led some educators to propose that entrance-age requirements for girls should be more lenient by several months in order that boy-girl progress in the early elementary grades might be more nearly uniform than it usually is. It is possible that future research will suggest similar adjustments in terms of the body build or general physical development of children, their emotional development, social background, or "readiness" in general. The self-confidence and future poise of children is profoundly influenced by the self-estimate which takes place during the kindergarten year in the society of peers.

The social development as well as health of the child at this age is influenced, at least to some extent, by various "first" events which are characteristic of the kindergarten period. This would include the first loss of baby teeth; the first occasions for speech situations involving an audience; the first continuous relationship with a sympathetic adult other than a parent (or equivalent); first regular deviation from family-regulated toilet behavior; first significant exposure to community-wide infectious-disease hazards; and first explorations into literally hundreds of new ventures and experiences. When the child enters school, he is quite likely to revert to any tensional-behavior patterns he may once have had, such as thumb-sucking, nail-biting, toilet lapses, and the like. This could be due to his fear of the situation (the teacher, the other children, the huge building, the noise), to his feelings of rejection by the home ("they've sent me away to this place"), or to general lack of previous social experience.

By this age the child's handedness is established (90 per cent will be right-handed, and the left-handed child will need help in accepting his difference), as is eye dominance; yet neither the eyes nor the fingers are by any means ready for reading and writing except at the most exploratory and rudimentary level. The child's general rate of growth will be slower than it was in infancy and early childhood but he will be constantly changing in his interests and abilities as the uneven development of motor skills proceeds.

The 5 year old is typically energetic, restless, active, vital, and enthusiastic. Although both his energy-span and attention-span are short, requiring frequent change of pace and activity, his teacher thinks of him in terms of perpetual motion. She also sees him as a chronically curious, inquisitive child, with a rapidly developing intellect and a passion for improving his controls and perfecting his skills. Nearly all of his thinking is specific and concrete, although he continues to be interested in fanciful, imaginative play and he is not yet very sure where the line is drawn between the real and the make-believe.

Locomotor and manipulative activities, especially those which are associated with large-muscle development (wheel toys, large blocks, climbing apparatus, pounding toys, and push-pull games), therefore constitute a large portion of the kindergarten program. Work habits and social lessons are developed gradually as the children learn to share, to take turns, to play together, to clean up and put things away, and (especially the more quarrelsome boys) to settle arguments by socially approved means. The original "I," "me," and "my" of the beginning kindergartner gradually softens into more frequent "we," "us," and "our" as the year moves along. This slow but steady socialization process is one of the major benefits of kindergarten training.

In the kindergarten are numerous opportunities for health and safety education. Safety in going between home and school is a frequent topic; so is training in personal hygiene (using a tissue or clean handkerchief, covering mouth and nose, keeping fingers away from the face), and attention to the child's needs for sleep and rest. Milk-and-juice period is a tangible example of lessons in diet and foods, and the teacher checks up on such matters as the child's breakfast habits and usual food choices.

The kindergarten program aims to develop the child's vocabulary and conversational skill, in preparation for later reading. Stories are read and told. The names of common objects are occasionally printed in manuscript. The teacher has a conscious plan for the development of language-arts readiness as each child furnishes his cues in his own way and according to his own schedule. Similarly, the child's readiness is developed in number work, in science, in the creative fields (music, art, rhythms, dramatics), and in that field usually called the social studies, which deals with human relationships. Exploratory trips into the school neighborhood and the community serve to broaden the child's horizons and stimulate interest in the larger world.

That approximately two out of three children in the United States have no opportunity for public kindergarten experience is a very real handicap both to them and to the adults who will subsequently work with them. Research evidence suggests rather strongly that children who have attended kindergarten tend to make relatively better progress in the first five grades, to "repeat" first grade less often, to excel in reading rate and comprehension, to surpass nonkindergartners in the rate and quality of handwriting in the first grade, to get along better with other children and in groups, to excel in oral language, and to receive higher teacher ratings on traits such as industry and initiative.[7]

Among the values of kindergarten experience are the promotion of health and safety, experience in working alone in the presence of others, experience in working with others in groups, and broader opportunity for contacts with other children and adults. The child prepares for future elementary school work through his exploratory contacts with the "3 R's," and he has a variety of experiences with all sorts of materials, thus revealing and developing his interests and aptitudes.

Perhaps even more important than the utilitarian concept of preparation for formal schooling is the concept that kindergarten serves the mental health needs of the child. Although some kindergartens are little more than junior-size first grade classes, with a formal and even austere environment, the majority are truly what their name implies, "gardens for children." Happiness and pleasure are more likely to be emphasized in this year than in the years to come. Scarcely ever again will the school child be so free to make his own choices, to explore at will, to express without particular restraint his feelings and his needs. It is difficult to assess the potential value of such experience in the development of a sound personality and a healthy attitude toward "school."

Meeting the many needs of 5 year old children is a task which requires an extraordinary person in the role of teacher. Most comfortable and successful in this role will be the adult who has a great deal of warmth and natural affection for children, much imagination to meet the many and varied needs of the youngsters, strong physical stamina to keep pace with an atmosphere of nearly constant activity, and an endless supply of patience and good humor.

The 6 year old. Since so small a proportion of children in today's elementary school have had previous kindergarten experience under the school's sponsorship, many of the comments in the foregoing kindergarten section would be applicable in a discussion of the 6 year old entering first grade. This is true particularly with respect to discrepancies in preschool readiness; the child's introduction to new social experiences; the first impact of self-estimate upon personality; the child's exposure to certain health hazards; the temporary reversion to escape mechanisms under tension; and the general procedure for inducting the child into school life.

The 6 year old is growing rather slowly in height as compared to former years but he is beginning to broaden out and as a result to gain more weight. These features, although depending in large measure on the child's build tend to characterize the following 2 or 3 years. The large muscles of the arms and legs are better developed than the small muscles of the hands and fingers, and fine work such as handwriting continues to be a very taxing process until later in the school year. Hand-eye coordination is incompletely developed, which requires much caution by the teacher in initiating formal reading on any extensive scale. The children tend to be still somewhat farsighted. Since the eyeballs are changing in shape and size, the teacher should be alert to the way the child uses his eyes in order to detect evidence of strain or poor vision. The loss of deciduous teeth is well under way, with the result that some children need guidance in their reaction to the discomforts entailed and possibly to the sight of blood; even more need help in adjusting to the social effects of their grotesque appearance. Permanent teeth are beginning to appear, with some discomfort, which may influence the child's school behavior. Dental hygiene is a necessary part of the curriculum.

The boys and girls continue to play together during this period, although their interests gradually separate and "boys' games vs. girls' games" will emerge as a concept during the year. The boys at this age seem to get along better with their fathers than their mothers; and since practically all first-grade teachers are women it is possible that the general academic slowness which differentiates boys from girls at this age is aggravated by the necessity of tolerating a woman teacher.

Other physical characteristics of the 6 year old are, in a sense, more sophisticated versions of the 5 year old pattern. The child has great energy and vitality, and as in kindergarten, he finds it hard to sit still. He still wants large-muscle activities, and his motto seems to be "activity for activity's sake." Active, boisterous games (hopping, skipping, running, jumping, bouncing, climbing, bumping) are needed, since he is developing, and enjoying, his sense of equilibrium. The school program must, therefore, provide for a great deal of physical activity, interspersed with periods of rest and quiet to accommodate the child's tendency to fatigue. Since the child's attention-span is still quite short, the entire program, especially in the first half year, must be arranged in terms of well-balanced short periods.

The child at this age is highly susceptible to respiratory infection as well as the common children's diseases which are prevalent in the early school years, and the teacher can expect a number of periods of absence. Children convalescing from serious or prolonged illness should be protected against too-rapid return to their former level of activities. Training in personal hygiene is important, and the teacher must be ever vigilant for signs of illness. Postural defects often are present and may be aggravated at this age, so that proper adjustment of furniture and careful training in posture habits are essential in the primary grades.

The intellectual development of the child continues at a rapid pace. Social education continues to center around the family, the home neighborhood, the school, and the community. Safety education, fire drills, playground safety rules, and similar experiences take on new meaning for the child. Vocabulary development is fostered through a great variety and quantity of interesting experiences. The child is intensely interested in stories, especially those about children, animals, and family life. Manuscript writing begins with the child's own name and words taken from class experiences. Various clues including vision tests, help the teacher to know when the child is ready to begin the all-important enterprise of reading. Number concepts are developed informally and through practical number situations. Plants, animals, natural phenomena, and bodily growth and care serve for much of the content of science education. Singing, creative art, dramatics, and rhythmic activities are necessary for the child and important factors in his emotional growth.

The first-grader is likely to become somewhat assertive and aggressive, an aspect of his increasing drive toward independence. He is inclined to change rather quickly in his behavior toward other children. He likes to do things for himself, dawdle at times as a manifestation of his self-sufficiency, resist rules, and be negative about things on occasion. Frequently children at this age will lie, cheat, or steal; often this reflects their eagerness to achieve, to be recognized, to win, to be "first." The 6 year old has tremendous need for praise and encouragement, and the teacher needs to help the child build up confidence in himself. This is all the more true if the school emphasizes comparative marking procedures.

There is reason to believe that the widespread use of the comparative approach to evaluating and reporting pupil progress has been a major reason for the emotional and academic maladjustment of many children. Virtually all scholarship and research in the various fields of personality development suggests that young children, in particular, are frustrated and confused by the system of placing them in academic competition with their agemates, and rewarding them with ill-defined but emotionally-loaded symbols such as A, B, C, D, F, or their equivalents. Snygg and Combs have stated the problems of competitive marking systems effectively.[8] Contrary to the assumption commonly held by parents, and even on occasion by workers in medicine and social service, the comparative marking system is an inadequate and unsatisfactory device for motivating children to learn. Its consequences frequently are disappointment and rebellion in the youngster who for various reasons earns less than the desired symbol of adult approval, a growing sense of inadequacy and resignation in the child who performs in the "average" range, and a false sense of values and accomplishment in those who receive the cherished symbols, especially where this is relatively effortless. Fortunate is the child who begins his educational experiences in a school where progress is measured on an individualized basis, where the concept of academic competition is kept under reasonable control, where success is encountered far, far more frequently than failure by children in all ability levels, and where the things learned are seen by the child as more important than the extrinsic symbols adults are prone to assign to them.

At the first grade level, the minimum formal requirements of the academic program are usually too high for about 20 per cent of children in a typical population sample. In underprivileged neighborhoods (or in poor situations where teachers are unable to provide the best possible guidance and attention), as many as 50 per cent of first grade children may be unable to cope with the full year's work. Often this is due to the simple fact that many children are, for legal and other reasons, admitted to school about a year sooner than they ought to have been. Mounting evidence on this score is leading school systems to adopt more stringent admission requirements (i.e., the trend is toward requiring the child to have reached six years of age by September 1 of the year he enters first grade). Where inadequacy of background and experience, rather than underage, is the reason for a child's slow initial progress, not stricter admission requirements but a modified program in the early years is needed. Where long range lack of academic potential is the reason for a slow start, a modified program all along the line is the necessary response of the school.

These kinds of adaptation on the part of the school are most likely to occur in communities where enlightened school leadership has developed broad and flexible policies over the years. In such communities, teachers adhere less rigidly to the useful but oversimplified guidelines that the "graded school" concept is based upon. Here we would expect to find less concern for grade-level-expectancy standards in the traditional sense, but more concern that each child should move forward as rapidly as possible but no more rapidly than is reasonable and feasible for him. The ultimate manifestation of such an enlightened attitude is the adoption of a "nongraded" school pattern, as described by Anderson[9] and Goodlad and Anderson.[10]

The 7 and 8 year olds. Although there are some important differences between typical second grade and third grade children, the two ages can be discussed together because of the essential unity of the later primary years. It is a period of remarkable expansion on many fronts, and in many ways marks the end of a childhood period. The step between third and fourth grades is thought by many educators to be one of the more dramatic milestones in the child's career, comparable with the jumps between kindergarten and first grade, and between sixth and seventh grades. Most seem to agree that the child, by the time of his entry to the fourth grade, should be permanently settled insofar as promotion and grouping are concerned.

In this period the child's growth in height and gain in weight continue about as in the preceding year with weight gain relatively greater due chiefly to increase in amount of muscle and stockiness of bones. He needs a school program which includes active games and other motor activities built into the daily routine, appropriate to his increasing strength and endurance. The child is still losing teeth, although he has by now lost most of his earlier self-consciousness about dental appearance. The eyes are quite well developed, so that near work is possible; however, near-sightedness may develop around 8 years of age and so unusual positional use of the eyes, or other evidences of strain, should be watched for. Small muscle manipulative skill is rapidly increasing, but the child becomes restless if required to engage in extended writing or other manipulative work. Legible writing becomes quite attainable toward the end of the 8th year; and along the way the child, eager as he is to improve, does a great deal of erasing and recopying as evidence of his serious dedication to the job. In fact, eagerness is a characteristic of the 7 and 8 year olds, and motivation for learning is at one of its highest peaks. The child has energy and vitality; he is proud of his skills as they develop; his curiosity about people and things is expanding at a rapid pace; his self-confidence builds ever upward until by 8 he reaches a point where he feels ready and willing to try anything. Because achievement and mastery have become important to him, the teacher plays her part carefully; she guides him into interesting tasks which are within his power to achieve; she helps him to gauge the limits of his abilities and sets up exercises for their strengthening; she steers him into many new interests to satisfy his appetite for learning.

Like the 6 year old, the 7 year old is still uncertain about property rights and personal ethics, and he may occasionally cheat or steal; he is also somewhat of a worrier and inclined toward occasional negative and withdrawn behavior. These "ups and downs" in his moods and response patterns gradually work themselves out, and by a year or so later he is more likely than not to be chronically exuberant and buoyant. Children with hobbies and self-initiated interests apparently find it easier to survive this two year period than those who do not. The teacher serves as a "home base" and a friend-in-need (with occasional exceptions, to be sure!) to whom the child turns for support and friendship.

By the age of 8 the child is just beginning to enter the stage when peer-group associations have great importance. The child moves toward this stage by occasional limitation of friends, by adopting more discriminating means of selecting his companions than during his earlier, democratic years, by an increasing interest in group games, and by becoming more exclusively interested in the company of his own sex.

Social learnings in this later primary period expand beyond the life of the community to life in other parts of the United States and in the world. Geography and history, communication and transportation, and topics related to the economic life of the community tend to excite the child's interest. The program in the language arts moves ahead rapidly in these years: by the end of the third grade many children have achieved a good quality of writing, a sizable writing vocabulary (perhaps 750 words), a good silent reading rate (perhaps 100–125 words a minute), and a sizable reading vocabulary (1500–3000 words). They will also have begun to use a dictionary and to study fundamental rules of grammatical usage. Arithmetic understandings proceed at a comparable rate, and in such fields as science the children acquire a fairly incredible fund of information and practical knowledge about the natural world, the heavens, and other studies once open only to students in secondary schools and colleges. In music this is a rich period during which group singing, rhythms in response to music, the uses of simple and complex instruments, and the reading of music are highlights. The advanced state of manipulative skill enables the children to derive deep enjoyment from creative art; and in the 2 year period many children pass from symbolic art into a period of more realistic representation of the world around them.

It is to be hoped that the child is blessed, during this period, with teachers who value the creative arts for the intrinsic pleasure they give to children, and who, therefore, do not seek to impose adult standards and formal, technical instruction upon them. Probably the basic reluctance (and/or inability) of the typical American adult to derive pure pleasure from music and art has its origins in the dull, ritualistic, uninspired, and unimaginative teaching of art and music which had this country in its grip for so many unfortunate decades. Probably an easy, rule-of-thumb measure of any given school's true worth would be a photographic record of the expressions which appear on the faces of its second and third grade pupils when the signal for a music or art period is given. Any response short of enthusiasm must, on the basis of what is known about children's interests and feelings at this age, constitute an indictment.

The 9, 10, and 11 year olds. When the child enters the fourth grade he begins a period of relative calm and stability. Some writers call this three year period the middle childhood plateau of slow, steady growth while others refer to it as the age of reason. It is a time of social orientation, with the peer group becoming increasingly important: both boys and girls become active in gangs, secret clubs, scouts, and similar organizations. Team activity also fills this social need, and provides an outlet for the strong competitive drive. In the psychoanalytic literature psychiatrists stress the latency or "absence of sex-drives and the emergence of ego strengths as the primary characteristics of children in the age group 9 through 12." [11]

The terms growth and latency as used above do not apply to physical progress during these years, for growth in height and muscle size, and particularly gain in weight begin to accelerate during these years. This is much more strikingly so in girls than boys because girls characteristically enter their prepubescent spurt during this period while boys usually do so at its end, as described in Chapter IV. By the end of the period the advancement of girls is usually much more apparent than it has been previously. Some of the girls may be taller and heavier than the boys, and the compensatory bullying and teasing of the boys poses special social problems for them.

The onset of puberty markedly affects behavior and interests, as well as general morale: discomfort (e.g., of outgrown clothing and furniture) and uncertainty cause moodiness; school work follows an uneven pattern of ups and downs; social affinities are changing, to correspond more nearly with maturational levels. For the most part sex antagonisms become acute during fourth and fifth grades, with the first signs of boy-girl interest appearing usually in the sixth grade. In classes the boys and girls will resist sitting near the opposite sex, and on the playgrounds most games are played separately. This is a period when the boys are particularly noisy, rough-and-tough, and generally casual about danger. As a result it is a period for frequent accidents on the playground and even in the school building. Safety-consciousness develops only gradually, and such topics as bicycle safety are stressed in the classroom. Tidiness and neatness probably reach a low point in the fourth and fifth grades. Girls during this period fluctuate between their earlier interests and habits and the more feminine interests which they gradually adopt as their secondary sex characteristics develop and they begin to identify themselves with more mature girls.

There are many reasons for emphasizing health training in the intermediate grades. This is often a period of dental neglect, with the need
for orthodontia appearing as early as the fourth grade. Appropriate guidance should be given children wearing braces to help them adjust to the
physical awkwardness and possible social stigma; children tempted to
remove their braces in school must be watched. The eyes normally have
reached functional maturity and the child can do concentrated close
work without strain. However, children with visual defects need supervision on the wearing of glasses, and should be seated in the most ad-
vantageous visual position for them. The same is true for aural defects.
Bad posture, often symptomatic of other physical or emotional difficulty,
needs to be watched for and corrected. The great interest of children in
food and eating, combined with their tendency to have wider food tastes,
makes it very practical to teach food and health rules in the intermediate
grades. The frequency with which true obesity begins to appear in these
years has been referred to previously. The child's increasing independence in the home makes it less than likely that he will regularly have
the 10 hours of sleep which he needs: again a cue to the school to emphasize sleep requirements in its health lessons.

Smaller and less well-developed children are likely to compete fiercely
with stronger and more mature children unless means are found for satisfying their competitive urge in situations within each child's power limits.
Unfortunately the typical elementary school athletic program, as well as
such groups as the Little League, violates this principle by affording practice opportunities only to those in least need of it: rarely does the program give the less fortunate child his fair share of coaching and game
participation. All children at this age need extensive opportunity to develop body control, strength, endurance, and playing skill. Furthermore,
this extends to games and activities utilizing the small-muscle manipulative skills which are increasing so rapidly at this age.

The child in the intermediate grades is past the peak incidence of infectious diseases, and his school attendance average is highest during this
period. Intellectual maturity, which correlates closely with physical maturity, is stimulated through reading (wide and extensive reading is now
possible) and through the many hobbies and activities in which the child
of this age engages. A longer attention-span enables the child to pursue
his interests in how things are made, how people live and work together,
how things came to be as they are, and how interesting people, real or
fictional, have overcome barriers to their success. Hence the 9 year old
has a passion for comic books and for adventurous tales on the radio and
TV; the 10 year old develops a leaning toward stories about patriotic

and athletic heroes, men of science and adventure, and boy heroes with whom he can identify; and the 11 and 12 year old continues this reading pattern with even more gusto.

Beginning with the fourth grade it is increasingly possible for the school to develop the intellectual bases for good citizenship and democratic self-responsibility. The child is concerned with individual justice, and better able to understand right and wrong. He is anxious to be treated in an adult way, and he seeks clues (through the study of laws and government, for example) to workable patterns of behavior control which he and his peers can use. The analogy of "rules of the game," carried over from his sports interests, is constantly influential in his non-game behavior. Increasingly he abides by group decisions as his prestige and his social relations come to depend upon cooperative behavior. The social studies are extremely popular with children of this age.

The curriculum of the intermediate grades is based upon the deepening interests and the skills-proficiency of the children. The social studies gradually shift into historical and geographical topics. In the language arts, increasing attention is given to the functional utilization of the basic skills in reading, handwriting, spelling, and expression which have been developed in the primary grades, although fundamental skills must be further developed and remedial instruction will be necessary for many of the children. Arithmetic instruction assumes increased importance and a larger share of the school day; and science, the subject area of greatest interest to children at this age, covers an astonishing variety of topics as children satisfy their curiosity about their environment and acquire a "scientific" way of thinking.

In music, instruction in band and orchestra instruments may be begun in the fourth grade for those who have both interest and aptitude; class use of simple instruments (melody flutes, rhythm instruments) often precedes this step. In addition to more skillful note-reading and singing, both individually and in groups, the children will readily indulge in folk dancing, square dancing, and listening to good music. Similarly, the child's art development moves ahead during these years. The child does much experimenting with materials, and he is increasingly accurate in representation. Much of the art and music program takes place in the setting of other learnings. Dramatic play is popular with children of both sexes.

Individual Differences and the Needs of Children

If all men were created biologically equal, and if the child rearing environment in each home and community could be kept within a uniform pattern, many of the practices which can be found in the public schools would then make more sense than they do under the uncontrolled circumstances of actuality. Every child that has ever lived has been different from all others in his physical inheritance, in his social circumstances, in his goals and motivations, and in his personality. His intellectual potentiality (now conceived as multifaceted) is established at birth, but like his physical potentiality it eventually reaches only those levels, usually short of the possible upper and lateral limits, which his opportunities and his experiences would permit. By the time the child reaches school, for example, his nutritional history may have already affected his eventual height, weight, and body pattern; his linguistic history may have already established the basic pattern for oral communication; his emotional history has already contributed to his basic personality; and life with his parents, siblings, and neighbors has already given him a deep-rooted self-concept and a system of social beliefs. He has already learned certain fears, developed certain tensions and anxieties, acquired certain preferences and prejudices, and built up a store of facts and ideas which make his educational needs different from every other child's.

Most schools, therefore, are naive and impractical in their overdependence upon the concept of "average" or "normal." Rigidity in the classification and grouping of children implies a blindness to the real needs of the nonaverage child. Motivational devices based upon competition are inequitable and illogical. Overdependence upon certain teaching approaches (recitation, paper-and-pencil tests, academic studies) gives a perpetual advantage to certain children and penalizes those whose experiential needs are best filled by more varied activities (excursions, construction projects, creative and aesthetic experiences). Differentiation and individualization of instruction must be arranged if each child (the slow-learning normal, the slow-learning below-normal, the physically handicapped, the gifted, the socially handicapped) is to find within the program the ingredients essential to his maximum all-round development.

Meeting Basic Needs

Studies of child development, bringing ever more sharply into focus the tremendous complexity of the human personality, have in recent decades given new and more significant meaning to the role of education in shaping the child's future. In sharp contrast to a day (not yet far enough removed) when prevailing practice assumed that children had to be forced to learn, one finds today a teaching corps which respects the child's personality and attempts to make learning an exciting, vital, rewarding experience for him. Today's teacher works towards the satisfaction of each child's need for (1) a sense of his own personal worth and (2) a satisfying and productive relationship with others. She realizes that these goals will be achieved only if the child acquires a great many basic skills of learning and living, if his curiosity and interest are constantly stimulated, if his potential powers — physical, social, intellectual, emotional — are developed to the fullest: in short, if his schooling challenges the best that is in him. She also realizes that the school must provide an environment of warmth and security, where such phrases as "I belong," and "I did it," and "we're working together," and "let's help Tommy," and "thanks a lot, Miss Jones!" are frequently heard. She knows, too, that learning takes place best in a program which features creative experiences and which provides good balance between a variety of purposeful and pleasurable activities.

The Elementary School Curriculum

The curriculum means all of the educational experiences which the child has under the supervision of the school. The rather remarkable changes in curriculum theory and practice which have taken place in the twentieth century make an understanding of current trends indispensable to an understanding of the child's school life.

The curriculum of a quarter-century ago was essentially a collection of independent subjects, each with its allotted share of school time and each taught without much relation to its sister subjects. Thoughtful and scientific consideration of the actual values inherent in each field of study, however, has led over the years to the elimination, or reduction, of certain material in most of these fields. The development of more efficient methods of teaching the various subjects, coupled with more realistic grade placement of abstract and difficult topics, has led to certain economies of time and effort. Thus, much of the earlier content of the curriculum has been reduced. However, the total of these reductions is insignificant by contrast with the vast number of new topics and new emphases within each subject, and with the great number of new subjects added to the curriculum. One need only examine current offerings in science, in literature, in health and safety education, in the social studies, in the creative arts, in human relations, and in physical education to appreciate this point.

There has been a trend toward the grouping of separate but related subjects into broad fields of study, the two most common examples being the social studies (history, geography, civics, and related fields) and the language arts (reading, writing, spelling, grammar, literature, etc.). These larger fields are assigned proportionately larger blocs of time within the school day. This enables the teacher to arrange a flexible program which is potentially more responsive to the developing needs and interests of the children. The broad-fields approach is probably the most widely accepted plan in use today.

Many schools, carrying the underlying theory a step further, have attempted to organize the curriculum, or a major part of it, around common problems of living. In such programs the work at each grade level is planned in terms of life-centered problems (e.g. securing goods and services, dealing with plant and animal life, communicating with other people) which are known to be of interest to children at that age. Drill in the fundamental skills of writing, calculating, and reading is included to the same total extent that it appears in other curriculum designs, but on a more flexible schedule and related to the emergence of need for use of the skills involved.

In general, curriculum trends in the United States today suggest that the life-centered curriculum will find increasing favor, perhaps through further modification of the broad-fields approach. This will be especially likely as evidence is accumulated to demonstrate that children actually do acquire fundamental competence in the 3 R's through such programs. Research thus far available offers much assurance to this effect: schools with the richest and most flexible offerings are most successful in developing basic skills and academic competencies. Unfortunately, these are also the schools which cost the most money. Hence the periodic criticisms of "frills" in the public schools.

The Prime Importance of Mental Health

The child in the primary grades is essentially a newcomer to an established situation, and the solicitous behavior of his parents, teachers, and others impresses expectancy standards deeply upon his consciousness. Whether or not he can measure up to these standards and gain acceptance becomes a real concern to him. Therefore the teacher provides many opportunities for him to experience success, to learn that he is "all right" and that he is capable of satisfactory performance. This is a time for helping the child to accept himself; and this task is of course easiest for the teacher whose own mental health is so solidly established that she is capable of seeing and appreciating the virtues of each individual child, whatever his limitations may be. It is also a time for striving earnestly to know, and to like, the parents and others whose personalities are inextricably intertwined with the child's own growing personality.

In the intermediate grades many of the child's problems stem from the gap between his actual development, uneven and incomplete, and his developmental aspirations. Feelings of anxiety and rejection may arise from his inability to conform to adult standards and comply with adult demands. Children are chronically pessimistic about their physical and social attractiveness, and those with actual handicaps — physical, social, economic, and intellectual — are likely to find the going somewhat rougher as the discriminatory pattern of choice in friends begins to supplant the earlier and more democratic pattern of the primary grades. For the classroom teacher this implies that many devices must be used for studying and understanding each child and his self-concept. She needs to know how the child spends his time, both in school and out, and how he feels about his family, his friends, and the things that happen to him. She then plans a program which helps children to look objectively at their own problems to sympathize with the problems of others (e.g. through sociodrama), and to concentrate on positive elements. She arranges many different group activities which satisfy the child's need to "belong."

Meeting Noninstructional Needs

The modern elementary school provides a great many services which, although they may relate directly to the child's learnings in school, are largely noninstructional in their nature. These services are mostly of four types: provisions for the child's physical safety, health and medical services, food services, and transportation services.

Provisions for the child's safety include regulations governing in-school, playground, and in-transit behavior. Both health and safety are served by the maintenance of healthful and well-planned physical surroundings. Pedestrian and bicycle safety regulations are carefully explained and enforced, as are regulations governing the use of equipment. The school attempts to minimize safety hazards (slippery corridors, steep stairwells, protruding hardware, and so forth) and to equip its playground with safety-approved equipment. Because of the high frequency of accidents on and around swings, for example, many schools have installed safety-belt seats or eliminated swings in favor of less dangerous apparatus. Teachers are usually assigned to playground and corridor supervision, and pupils engage in playground patrol and similar activities.

The provision of a school nurse is fairly common, sometimes within the school district budget and sometimes as a service provided by city, county, or state agencies. Except in the larger cities, and even then on a very limited scale, few school districts have an adequate arrangement for regular medical and dental inspections and service, and especially for emergency care. Coordination of the school's health services with health services privately provided is usually less successful than it ought to be.

Nearly every school today finds it necessary to make provision for the serving, or at least the supervision, of noon lunches. The rise of the consolidated school district, with large numbers of children transported considerable distances by bus, is a major reason for the growth of school cafeteria service. In congested urban areas with dangerous traffic conditions, lunch-at-school saves the child 2 trips each day. In less-privileged neighborhoods, the school cafeteria is visualized as an assurance of adequate diet for the child. Therefore the school, for these and other reasons, finds itself very much in the restaurant business. Whether or not this trend toward replacing the home, as in the case of feeding children, is altogether desirable is a source of great concern to some educators. They point out the great expense of equipping schools to serve food; the tremendous demands upon the principal and teachers in supervising this additional activity; the attitude of many parents who, though entirely capable of serving a good lunch to their children in the home environment, are all too willing to shift this responsibility to someone else; and the many hidden costs (in staff energy, if nothing else) of lunch programs which may cause the curriculum itself to suffer.

Similar doubts are raised concerning the wisdom of the present trend toward school-managed transportation services. Again, the consolidation of smaller school units and various urban safety hazards explain the legitimate need for arranging transportation; but whether the tremendous expense (in both dollars and personnel) involved is justified in a great many instances might well be debated. Although one would scarcely succeed in counteracting this trend by mention of young Abraham Lincoln and his hardy boyhood, it is at least tempting to suggest that today's child has relatively few opportunities to toughen his leg muscles as he steps in and out of his publicly-financed taxi.

Some Implications for Policy

Implicit or expressed in the preceding descriptions of the four elementary school age periods were a number of problems which are rooted in, and associated with, certain administrative practices and policies in the schools. These can be summarized as follows:

(1) *Admission practices and policies.* Because children vary so greatly in their biological inheritance, in their preschool development, and in their rates of learning, a uniform and inflexible entrance-age and admission policy cannot meet the needs of all children. The trend is toward raising minimum age standards (6 years old before September 1, for admission to first grade) and toward screening procedures which enable individual adjustments to be made.

(2) *Incentives to learning.* Extrinsic motivational devices (marks, gold stars, prizes, etc.) are in strong disrepute. Their overuse has contaminated the purposes of education and impaired many of the intrinsic values of

learning. The competent teacher builds in her students an appreciation of the ways in which learning will improve living. Self-development is a more virtuous goal than winning a prize.

(3) *Promotion practices.* The basic dilemma of today's teacher is that an artificial and archaic system of grade classification conflicts with the basic philosophy and psychology by which she operates in the classroom. The only straightforward solution is the abandonment of grade labels and of the promotion concept which attends them.

(4) *Policies governing pupil behavior.* The predominance of activity and the emphasis upon democratic relations implies a changed attitude toward discipline in today's school. However, this is far from saying that children should be disorderly, irresponsible, or thoughtless of others in the school; on the contrary, the attainment of self-discipline and group-discipline of a high type, consistent with democratic ideals, is a prime objective of modern education. A school ought to be a demonstration of the way people should live and work together.

(5) *The child's classroom environment.* Richness of program is negated if the school building is overcrowded or unsuited to the needs of the curriculum. Individualized instruction is impossible if materials are unavailable and if classes are big. Even 25 children are said to be too large a number for one teacher. Thoughtful guidance and intelligent teaching can hardly be expected if the teacher is a mediocre person.

(6) *Supplementary services.* It is impractical to discuss the care and training of slow-learning, handicapped, maladjusted, and gifted children if specially trained personnel are not available to supplement the regular teacher's efforts. Library services, instruction in the creative arts, health and medical services, and other auxiliary benefits are virtually lost without the special help of professional allies.

SECONDARY EDUCATION AND THE PROCESSES OF ADOLESCENCE
MORRIS L. COGAN

Adolescence and the School

If the secondary school is understood to include the junior high school grades, then the period of secondary education is coterminous with most of the phenomena that characterize adolescence in our culture. What are some of the developmental patterns of adolescence and what are some of the implications of such phenomena for the schools? More specifically, what direction, what guidance can educators find in the chapters of this volume, chapters dealing with the rhythms, the patterns, and the variations of child growth and development? And reciprocally, what guidance and direction can educators offer to the nurses, the doctors, the social workers who, like the teacher, attempt to focus their professional energies on a well-defined segment of the child's life, only to find that such a life is not segmented and that willy-nilly the physio-

logical must be taken into account with the psychological, and that educational factors may be related to sociological, emotional, or somatic
phenomena?

It is, for example, more than merely interesting to the educator to
learn about the extremely wide range in the normal variations of adolescent height, weight, and height-weight ratios. If the educator takes
this information into account it may have an impact on such a prosaic
question as the size of furniture to provide in the secondary school, or
it may have wide ramifications in the planning of the total curriculum,
which should perhaps reflect a concern for the teen-ager's acceptance of
normal variations in his own and his peers' development. The discussion
of physical growth and development during adolescence, as described in
Chapter IV, is highly relevant to many of the problems of the adolescent
in school.

Before discussing some of the phenomena that characterize the adolescent in school, it may not be amiss to propose certain cautions. It
should be noted that although this section may treat of certain general
patterns, these generalizations are of limited applicability. They should
not be applied, for example, to the individual in any prescriptive sense.
For work with an individual child these typicalities may offer a crude
outline; the work itself must be individual, and interpretations must be
situational and personal.

The Transition to the Secondary School

Adolescence is not only a transition biologically and socioculturally,
but it is also an educational transition. The pupil who enters the secondary school commonly comes from a small elementary school characterized
by an almost maternal knowledge of and preoccupation with the pupils;
he enters a larger school that is alien in many respects. He must come
to terms with a more impersonal, more formalized instructional system
organized into departments, a system that has certain virtues but that
certainly makes heavy and varied demands upon the young people it
seeks to educate. These boys and girls, accustomed to a grammar school
related to the immediate school neighborhood, now take their places in
a school that frequently has strong connections with outside agencies
and with the larger community, which often become adjuncts to the
classroom and sometimes true extensions of it. Where the elementary
school makes known to the pupils a set of expectations established by a
few teachers who communicate the sanctions of a small, relatively self-
contained school society, the secondary school has boundaries close to
the college, or to the first job, or to marriage, home, and family. These
institutions steadily press forward in the adolescent's concerns as he

makes his way through the secondary school, giving values to the secondary school experiences vastly different from those of the elementary school. As a result, the transition to the secondary school may be accompanied by psychosomatic illnesses, by an apparently inexplicable falling-off in school performance (as though the child had suddenly become dull), by truancy, physical exhaustion, and/or by asocial or antisocial behavior. Those who work with children need to be alert to some of the underlying phenomena of the transition from the elementary to the secondary school.

Developing Standards of Conduct

What does the child bring to this new school? He has acquired the fundamentals — the basics of communication, the beginnings of quantitative thought, some of the rules and regulations of living in a school society. He is now ready to increase and deepen his knowledge; he is ready to undertake independent thinking, to move into the domain of abstract ideas, to make judgments, to establish ideals and standards. "The 10-year-old has acquired a handy set of regulations . . . of playground fairness and justice. . . . The child of 14 may be beginning to feel the need for a moral ideal which will be in conformity with his own nature and not simply a practical way of keeping out of trouble." [12]

This is one of the strong, constant themes of youth in the secondary schools. To speak of a striving for a satisfying morality as characteristic of the boys and girls who are in secondary schools, in a period when the phrase "juvenile delinquency" has almost the status of a single word, would seem to be flying in the face of common sense. Yet on second thought it can be seen that although many delinquents have rejected parts of the morality of their adult society, they have at the same time forged a code of conduct, personal and social, to which they do give deep allegiance. The young delinquent is not often amoral; he commonly has strong convictions as to what is right and wrong. It is the failure of society that the delinquent has rejected society's standards and has adopted some other set of values instead.

It seems safe to say that the pupils of the secondary school are increasingly aware of moral and ethical ambivalences. The question of the basis of right conduct is complicated in the United States because the validation of important areas of morality is often left to the individual, who is expected to carry on some sort of personal examination, an internal dialectic, perennially constructing and reconstructing the moral basis of his life. The particular problems accompanying this process of personal validation would tend to appear with diminished frequency and intensity in societies in which a standardized morality is accepted by un-critical youth.

The secondary school pupils in America, then, may be expected to seek moral truths and, in the quest, to find, to accept, to reject, and to question "truth," and to start the quest anew. This is one of the prime factors to be considered by those with responsibility for adolescents. If the child is rewarded for exhibiting a sense of individual moral judg-ment and at the same moment punished for having explored different modes of moral conduct and for tentative nonconformities, he is put into a baffling dilemma. It would seem clear, therefore, that both school and society should take such dilemmas into account in guiding and judging the adolescent.

The behavioral components of the quest for morality are worth noting, if only for the fact that they illustrate so well a large class of actions that would otherwise tend to appear incoherent, anarchic, or contra-dictory. Among these behaviors may be listed the exploration of various modes of conduct; fervent but quickly changing personal allegiances; and verbal (and thus vicarious) manipulation of such morally sensitive areas as marriage, courtship, peer group standards, and the like.

Toward an Identity

Since the secondary school student is engaged in multiple transitions — from sexual immaturity to full reproductive powers, from the family and immediate neighborhood to the larger community and to the world, from dependence to autonomy — it is no wonder that much of the energy of the adolescent is turned to an effort to establish an identity, a more or less stable picture of himself, a picture in which the parts are integrated and comprehensible.

The optimal fulfillment of the ego and integrative needs of adolescents requires that they have rich experiences with reality, so that relationships may be comprehended and dependable generalizations established. Such organization of the "mental outcomes of experience," says Prescott, may aid in the achievement of a unified personality tied together by a "set of fundamental life values." [13]

The role of the school in meeting this need for the establishment of the unified personality is a difficult but crucial one. It is difficult because the provision of real experiences is often impossible in an institution that achieves economy of instruction by segregating its pupils from "reality" and instructing them through language, itself a major symbolism. Yet, within this context, the young person must find a portion of the answer to some of the questions that plague him: "Who am I? Am I a person who is of some account in the world? Am I child or adult? Have I or can I develop the ability to earn a living, make a successful marriage, hold friends?"

Some of the behaviors of young people who are trying to answer questions of such moment to the integration of their personality are apparent in school. They often seek the security of allegiance to a stereotype, to a gang, a club, a cult, a friend, or a hero. They seek and value highly the security of having one or several "best" friends. They may also build up for themselves certain ideas not only about the kind of person they are, but also about an ego-ideal, the kind of person they would like to be. Havighurst and his colleagues have noted several common models for the ideal self: "The age for choosing a glamorous person is about eight to sixteen. The choice of an attractive, visible young adult may start at eight or ten and continue all through adolescence, or it may give way to a more abstract ego-ideal in the form of a composite imaginary person. The final and mature stage of the ego-ideal is the composite of desirable characteristics, drawn from all of the persons with whom the individual has identified himself during his childhood and adolescence." [14] It is interesting to observe in passing that the individual's socioeconomic environment may influence his choice of ego-ideal, it having been noted by Havighurst, Robinson, and Dorr that youth in the lower socioeconomic brackets tend to identify more often with glamorous persons than do youth in the higher income brackets.

Since the adolescent is in the process of formulating a morality, an identity, and an ego-ideal, it is important for those who have to deal with him to recognize that his behavior — his reaction to fact, his opinions — may be bizarre, exaggerated, and vacillating. Thus one may witness the spectacle of a young man of 16 simultaneously asserting (a) that marriage is an outmoded institution, (b) that he must be permitted to "go steady" with the girl he loves madly, and (c) that the story of Romeo and Juliet is manifestly absurd because both of the lovers are far too young to be truly in love. It would seem important, then, to understand that some of the very behaviors that appear to the adult to be dictated by whim, by vagary and unreason, appear to the adolescent himself to be dictated by logic or by some personal, transcendent revelation of absolute truth. The adolescent perhaps usually underestimates the complexity of life, and often falls prey to facile, oversimplified explanations of his own conduct and that of others. He is in fact trying on many different roles for size, with strong commitments to a given role at a given moment. His puzzling characteristics have their rationale.

Social and Sex Roles

The physiological changes that mark the attainment of puberty and the beginning of sexual maturity have their counterpart in certain behavioral changes that accompany the adolescent's attempts to come to terms with his developing sex and social roles. The problem of dependable sex knowledge geared to the adolescent pupil's level of maturity is often handled by default in the secondary school. One of the reasons for this is that the entire topic of sex in the United States is emotionally explosive, and the schools are unclear as to whether the responsibility for sex knowledge rightly belongs with the parents, the doctors, or the teachers.

Whether the schools accept or reject the responsibility for sex instruction, it is quite clear that the school is inescapably a portion of the arena in which sex roles are developed. The children need intellectually and emotionally convincing experiences from which they may secure dependable facts and through which they may arrive at relatively relaxed attitudes concerning their own bodily functions and growth patterns. One of the developmental tasks facing this age group is the need to achieve new and more mature relations with peers of both sexes. Not only is it important for the secondary school pupils to come to see girls as women and boys as men, but they need also to acquire certain complicated social skills, including the ability to work with others, to lead without dominating, to perform the "socially approved adult masculine or feminine social role." [15]

Many educators, in trying to help the adolescent attain more mature sex and social roles, have turned to the schoolman's perennial panacea: a course — in hygiene, or biology, or "social and family living." There would seem to be some reason for suggesting that for such purposes educators might well use literary, artistic, and esthetic experiences more, and courses in biology less, or that the esthetic resources of the curriculum be better utilized, if only in parallel with the courses in biology. Pupils need to see sex and social relations more as integral to the rest of human development and aspiration, and perhaps less as processes divorced from human exemplars. In the hands of competent teachers, literature and art would seem peculiarly well-suited to help the adolescent assume the roles required of him.

The Peer Group

A very evident part of the process of adolescent development is a shift in the kind of group to which young people give their allegiance.

The most obvious transition occurs as boys and girls move from the child's world to the world of the adult. It is to be noted, however, that in crossing this bridge, the adolescent proceeds in company with his peers, not with his parents or with other adults. With the best will in the world adults cannot make this journey a second time, and their sons and daughters must make it in company with the sons and daughters of other adults. If this is so, then it might appear reasonable to anticipate that the secondary-school youth will in many respects take his standards and attitudes from his peer group rather than from his parents or teacher, and in fact during the adolescent years the "most potent single influence . . . is the power of group approval. The youth becomes a slave to the conventions of his age-group. . . . Yet this conformity seems limited to the externals of life. In their inner life adolescent boys and girls are still individuals, and sometimes individualistic to an extreme." [16] Conformity with peer group standards and the parallel maintenance of inner individuality are likely to increase the puzzlement of teachers in dealing with their pupils.

J. E. Horrocks points out that it is crucial for the adolescent to be accepted by his age-group, and that such acceptance is easier for the conforming adolescent because deviations from important standards of behavior, dress, or values are sharply rejected by the group.[17] Knowledge of the potency of peer-group standards can, however, be harnessed by the teacher for the development of a classroom morale that serves in general to support the class work. If this is achieved it will be the hardy individual who will run counter to the direction of the teacher's endeavors. The inner individuality and the often poignant inner life of the adolescent also offer instructional opportunities to a sensitive and perceptive teacher.

Character Development and School Experiences

All through the history of American secondary schools there has been a persistent thread of concern for character development, for civic competence, for moral and ethical excellence. The emphasis on character *qua* character was rather faint, however, in the period from the 1920's to the '40's. The contemporary scene, on the other hand, is marked by the heated exhortations of various groups seeking to turn the efforts of the schools more directly to the teaching of moral, ethical, and religious values. Educators seem to find it increasingly difficult to do more than offer lip service, however, to the idea of a direct didactic approach to character development. Among the reasons for this is the self-consciousness of some educators in the face of the task, since they are fully aware that direct teaching in the field of character development has not been very successful. Other limiting factors are (1) the delicacy of the task involved in teaching morality without directly teaching a religion, and (2) a perhaps unconscious reluctance to undertake a job the major framework of which is clearly set by family, social, and cultural forces of such magnitude as to make the efforts of the school appear puny at best. Nevertheless it seems likely that school experiences will have some impact upon character development during adolescence. Where the school succeeds in reinforcing the general direction of character development started in the family and in the community, then it seems likely that classroom experiences will serve to support and intensify the trend. If, in addition, certain children from the lower socioeconomic strata enter a school dominated by middle-class values and aspirations, some of these children may internalize the new values. It should be added, however, that there is not much reason to anticipate that the present secondary school will have a major impact upon the character development of its pupils, unless it can create real situations in which the children must exercise choice, assume ethical responsibilities, and make important decisions in terms of right and wrong.

Whatever may be the true extent of the influence of the school upon the character development of its students, it seems clear that these students need help. Their ideas about honor, crime, loyalty, and the like have largely been bound up with specific situations, with concrete instances that are relatively unambiguous, that can be dealt with directly in terms of a straightforward code of conduct. In the life of the secondary school, however, these situations become more and more complex and ambivalent. For example, the 10 year old child who can solve most of his ethical dilemmas through recourse to a fairly direct "playing field" set of rules now finds that he is encountering behaviors that cannot easily be categorized as right, wrong, good, or bad. The complexity of this ever expanding area of ambiguity and the struggle of the adolescent to build an integrated character for himself within this new, adult context of nuances instead of black and white categories, of interpretation of behavior rather than interpretation of rules, is well illustrated in Huckleberry Finn's moral development as he wrestles with the problems of slavery and with his part in Jim's escape.

The character traits most admired by boys and girls change gradually over the years. At age 11 to 12 boys generally prize skill and leadership in games, and fearlessness and readiness to take a chance. At 14 and 15 the qualities valued earlier are being challenged by a growing admiration for social poise and grooming.[18]

A research study of some of the character traits of a sample of 16 year olds indicates that at that age the concepts of honesty and truth-telling are "uniformly and rigorously accepted." It is interesting that although adolescents seem to possess strong moral courage in the defense and protection of their own rights and the rights of others, this courage is diluted by doubt and fear when the adolescent's status with his peers is at stake in a moral decision. This evidence again attests the importance of peer-group standards in adolescence. The boys and girls in one research sample had not succeeded in clarifying their loyalties: "The least developed aspect is loyalty to ideas, principles, and values." On the other hand the sense of responsibility seems to be highly developed, these youths apparently taking very seriously their duties to home, to school, and to job. The author concludes that these 16 year olds show strong agreement with "obvious middle-class codes of conduct in stereotyped language requiring little thought or analysis . . . but exceptions and inconsistencies appear when these values are represented in specific situations." [19]

Adolescent boys and girls in school need experiences that will help them move from childish, oversimplified, stereotyped life values to a more mature outlook from which human beings and human values are seen as complex, and often in conflict. The teacher who wants to help his students in this area needs to give some thought to the kind of problems he sets for them. The high school students who are set to the task of mastering the dates of the battles of the Civil War or the events of the plot of *Othello* will not have the opportunity to come to grips with the complicated questions involved in the economic, political, ideological "rights" and "wrongs" of the Civil War or with the violent internal struggles of the passionate Moor faced with apparent proof of his wife's infidelity.

Prescott[13] (pp. 102–104) has sketched in some of the dimensions of the role of the school in the attainment of emotional maturity. He suggests that the school should undertake to reeducate pupils showing deviant emotional behavior and provide emotional and esthetic experiences designed to encourage culturally satisfactory individual modes of affective behavior. He points out the utility of training in esthetic expression as a way of helping individuals to maintain morale, relieve their tensions, identify with a cultural group, and become generally more sensitive to beauty. Where the schools have attempted to meet the need of adolescents for spiritual, emotional, and esthetic experiences their efforts have sometimes been hampered by a lack of teachers competent to select and organize a suitable curriculum. The impoverishment of school offerings in esthetic learnings is often attributable to the community's acceptance of severely utilitarian aims of education, to the exclusion of emotional and esthetic outcomes. The whole question is further complicated by an unresolved conflict as to whether or not the real function of education is to train children in only the intellectual and rational processes, which are assumed by many to be antithetical to the emotional processes. That the best answer probably lies in an integrated position in which the claims of the intellect and of the emotions have been reconciled does not seem to help the situation in the schools, and most of them continue to do something less than justice to this problem. The education of the emotions has too often been relegated to the extracurricular activities; it should be central to the literature, the science, the mathematics, and the social studies of the curriculum.

Mental Development in Adolescence

By the last 2 years of high school the pupils have reached or approached closely their peak of mental progress, although the acquisition of knowledge and the mastery and use of interrelations continue much longer. There is some difference of opinion as to the proportions of full mental development that are achieved at various ages. Jones and Conrad find some evidence that "50 per cent of adult [mental] status is reached shortly after 11 years; the remaining half of mental growth [development] occurs during adolescence and the early part of post-adolescence." They note, however, that other writers conclude that only a very small proportion of mental growth occurs after $10\frac{1}{2}$ years.[20]

Nevertheless it seems fair to say that young people continue to make substantial gains in test intelligence through high school and college. The ability to retain learned materials increases steadily through the high school years, as do motor learning, the ability to concentrate, and the ability to deal with abstractions and symbolic processes.

The early stages in the development of problem-solving ability are characterized by a "lack of circumspection, conventional beginnings, slight and inconsequential variations from one attempt to another, frequent relapses into a former routine, and tardiness in profiting from errors," and develop to "greater prevision, more adequate analysis of the design, less conventionality and automatism in procedure, more radical reconstruction of plan in successive trials, all of which led to greater promptness in profiting by mistakes."[21] It seems safe to say, in view of even a very brief review of the characteristics of mental development, that the secondary school pupil is rapidly approaching a peak of mental ability and that the school would do well to "stretch" him, to set him to tasks for which he is well motivated and which will call for all his powers.

Language Development

It seems impossible to arrive at any accurate estimates of average vocabulary for the various age levels. There appears to be a steady increase in the proportion of abstract nouns, and in the use of longer sentences with more and more subordinate clauses, as the child matures.[22] The average length of response "is a highly sensitive index that reveals developmental trends from infancy to maturity, and also reflects sex, occupational, and intellectual-group differences with remarkable consistency."[23] In addition, the older and more intelligent the child is, the more highly differentiated the language structure is in general, i.e., the higher the ratio of types of words to total words used.

The adolescent need for language is one of the remarkable phenomena of this period. Often accused of being addicted to the nod, the grunt, or the monosyllable as the answer to a classroom question, this same taciturn youth appears to be able to maintain interminable conversations and discussions with his peers. The secondary school youth not only uses language, but he is so impelled to communication and to linguistic processes that he *makes* language — club passwords, shibboleths, "pig Latin," and all sorts of neologisms to express the ideas that fill his mind.

The need for new vocabulary is related to the adolescent's extended experiences, his entrance into larger societies, his manipulation of more complex interrelations of ideas, and his essays in the interpretation and communication of new experiences. But to anyone who has observed the language development of secondary school youth it becomes clear that they need more than just vocabulary. They need and the school must supply the vicarious and the actual experiences that will give meaning and substance to the new vocabulary, a vocabulary which for adolescents is less learned than created. They need to explore minds, their own and others', they need new words for new worlds, for new ideas and new combinations of familiar ideas. And finally they need metaphor — metaphor in the radical sense of the figure, the symbolization by which they may indicate the properties and the similarities of ideas that are too complicated, too fragile, or too pristine to be understood or communicated by the word alone.

Reading

The change from the elementary school to the secondary school is also a change from simple, stereotyped reading materials, from relatively naive recitals of uncomplicated incidents and predictable people, to elevated speech, unfamiliar rhythms, and complex patterns of human relations. The stories and novels of the junior high school years often seem static after the eventful reading materials of the earlier school years. It is perhaps at this transition point that the skill of the teacher will figure with some importance in the development of adult reading habits.

There are some circumstances that may serve to help the secondary school develop satisfactory reading habits, skills, and appreciations among adolescent pupils. The interests of the pupils can be taken into account in the planning of the secondary school reading program. The teen-ager is entering an adult world and he wants to read about adults. This fact is often neglected by teachers who, seeking to use the motivation of established reading habits in achieving a gradual transition to adult reading, confuse the pupils' developed interests with their developing interests. As a result it is not uncommon in the seventh, eighth, and ninth grades to see pupils reading pretty much what they had been reading for the past year or two, except that they are possibly reading more of it in a given time. Perhaps this is an overcorrection made by teachers who are familiar with the damage that can be done by throwing 13 and 14 year olds too precipitously into an intensive reading of certain adult classics.

In a brief review of certain aspects of the reading interests of secondary school pupils, Horrocks[24] has shown that adventure stories rate high for both sexes in all grades, and that comic books and regular magazines continue to hold first place as the best-liked media. Some studies point to an increase in nonfiction reading in the upper grades and to a gain in the appeal of literature dealing with abstract qualities over more purely narrative literature. It seems probable that the tenth grade marks a rather decided change point in reading interests.

Many adolescents are avid readers of the newspaper, and although the comics are most frequently read, the front page and the sports section are high among the favorites. With increases in age there tend to appear increases in the frequency of reading of the editorial page, and the entire paper is read more thoroughly.

Contrary to popular supposition, "high school boys enjoy poetry when it appeals to their chivalry, love of adventure, humor, and idealism." Older children respond best "to interesting action, characters, and problems." Boys seem to prefer heroism and adventure, while home and school situations appeal to girls. Both sexes enjoy stories dealing with humorous situations and with qualities of "kindness, faithfulness, and loyalty." Interest in fiction rises rapidly from age 9 to 18.[25]

In view of the language developments of adolescence, the secondary school should be concerned with increasing the students' skills in recognition and use of new words, and in comprehension, interpretation, appreciation, and evaluation of what is read. As suggestions for accomplishing this more effectively, Orr and her colleagues[26] offer 8 ways of making provision for reading differences:

(1) grouping pupils by needs and by interests, with flexibility in changing from group to group;

(2) reading assignments differentiated by levels and by types;

(3) opportunity for practice of reading skills and techniques at all ability levels;

(4) free reading for the rapid readers;

(5) wide variety of materials for voluntary reading;

(6) provision for "self-directed activities by the group and by individuals";

(7) remedial work for those who need it; and

(8) challenging experiences for those of superior reading ability.

With provisions such as these, plus an adequate program of testing for diagnostic and evaluative purposes, there is reason to expect that pupils will grow in their appreciation of language for the communication of concept, mood, emotion, setting, or information.

Quantitative Thinking

Mursell[22] (p. 192–193) notes that the development of "relational thinking" is characterized by continuity. Some of the phases he notes are:

(1) early, prenumerical behavior, as for example aggregation in early childhood;

(2) numbers as the names of successive events;

(3) counting;

(4) grouping;

(5) standard arithmetical operations; and

(6) the transition from arithmetic to algebra.

The teaching of mathematics is, in general, quite unsatisfactory at the secondary levels. Various hypotheses have been offered to account for this. Prescott, for example, states that numbers are commonly taught before the pupils have had adequate quantitative experiences. This insufficiency of concrete experiences with numbers continues in the elementary grades and is compounded in the secondary school, with the result that many pupils come to dislike quantitative processes and tend to eliminate mathematics from their curriculum.[13] (p. 219) In research performed in 1954, some evidence was found to indicate that, on the average, eighth grade pupils tended to perform less of the required assignments and to engage in less self-initiated activity growing out of classroom experiences in mathematics than in either English or science.[27] Two of the factors operating to depress the level of productive work in secondary school mathematics may be that: (1) teachers of mathematics seem in general to be unwilling to devise creative pupil activities, e.g., original investigations involving quantitative phenomena, book reports on mathematical prodigies, the construction of mathematical models, the writing of original, realistic problems, etc.; and (2) teachers of mathematics seem in general to be unable to communicate either an esthetic appreciation of the symmetries and regularities of their subject or to convince their pupils that secondary mathematics is useful, in fact necessary for effective living.

The Secondary School Curriculum

Perhaps the major trend of curriculum development in the American secondary school has been toward a reorganization of learning experiences around the needs of youth. As a matter of fact, special educational needs of the adolescent have occupied so paramount a position in the concerns of educators that a special school, which came to be called the junior high, was devised about 40 years ago to facilitate the adjustments dictated by the special nature of adolescence. In a review of the status of the junior high school, Koos has noted that "a major and special responsibility [at the junior high school level] is the recognition of the nature of the child at adolescence . . . [but] adequate recognition is impossible without large-scale modifications of the programs and regimens common to the later years of the 8-year elementary school and the first years of the 4-year high school." [28]

This constant solicitude for the needs of adolescents is also to be found in the senior high school, although the reorganization of these last 3 or 4 years of secondary schooling has been far less radical than that of the junior high.

The secondary school remains an institution in which the major educative experiences are bookish and verbal, not "real" in the sense that an actual apprenticeship, for example, is "real." This is to say that the secondary school is most rewarding to the young people who are at home with words and books. This, it must be obvious, works a hardship upon those pupils who, in order to learn, need direct observation, participation, and activity, or who lack verbal aptitudes yet possess an esthetic or scientific bent, or enjoy special talents for dealing with quantitative or spatial relationships. When, for these reasons or others, the student finds himself consistently inadequate in his school work, it is not unusual for him to internalize this reiterated lesson of failure and to generalize from it. He then often becomes convinced that he is inadequate in life, that he has failed as a total personality. This picture differs drastically from the stereotype of the brash, overconfident high school graduate who has learned nothing in school and has never learned that he has not learned. Perhaps both pictures are overdrawn, yet the writer has often noted in the course of interviews with secondary school pupils that many who are not notably successful "academically" — especially those who are not enrolled in the college preparatory curriculum — feel themselves definitely inferior to their more scholastically successful peers. One girl in the commercial course, of outstanding ability and promise, remarked of her teachers, "Some of them are not so good. The college preps get the best." Then she hastened to add, "but of course they should."

The curriculum is notably out of step with certain adolescent developments. As the pupils mature they grow in ability to share in the planning of their school work. Yet from the lower to the upper grades there is probably an inverse relation between the pupils' ability to plan their school experiences and the extent of their participation in such planning. In addition, increments in the pupils' ability to think critically and to assume an active role in problem-solving are perhaps not often enough taken into account in classroom curriculum and method of teaching. The secondary school period should mark a sharp increase in the development of the pupils' experience in making judgments and decisions, and in establishing the criteria for the evaluation of their own work and progress. This process will tend to be held back if too much class time is devoted to rote and automatic learning.

In the final analysis, the curriculum is created anew in each separate classroom. The key element is not the syllabus, nor the course of study, nor a method of teaching, it is the teacher. Some thoughtful educators are becoming daily more impressed with the necessity for improving education not so much by tinkering with curriculum as by raising the general level of competence of teachers in service and of students preparing to teach.

Vocation, the Curriculum, and the Student

The changed conditions of living and working in a technologically developed nation will continue to influence the curriculum of the secondary schools, especially in the area of preparation for a vocation. Newton Edwards has pointed out that for many people it is becoming difficult to find "gainful employment of a kind that gives tone and zest to life." He goes on to add, "If the machine splinters personality, . . . leisure, properly conceived and utilized, can be relied upon to restore the organic wholeness of experience."[29] David Riesman has dealt with the same problem in *The Lonely Crowd*. If technological success continues to mean increased leisure and increased need for leisure activities to offset the disintegrating effects of meaningless, semiautomatic jobs, then the schools may find themselves in the curious position of preparing adolescents for vocation by preparing them for leisure. It should be borne in mind that the schools for the past 30 or 40 years accepted the worthy use of leisure as one of the objectives of education, but this endeavor will assume major proportions if Edwards and Riesman are correct in their analysis.

The secondary schools find it increasingly desirable to offer general vocational education rather than direct training for specific jobs. Such a policy seems justifiable in view of the increases in on-the-job training and in view of the difficulty in predicting either the kinds of jobs that will be available or the kinds of jobs for which the individual will be suited. Nevertheless, the adolescents who look to the school to prepare them for a vocation may begin to feel more and more insecure as they approach graduation, lacking the security of direct preparation for a specific job. Those who have to deal with youth need to know about these anxiety-producing circumstances and need to be prepared to interpret them.

Certain behaviors of adolescents become more comprehensible if one is aware of some of the phenomena accompanying the adolescent's choice of a vocation. The mere announcement of such a choice may contribute to the adolescent's inner security and to his status among his peers.[30] The selection of a vocation represents one of the major steps toward economic independence and away from dependence upon the parents.[24] [p. 727] The school clearly needs to use its curriculum, and its guidance personnel, to help pupils toward a more realistic appraisal of their own promise and of the availability and employment conditions of certain highly regarded jobs.

For those who seek to know and to help youth of secondary school age, it is perhaps important to conclude this brief treatment of vocational choice with a note of caution. Mention has already been made of the fact that certain selective factors operate to reward the verbally gifted pupils in many secondary schools and to punish pupils who are not academically gifted or who possess talents either not identified or not valued by the school. When this occurs it may also occur that such pupils establish too low a level of occupational aspiration for themselves. This may mean, for example, that a boy who plans to become a garage mechanic may be fully capable of successfully completing 2 or 4 years of special education and becoming a draftsman, a technical assistant, or even an engineer. An analogous situation obtains for large numbers of students who could successfully complete 4 years of liberal arts college work. The implications of such waste of human resources are becoming increasingly clear — to psychologists as well as to various manpower commissions.

"Normal Variation"

There is a pressing need for adolescents to learn the true meaning of the words "normal" and "average" as applied to the phenomena of human behavior and development. It is a cliché of sociology to state that adolescents tend to be conformist to an extreme. They distrust deviation; they often overvalue a local or cultural norm, an ideal of dress, appearance, physique, or even a group-determined standard of school achievement. Thus, two interrelated themes make a strong bid for inclusion in the curriculum: (1) the significance of words like "normal" and "average" when applied to the phenomena of human behavior and development; and (2) the meaning of conformity, individuality, "other-directed," and "autonomous," as developed by Riesman in *The Lonely Crowd*.

Some of the dimensions of the first topic have been indicated in Chapter IV, where the concept of "unusual but normal" in the physical development of children was discussed. This idea seems absurd to many young people, who confuse "unusual" with "abnormal." The adolescent needs to be cognizant and accepting of his own and others' growth patterns and variations in these patterns. The situation is, of course, analogous for the problems of conformity to stereotyped patterns of thought and to trends in ideas. The adolescent needs experiences that will permit him to develop his own set of values, his own individuality.

Some few teachers make a fairly successful effort to encourage their pupils to think and to read about norms, standards, conformity, over-conformity, autonomy, and the like. Most such efforts, however, appear to be doomed to failure because the curricular materials of, for example, the English teacher or the social studies teacher, who may be concerned with this problem, often fail to carry conviction. This is so because the textual materials chosen for this task are often poor, are often themselves the carriers of unexamined stereotypes. The "traditional" texts, the "classics," have often been discarded; the substitutes are frequently beautifully printed and lavishly illustrated examples of hack work that fail to carry the emotional, intellectual, and esthetic conviction of the works that have been displaced. When this occurs, those who are concerned with the education of young people can expect to find that these youths will not only blindly accept group, clique, or gang values, but that this pattern of behavior will continue into adulthood, and that as adults these persons will continue to look outside rather than within themselves for guides to their behavior.

Learning Outcomes and Interpersonal Relations

One of the most sensitive areas of adolescent experience in school is the interpersonal relations established between the pupil and the teacher. Jersild notes that pupils may encounter in school "a vast amount of treatment which, in effect, might well be construed as a kind of rejection." Pupils are often reminded that "they are not much good. The school dispenses failure on a colossal scale. . . ." [31] The force of this finding is not lessened by the fact that there is evidence to indicate that it is our entire culture that dispenses failure to the young.

In any event, educators are turning their efforts to what is truly a massive attempt to create a climate of learning characterized by only moderate anxiety, by warm, friendly, supportive behavior on the part of teachers and pupils. Where the activities of the classroom are marked by warmth and pupil participation, the general trend of research evidence seems to indicate definite gains in the learning of social skills, research skills, and ability to organize materials and to assume initiative. The outcomes in terms of specific subject-matter knowledge are at least as good as those found in the more teacher-dominated classrooms. Ironically enough, the attempt to improve the teacher-pupil relations may create problems of behavior among boys and girls who move from a highly permissive elementary school to a more formalized secondary school.

In summary, the secondary schools of America provide an important segment of the experiences of youth. The philosophy and the major objectives of the public secondary schools are drawn from and contribute to the fabric of the nation. In attempting to carry out their functions these schools establish certain institutional conditions and certain interpersonal relations that form a part of the cultural matrix in which young people grow to individual, social, and cultural maturity. Those who are concerned with the individual, social, and cultural well-being of youth must study the schools and take their effects upon youth into account; anything less will inevitably lessen the worth of the efforts they devote to the welfare of young people.

PROBLEMS IN ADJUSTMENT TO SCHOOL
DONALD C. KLEIN

A number of investigators have presented data reflecting a startlingly high incidence of major and minor adjustment problems among children in kindergarten and the elementary grades. Most studies have relied upon teachers' ratings in lieu of any satisfactory objective evaluation. One such study, an extensive investigation by Wickman in 1928, does not differ markedly in its findings from more recent ones. Wickman found minor difficulties in almost half the boys and a third of the girls. Serious disturbances were described in 10 per cent of boys and 3 per cent of girls.

Other data tend to substantiate findings based on teacher appraisals. Observations in a number of classrooms from kindergarten through sixth grade show that between 10 and 30 per cent of children manifest emotional tension, difficulties in interpersonal relations, withdrawal symptoms, and other indications of unsatisfactory emotional adjustment. Clearly, the topic of school adjustment is an important one.

Faced with multiple and often conflicting demands and value-orientations, interested increasingly in education of "the whole child," and confronted by increasing numbers of these "whole children" in large classroom units, our schools are searching for workable philosophies and policies. Given strong community support and sanction, schools can become a fruitful area for action-research, and educators will no longer be forced into the position of overgeneralizing from single research studies or from personality theories as they are announced in their most preliminary formulations.

A recent publication by the American Orthopsychiatric Association is especially encouraging in this respect.[32] It brings together twenty-six projects in which specialists in mental health have been testing approaches to school adjustment problems, often with the active collaboration of educators as members of the research or service team.

Factors Affecting Teacher-Pupil Relationships

Dilemmas of the teacher. For the individual teacher faced with a crowded classroom, a varied subject-matter to be mastered in a few short months, the special needs of certain individual children, and often the conflicting expectations of parents and others, the problems of education generally and of school adjustment specifically are neither hypothetical nor philosophical. Despite the urgency of immediate practical solutions, however, the theoretical problems cannot be entirely set aside until research has been completed. The teacher repeatedly asks whether she can devote time to the problems of individual children, often wonders whether some of her charges are given adequate attention, and occasionally must suffer gnawing doubts about her ability to meet the demands of the average school day. These questions become ever more acute as educators become increasingly aware of the complexities of personality, of classroom dynamics, and of the significance of school experiences in the development of healthy individuals.

It is customary in discussions of pupil guidance to devote much attention to the needs of children and to the ways in which the teacher can meet these needs. Indeed schools today are, in the main, imbued with this kind of concern for the well-being of the child. One is impressed with the general atmosphere of happiness and relaxation among children in most schools. It is the teachers now who oftentimes seem soberly serious and even a little harassed as they go about the deadly earnest task of making the school experience rewarding and enjoyable for their charges. There is probably a parallel here to the anxious concern which many of today's parents bring to the job of child-rearing.

The prescription for good child guidance in school or home is easy to express, easy to comprehend, and devilishly hard for fallible human beings, professional or otherwise, to attempt to carry out without at least some feelings of inadequacy.

Any child needs an adult — parent or teacher — who has affection for him, who tries to understand his needs, who will be responsive to the most important of these needs, who will be as consistent as possible in relation to him, who will limit his behavior, keep harm from him and him from harming others, and who will establish clear-cut and appropriate limits to the behavior of the child at various stages in his development. In short, someone who will respect the child. Why does such a relationship not develop between some children and some teachers?

Sources of tension. It is well known that children often bring to school certain ways of looking at and responding to both authority-persons and peers, ways which have been overlearned at home in response to parents and siblings, and which are inappropriate to the new setting. While it may help a teacher to realize that the child feels hate not really for teacher but for mother, it is only within herself that she can find ways of meeting the onslaught and helping the child.

On the teacher's part, she may feel that a child's behavior is directed against her personally. No doubt, too, most teachers are apt to be less at ease with certain children, and feel less warmth. However objective the teacher may try to be, personal needs and inner emotional states will at times enter the picture. Some teachers feel uneasy about such personal involvement, which they believe is inconsistent with their professional role. Resulting tensions may further distort teacher-child relationship.

From the teacher's viewpoint various satisfactions are involved in the education of the young child. When the pupil fails to respond and develop, for whatever reason, inevitable strain occurs in the teacher-pupil relationship. It is certain also that such factors as job insecurity and marginal status in the culture are additional factors influencing the emotional relationship between teachers and pupils.

Other factors may be found in tensions within the school building, within the school system, and between the schools and the community generally. Neither teacher nor child can be immune to such tensions. Stanton and Schwartz have in recent years carried out a study of similar tensions within a mental hospital community, and have found clear relations between such tensions and marked exacerbations of patients' illnesses.

No doubt certain endangered children are more apt than others to develop emotional disturbance in emotionally charged situations. Tenuousness of inner controls, personal rigidity, or a position on the fringe of a group, are only some of the factors which cause more obvious upset in one child than in another. Very often such children appear to be the cause of classroom difficulties, and they are occasionally used as convenient scapegoats by their peers. It is important to realize, however, that individual disruption may be merely symptomatic of more basic tensions in the group as a whole, to which all the children are responding in their own ways and with their own resources.

School-home relationships. In their work with disturbed children school guidance personnel are at times blocked by their inability to secure parental cooperation. It is not an exaggeration to say that the most important aspect of any over-all program of school guidance is the development of effective school-home collaboration.

Such collaboration is often not possible when efforts are begun only at the point where a child has become a problem in the eyes of the school. At such times parents are apt to feel criticized, and then out of their own guilt to react with attack against the teacher, the school system, or education in general. Increasing numbers of schools are finding ways of making routine home contacts with all parents before entry of the child into school.

In general, it is not possible fully to understand an instance of school-home conflict apart from the entire context of school-community relations. Probably some degree of tension is inevitable because there is so much investment of interest and personal involvement in the children on the part of people responsible for them. These people have different perspectives, which are the result of their quite distinct social roles vis-à-vis the children. Often the tensions produced lead to unfortunate difficulties in communication. They generate specific pressures and issues which sometimes are settled unilaterally by administrative decisions on the part of the schools. With these actions the tensions seem to disappear, but they are only suppressed. Inevitably they reappear, often in aggravated form, blocking effective cooperation with respect to the child's problem or bringing with them new issues.

Broadly, it is more effective to seek to understand the reasons behind any specific parental pressure or criticism. The answer does not usually lie entirely in the parents' personalities or the tensions of the family. With increased understanding may also come suggestions for ways to reduce school-home tensions, improve communications, and bring more parents into effective collaboration with the school program.

In view of the complexity of the field, it behooves all those engaged in work with children and their families to bring together their knowledge and their resources for joint attack upon the problems of individual pupils and groups of children. The team approach is no more than a catchword, however, until the members have worked out a relationship in which their interdependence is clearly understood and valued. At such a point they will be able to diagnose more adequately the needs of children against the background of the complicated field of forces presented by the family, the school system, the other agencies of the community and the community itself with its diversity of attitudes and values. Fortunately, educators, health personnel and others working in communities are becoming aware of recently developed methods for understanding and dealing with factors which block group development. As the result of the work of Kurt Lewin and his students, group dynamics and human relations institutes and laboratories have been springing up in almost all regions of the country under the auspices of the National Training Laboratories, a part of the National Education Association, and universities. The first such program for public school administrators was inaugurated at Bethel, Maine, in the Summer of 1958.

In view of the importance as well as the complexity of the foregoing considerations no attempt will be made here to deal directly with matters of specific pupil-adjustment patterns, teacher-pupil relations, the ideal teacher, etc. The focus, instead, will be upon segments of school activities pertaining to general problems of adjustment, on ways of viewing various programs in terms of their objectives, and on the need for much more research in this area utilizing the combined orientations of psychiatry, psychology, education, the social sciences, and public health.

As various problem areas have been recognized, special programs have sprung up. These programs often involve either the use of separate classes, or the employment of specialists from education or other fields, or both. Thus many school systems now undertake remedial work in reading and other skill areas, have guidance programs for emotionally disturbed children, provide special instruction for the retarded or intellectually gifted pupils, and maintain programs in physical health.

From their variety, it appears that the special programs developed by schools throughout the country have arisen unsystematically and in response to diverse local concerns and pressures. Nevertheless, on closer study the various efforts devoted to better school adjustment seem to stem from three major orientations — *remedial, preventive,* and *group* or *classroom maintenance.* As will be seen, education as a whole is properly concerned with all three, and finds it hard sometimes to reconcile one with another, particularly on a classroom level.

What is the essential purpose of any special program? Is it *remedial* in nature — that is, does it attempt to treat some disturbance in the intellectual, emotional, physical, or social sphere? Is it *preventively* oriented, seeking to deal with conditions in the educational program which have been found to contribute to disturbance in one of the above four spheres? Is it established for the purpose of *classroom maintenance* and teacher morale, removing from the main stream of the school certain children who, through their heterogeneity or their deviant behavior, add to the stresses of the already harried classroom situation?

Remedial Programs

Certain remedial or treatment programs have developed secure traditions in American education. For the elementary school child the acquisition of basic language and number skills (reading, writing, arithmetic and, in some places, speech) seems essential to later school accomplishment. Yet, despite the best of instruction, a substantial number of children become underachievers with respect either to their grade level or to their own individual capacities. Many of the latter remain undetected unless given individual study by psychologists trained in the use of individual tests of intelligence, achievement, and personality.

As in medicine, the treatment of a problem must rest not only upon the recognition of the symptom, but also upon careful appraisal of the etiology of the condition. It is scarcely necessary to mention the existence of an interrelationship between emotional adjustment and degree of intellectual achievement. Yet the precise nature of this relationship in any one child is often most obscure. Psychiatrists and others who have worked with disturbed children in psychotherapy are most inclined to consider the possibility that reading deficit, for example, is a reflection of more central personality disturbance, the latter deflecting available emotional resources from task spheres. The classroom teacher or remedial reading specialist is perhaps more inclined to view a reading or other skill deficit as a handicap which may lead to increasing spirals of alienation from school, and thus to personality disturbance. McLelland has carried out an extensive and thoughtful review of the general problem of underachievement in our society, which emphasizes the interrelations between motivation of the student and dominant values held by the culture.[33] Whatever the nature of the causal relationship in any particular child, many children can and do benefit from skilled remedial instruction. It is likely that many of these children benefit as much from the sympathetic interest and attention of a single interested adult, in an individual or small-group tutoring arrangement, as from the specific word-attack skills, vocabulary building, or phonetic understandings, which form the content of such encounters.

Preventive Work

Many school efforts are conceived on a broad preventive basis. Indeed, education as we know it in Western civilization affords probably the most fruitful resource for the developing mental health field. Experience in at least two school systems — Wellesley and Weston, Mass. — for the past 8 years has demonstrated that mental health specialists and educators can join together effectively in studies and action programs aimed at the detection of incipient disturbances in clusters of children going through common experiences, or having common characteristics, which might impair personal integration and school adaptation.

Effective preventive work must depend on the most careful and rigorous study and planning. In work with mentally retarded children, for example, it is not naive to ask "What is the problem?" even when there is so obvious a handicap as mental retardation. A statement of the problem must go far beyond the physical, social, emotional, or intellectual description of the child. The statement must include a consideration of the child in the situation, the life-space of the child as it exists in the child's own mind, and an examination of what later problems, *if any*, educational or otherwise, are created by existing educational arrangements. This approach should lead to careful follow-up studies of retarded children who have already gone through the school system. No doubt, adequate fact-finding would include information gained from cooperative inquiries with other community resources — parents, pastors, employers, etc.

As in modern industry, which is increasingly utilizing psychology and social science in coping with personnel problems and human relationships on the job, schools are beginning to recruit educational and clinical psychologists, social workers, and psychiatrists. In addition to turning to them for help with the assessment and guidance of problem children, educational administrators should encourage them to take up some of the pressing problems involved in the preventive orientation of the schools.

Non-typical groups of children. The preventive orientation seems to include at least three major subdivisions: (1) problems which arise because of peculiarities of special clusters of children; (2) problems which arise at certain crucial points in the life cycle; and (3) problems which arise because of the stresses imposed by the educational arrangements themselves.

In addition to the mentally retarded, schools sometimes become concerned about the effects on gifted children of exposure to an educational program pitched to a wide range of talents but inevitably geared to the majority, those within the normal range of intellect. Here again, there are many opinions but only a few facts and the latter seem often ignored. Terman's famous research provides us with the most thorough longitudinal study of gifted people from childhood into adult life. There is nothing in the reported data to suggest that gifted children who were accelerated in school became social misfits as adults. Nevertheless, many educators, from their observations of children, have become convinced that acceleration leads in many cases to marked difficulties in social integration in adolescence. Some may feel that speed of educational progress in elementary grades is much less important than the opportunity for development of social skills through carefully guided peer contacts. Some schools have attempted special enrichment programs through guided self-study, or the use of special contacts with children from higher grades regarding some subjects. It is not always recognized that many teachers have been deeply troubled about the gifted child; they have felt that they were slighting the advanced child who rarely makes undue time-demands on the teacher, and wondered what later problems of motivation, orientation to intellectual pursuits, etc. might develop in upper grades and at the college level. Here again objective observations are needed, based on the best opinions — hypotheses — currently available. It is also necessary to recognize the formidable pressures in our society against special education for highly endowed individuals arising from American ambivalence towards education and mistrust of an educational elite.

Except for art and music, superior abilities are very rarely given particular attention in most elementary grades. Even art and music, and sometimes crafts, are generally provided as exposures for all children. Nevertheless many teachers are alert to special interests and experiences of their children and utilize them in order to add interest to the day, enrich the experiences of other children, develop class pride, and aid in the social adjustment of a particular child. In regard to the latter, Osborn has carefully documented in a summer camp context the efficacy of providing a social isolate with special skills which may give him a higher value in the eyes of the peer culture.

Common stress situations. A preventive program is also concerned with difficulties which may arise in groups of children, not because of special characteristics of the children, but because of the more or less stressful situations through which many, and sometimes all, children pass. For example, a universal life challenge occurs at the time of school entry. This phase of school adjustment is considered to be primary, not only in time but also in importance, and will be discussed in some detail.

The advent of school marks one of the highly significant growth-points in a child's life. The child has already mastered certain basic skills of manipulation and locomotion, has assembled these skills into more complicated operations involving simple creative and artistic goals, and has established some rudimentary skills in social relations with peers and with children older and younger. The child at the kindergarten age is now considered "ready" to work in three major developmental areas: (1) separation from the mothering person; (2) task orientation; (3) adjustment to the peer group.

(1) *Separation from the mother.* Entry into school is in a sense the culmination of a process of separation from a mothering person. This begins at birth itself, and continues through the weaning period, the establishment of contacts with the father, other adults, and children in the immediate vicinity, and often through the time when mother's attention and affection is drawn to a younger sibling. At the first contact with mother and child the teacher may often be able to note evidences of what patterns of adjustment the child has begun to develop in response to the separation crisis. Skilled teachers have noticed wide variability of patterns and have developed their own personal cues signifying the child's degree of readiness for the new circumstance of separation confronting the child.

Since separation is an event that involves at least two persons — child and mother — it is in most instances, and perhaps all, a kind of emotional crisis for both. To the mother's feeling of partial loss of the child are added her identification with the child as a small, helpless creature in a formidable world, and her own feelings of inadequacy in the parental role. School and teacher loom as representatives of the outside world who may be expected to detect whatever flaws there have been in child-rearing. Some preliminary study indicates that for most mothers the usual period of initial adaptation to the separation takes 4 or 5 weeks.

(2) *Task orientation.* Gruber[34] describes task orientation as follows:

The general psychological development in children between the ages of 4–6 . . . involves a conspicuous movement on the part of the child toward adult modes of behavior. At this time, the child leaves behind the more narrow and confined types of activity directed towards the acquisition of the various skills and the mastery of the infant modes of functioning, and begins to display a more integrated and broader mode of functioning, indicative of *greater maturity, emotional control, perseverance in constructive activities* and interests in social participation. . . . Task orientation refers to the expression of those traits by children who are about to enter kindergarten. (*Italics mine.*)

Gruber made ratings of task-orientation of 50 children during the spring preceding kindergarten entry in the following fall, on the basis of observations of behavior in a doll-play situation. These ratings were found to predict, with moderate accuracy, subsequent school adjustment as assessed by observation of classroom behavior, teachers' ratings, and peer ratings. These children have since been followed through the first 6 grades. Those children who showed initially high task-orientation have maintained an almost uniformly high adjustment to school. Those children with initially low task-orientation have done relatively poorly as a group, both as to achievement and as to classroom behavior, but there has been a gradual improvement over the years. A larger middle group showed greater fluctuations from grade to grade in both positive and negative directions. Here too, however, the trend has been in the direction of improved adjustment.

There are wide individual differences in task-orientation among kindergarten age children. Kindergarten teachers usually recognize this, and present a varied program geared to the level of the individual child. It is sometimes desirable to allow a child to repeat kindergarten in order that he will be better able to meet the more work-centered demands of the grades. However, parents usually need much support before accepting such a recommendation. To the shame of "failing" kindergarten is added the guilt of the parents, who feel they have failed in their job during the preschool years.

There are also vast differences among kindergartens in the teachers' expectations with regard to the behavior of children. Some look to the rigorous demands of the first grade and attempt to prepare their pupils with increasing doses of Spartan discipline. The emphasis is on ready response to directions, a high degree of impulse control, and the suppression of interpupil tensions in the cause of group order. Others hope to extend the pleasures of preschool play just a little longer, hoping that a golden year at the beginning of school will compensate for the rigorous years to come. Those few who insist on keeping very close to either line might find, on self-examination, that their orientations are based more on personal reactions to their own transition from play to work than on the realities of the immediate situation or the actual needs of their pupils.

(3) Adjustment to the peer group. According to Riesman in *The Lonely Crowd,* ours is the age of "other-directedness," wherein the expectations of those around us are apt to take precedence over a well-developed inner code of behavior. He points out that many people are faced with the necessity of avoiding undue expression of aggressiveness; to appear to cooperate with our fellows and actually to do so, while at the same time engaging in active competition with them. Some psychotherapists, too, have noted a shift in the core conflicts of their patients from the sexually-based disturbances of the late 1900's to a greater incidence of problems concerning the management of hostility and aggressive impulses. We live in an era when external standards and controls repeatedly break down on a global level, and the control of aggression becomes a problem of sheer survival. Small wonder then that children's adventures in self-assertion and rebellion are often viewed by parents, teachers, and the community at large as the precursors of delinquency and destructive havoc. These pervasive anxieties are no doubt sensed by many children, and become compelling forces in the early socializing experiences of the school. Teachers, even those few who do not share these concerns, cannot hope to dispel them in their pupils. They can, however, provide a situation wherein there are clear-cut and consistent limits, not overly restrictive, to self-assertion and aggression.

The early school experiences are of incalculable value in providing opportunities for social learning vis-à-vis both extrafamilial adult authority-figures and compeers. Some children are badly equipped to take advantage of such opportunities when they first enter school. In a few instances children are struggling in a morass of tensions and anxieties relating to extremely malign intrafamilial relationships. In a surprising number of cases, however, the child is laboring under the disadvantage of inadequate or one-sided training in social "skills." Sullivan[35] expresses the latter problem in the following way:

People going into the juvenile era [i.e., approximately from 6 to 10] are all too frequently very badly handicapped for acquiring social skill. Take, for example, the child who has been taught to expect everything . . . [or] . . . the petty tyrant who rules his parents with complete neglect of their feelings. Take the child . . . who has been taught to be completely self-effacing and docilely obedient. . . . All these children, if they did not undergo very striking change in the juvenile era, would be almost intolerable ingredients, as they grew up, in a group of any particular magnitude. . . . In this culture, where education is compulsory, it is the school society that rectifies or modifies in the juvenile era a great deal of the unfortunate direction of personality evolution conferred upon the young by their parents and others constituting the family group.

Social psychologists, especially those interested in small groups, have in recent years been developing techniques for the observation and measurement of social interaction. Bales' interaction profiles and the interpersonal dimensions of personality developed by Leary, Freedman, Coffey, and their co-workers, are extremely promising developments in this area. With such devices it should be increasingly possible to make meaningful descriptions and comparisons of children's social behavior, to do normative studies at the several age levels, and to begin to determine the true value of various educational approaches to social learning.

It is well known that during the first years of school the peer group increases sharply in importance as an influence in shaping behavior and affecting self-esteem. Teachers are in a most favorable position to observe this process, which Sullivan describes as "a simply astounding broadening of the grasp of how many slight differences in living there are" and which he calls *social accommodation*. Many educators feel that they are more or less barred by the children from being "in the know." As a result, they have turned increasingly to seemingly more objective tools, including sociometry, which provides a picture of linkages within a group by asking group members which others they would and, sometimes, would not wish to eat with, play with, sit next to, etc. Sociometry is occasionally used as an aid in making classroom seating arrangements. It is a valuable screening device in the detection of socially-isolated children, or those rejected by the group. Obviously such isolation on a sociometric test is not synonymous with poor personal adjustment, unless of course we wish to elevate extroversion and gregariousness to the position of adjustment norms. Social isolation may reflect emotional disturbance and even severe withdrawal; it may indicate lack of acceptance because of differences in social background, neighborhood, etc.; it may even, in more than a few instances, reflect a subtle process of scapegoating, wherein one member of a group is cast out as "the bad one," and thus made to blame by the other group-members for their own bad impulses, such as aggressiveness only recently brought under control. On the other hand social isolation may simply reflect a pattern of adjustment in which inner resources — an interest in reading and intellectual pursuits, an absorption with one's thoughts and one's inner reactions to outside persons and events — are paramount. Only careful study of the child's school and home adjustment can provide such discriminations. It is important that they be made. However, adults frequently are overconcerned about introversive tendencies in children and many introduce new situational strains by trying to alter the natural development of the child. A highly skilled and creative teacher vitally concerned with pupil adjustment recently described the strenuous and ingenious campaign she carried on to interest a very bright, self-sufficient girl in some of the other, less bright, children in her class. The goal was partially accomplished when a pretty, talkative, and apparently vacuous girl was seated next to the object of concern. The latter could no longer become absorbed in reading and studying, and ultimately — possibly in desperation — made some effort to respond to the persistent, if somewhat insensitive, efforts of her neighbor. A kind of triumph of gregariousness over industriousness, or perhaps better of prattle over mind!

The social milieu of the child in the classroom does not exist, of course, independently of the teacher. Possibly the safest conclusion which can be drawn at present is that no single approach — teacher's observation or sociometry — provides a fully accurate picture of the classroom group. Sociometric devices, when used intelligently as aids to the teacher's own awareness, can be extremely valuable. When applied artificially by those untrained in their implications, and without an understanding of their limitations, they may become harmful to classroom cohesiveness or affect adversely the social adjustment of individual pupils.

Workers at the University of California Institute of Child Welfare made use of a sociometric device, the Reputation Test, to study social aspects of personality development of a group of children at the elementary grade levels. In the report of this study one is impressed with the complexities of social adjustment and peer group expectations. The latter are markedly different for males and females and vary somewhat at the several age levels. Study of individual protocols suggests that acceptance or rejection is not a simple matter of the presence or absence of a few desirable or undesirable traits. One highly-disliked girl, for example, was not depicted as having obviously negative or irritating qualities but simply was seen as a peculiarly colorless and "blah" individual.

The newcomer. The adjustment problems of children who move from community to community or from school to school within a community are in some places in our country apt to belong in the category of common stress reactions. The great geographic mobility in contemporary life is often associated with equally striking mobility up the social and economic ladder. Much more needs to be known about the ways in which families adapt to these shifts. Many children develop surprising adeptness in adjusting to new communities and new schools. For most there is, understandably, a period of weeks or months before the change is mastered.

It is generally agreed that the timing of such moves is often important. Children are better able to find a suitable place in the class when the whole group is in the process of beginning the work of a new grade, getting to know a new teacher, etc. However, few are able to meet the challenge without special help from understanding adults.

There are other factors within groups which, at certain periods in their development, make it harder for some classes to accept newcomers as compared with other classes at other times. Pupils who are in a phase of vying with one another for the teacher's limited amount of time and personal attention may resent the need of a new child for special help. A class leader who, in return for his special position in the adult's eyes, helps the teacher maintain class morale, may find a newcomer threatening unless he is drawn into the process of helping the new child find a place in the group. There is an almost limitless variety of intraclass situations which tend either to facilitate or hinder the integration of a new pupil.

Difficulties in integrating a newcomer may arise when the latter's background of training and experience differs markedly from the group's in ways which challenge certain of its important values. One such situation involved a 7 year old from an urban lower-class background who entered a small homogeneous class of upper middle-class children in a suburban community. When observed, the boy was not learning, was hyperactive, impulsive, and distractable, and seemed filled with anxiety. As he discussed, with some pressure of speech, his former neighborhood, the class laughed uncomfortably when he mentioned "cops" and used a number of other slang expressions. The school was about to refer the boy for special testing, both to appraise his intellectual abilities — which seemed below normal — and to assess the severity of emotional disturbance. Before the referral could be carried out the family moved to another district within the same system, and the boy was enrolled in a school with upper-lower and middle-class children and a more transient population. When next observed, about 1 month later, the boy was at the grade level in learning and showed none of the extreme restlessness and anxiety formerly seen.

Difficulties in adjustment to a new school are often found to be associated with difficulties of the entire family in adapting to the new community or neighborhood. A well-functioning PTA or other parent group can sometimes assist the child's school adjustment by simple neighborliness towards a strange family.

Sex differences in school adjustment. It sometimes appears to the harassed teacher that boys are simply not made for school, or *vice versa*. Boys are almost universally reported to show more school adjustment problems than girls in the social, emotional, and intellectual spheres. They are also the more frequent habitués of child guidance clinics. The

California Institute of Child Welfare found that children's own appraisals of themselves and their schoolmates give clear recognition of this sex difference, especially at the first grade level. At this point girls get more favorable mention in 9 items of the Reputation Test, boys in only 2. At the fifth grade, however, with additional items added, the girls are mentioned favorably on 12, the boys on 6 items. One might have suspected that the discrepancy between boys and girls in the reputation area would have increased over the years, on the basis that female teachers might tend to perpetuate an overvaluation of the feminine role and provide fewer appropriate outlets for boys than for girls. Quite the contrary, however. The bad reputation of boys — quarrelsome, bossy, gets mad easily, not good-looking, wiggly, untidy, fights, not many friends — is more pronounced at the first grade, at which point the girls are rated by boys and girls alike as quiet, full of fun, not quarrelsome, good sport, good at games, acts like little lady, and popular. By the fifth grade, boys are credited with more positive attributes and girls show a secondary shift in the unfavorable direction.

Though girls appear to make better school adjustments in the early grades, almost all studies (reviewed by Terman)[36] of nervous mannerisms, fears, and hyperemotionality indicate that girls are, but only slightly, more prone than boys to these symptoms. Terman contrasts such data with the many studies of classroom and home problems, based on teachers' and mothers' ratings, indicating a marked discrepancy in favor of the girls. He comments: "The only reasonable inference is that ratings of children by women teachers and mothers are biased in favor of girls."

Physical Health Services

The discussion of preventive activities in our schools must of course include mention of physical health services, which in many instances play a major part in pupil guidance and emotional health.

There have been many instances of severe classroom behavior problems and learning deficiencies which have yielded following correction of visual, auditory, or speech defects, reading disabilities, dietary deficiencies, or even poor sleep routines. There is increasing evidence, also, that physical growth failures may be associated with emotional and/or learning difficulties. School physicians and nurses, while available for emergency treatment of physical and emotional difficulties, are in many school systems essentially the core of preventive programs. Mainly these consist of regular physical examinations, periodic screening of vision and hearing, instruction regarding diet and other matters of physical care and conferences with parents and teachers regarding the total health needs of children as well as specific health problems.

Health education is a primary objective of health services in schools and should be participated in actively by physician, nurse, and teacher as well as by specialists such as trained health educators, physical educator or nutritionist. The role of each may be different but these roles should be coordinated, each supplementing the work of the other in particular ways. This can only be accomplished by such close contacts as health personnel staff meetings and case conferences. The physician's direct role will be largely that of using physical findings or reports of problems or illnesses to enhance understanding by both mother and child of what constitutes healthful living and how to avoid these developments when possible. For example, while dealing with the results of an accident the physician or nurse can drive home in an impressive manner how accidents are commonly caused and may be avoided. So also, a nutritional upset leads logically to discussion of diet. The physician can reinforce the influence of these episodes by securing the cooperation of the other members of the health team in more general discussion of these problems. The school physician can be most effective when he is able to keep in touch with the family physician and thus to utilize in the school the knowledge of the latter relating to the needs of a child.

The school health team, if properly trained in a broad public health orientation, can draw together all available resources, in the school milieu and the community at large, for the detection and care of physical and psychological problems and for the creation of an emotionally, as well as physically, healthy environment for the growing child. Such a team is able to serve as an effective interpreter of the educational program to those not familiar with the schools; it also can help the school make the best use of good medical advice in planning for the needs of palsied or other brain-damaged children, those with special handicaps, those convalescing from serious illness, and those with specific emotional disorders. While the knowledge of a child provided by the family physician or specialist is often extremely helpful, the school system with its own medical staff may well be in a better position to evaluate outside medical opinion with respect to the educational program. Often school administrators, against their own professional judgment, have followed specific advice from outside physicians which affects the child's adjustment to the school situation. In our society the educator is apt to defer to the physician in matters which appear to relate to the health of the child even when in his opinion the school adjustment of the child is clearly jeopardized. Closer collaboration of the two professions on as nearly an equal basis as possible would certainly lead in many instances to more suitable planning for the whole child.

Classroom Maintenance and Teacher Morale

The remedial and preventive approaches to school adjustment have been briefly reviewed. The third and perhaps most controversial approach — that of classroom maintenance and teacher morale — remains.

Role model of the ideal teacher. Little of a systematic nature is known about this subject, possibly because until recently teacher morale was taken for granted and any good teacher was expected to be able to deal with just about any child. Probably many teachers today still subscribe to a role model approaching infallibility.

Teacher fallibility. As a mental health consultant to teachers, the writer is sometimes struck by the professional frustration caused by the need for near-perfection, which is naturally more important for some teachers than others. Not so long ago women teachers were forbidden to smoke, to take a cocktail or to marry without losing employment. Now that they are allowed these pleasures, their main problem is simply that many of them are not supposed to have problems. The teacher properly feels a craftsman's pride as she sees children develop and prosper in her class. When the child fails to achieve to an expected level it is clear that the reason lies in one or more of only a few factors: Inadequacy of the material, inadequacy of the tools, inadequacy of the working conditions, inadequacy of the craftsman. The teacher who has a strong need for professional perfection unconsciously must inevitably blame herself. Outwardly she must maintain the appearance of infallibility, and is apt to redouble her efforts under increased tension, hesitating to call upon a supervisor or consultant for help; or she may seek flaws in the child, the home background, the crowded classroom, etc.

The most important point in all this is that when the professional role model of the teacher becomes less taxing, education can be freer to accept *explicitly* the idea that not all teachers are for all pupils or all teaching conditions. Different individual children or configurations of children within the classroom naturally affect individual teachers in various ways. Size of the group; degree of heterogeneity with regard to age, intellect, or socioeconomic position; presence of one or another kind of physical or personality difficulty — these and many other factors introduce additional real strain to the teaching job.

In a setting where teachers are expected to experience difficulties with some children under some conditions, pupils' school adjustment should be facilitated. Not having to deny difficulties or conceal inadequacies, the teacher would presumably be better able to reduce the classroom pressure in some manner. First, she can make use of supervisory help or seek the counsel of the school psychologist or other guidance specialists; second, she can consider, realistically and without guilt or need to rationalize, placement of the child in another classroom with a different teacher, a step which some educators are now making legitimate under the rubric of "lateral transfer."

Psychological removal of problem children. In a setting where teachers cannot acknowledge the possibility of teacher failure to establish a suitable relationship with any pupil, the teacher cannot deal realistically with such difficulties. She must seek for causal factors outside the classroom in order not to blame herself. Very often she unknowingly relies upon *"psychological removal"* of the *disturbing child,* that is, the establishment of a kind of barrier between teacher and child. The latter is differentiated from the other children by means of the troubling characteristic. He or she is no longer so much a child as a problem of one kind or another.

Use and misuse of specialists. The provision in many schools of specialists in various fields — reading, speech, psychology, guidance, etc. — may sometimes facilitate the process of psychological removal. It may be easier to perceive a youngster primarily in terms of his or her reading problem when there is a reading specialist at hand to take over this particular facet of the child's education. Certainly this is not an argument against provision of well-trained specialists. It is rather a suggestion that specialist services be appraised in terms of whether or not they add to or detract from the contribution of the classroom teacher to the over-all adjustment of the child. Perhaps the problem is similar to that in medicine, where in recent years there have been attempts to develop instruction in comprehensive medicine to compensate for the high degree of specialization which, many believe, has too often substituted for a concern with the total well-being of the patient.

Elementary School Guidance Programs

Some schools now provide child guidance facilities, staffed usually by psychologists and social workers supported by psychiatric consultation, which are intended to work with the emotionally disturbed child. As such facilities carry on their activities, teachers are helped to identify more accurately increasing numbers of disturbances which before had escaped notice, especially problems marked by symptoms of withdrawal, underachievement, and passive resistance to school. Facilities are often overtaxed and teachers sometimes meet with increased frustration as they become increasingly aware of children's needs but find themselves unable to get help with them.

Even with adequate facilities for appraisal and treatment of emotional disturbances, separate guidance facilities must continually seek ways to establish and maintain effective collaboration with the classroom teacher. The child under treatment usually remains in the classroom, and if this is not possible, ultimate return to the classroom is one important goal of the therapy.

Referrals. Guidance specialists and teachers alike should be concerned with the suitability and timing of referrals for psychological assistance. The writer believes that, in general, the most suitable referrals are for *minor disturbances* which have developed only a short time before. Obviously the guidance worker is then in a better position to screen out incipient severe problems for more intensive effort and can advise the teacher on the management of less serious difficulties. When the teacher is at her "wit's end," has "tried everything," and just "cannot make any headway" with a child, the guidance worker should proceed with much caution and only on the basis of ample study of the situation. Ready acceptance of the child for study may, instead of helping child or teacher, only lead to further difficulties in the classroom relationship. First, it confirms the teacher's fear that she has indeed failed and that her level of knowledge and skill is not up to the job of working with the child. Second, such confirmation may mean either that the teacher is not fit or that the child must be most abnormal to baffle her so. Third, it often accentuates or completes a progress of psychological removal of the child, perhaps begun when the teacher's efforts were first frustrated. The *problem* (i.e., the child) *is now out of the teacher's hands.*

Mental Health Consultation

Techniques of consultation have been developing in recent years for use by mental health teams with educators or other professionals concerned with the emotional well-being of those with whom they work.

Teacher-oriented approach. Stemming in the main from psychiatry and psychoanalysis, these techniques have often resembled either individual or group psychotherapy. The major focus of attention has been on the nonobjective or inappropriate reactions of the teacher to the child. Teachers have become aware of anxieties and hostilities aroused in them by certain children or classroom situations. Tensions vis-à-vis parents or superiors also have been pointed out.

One ideal of the good teacher certainly includes a high degree of self-insight and a considerable degree of objectivity with regard to child-teacher relationships. No doubt many teachers welcome contacts with psychiatrists or others who, through therapeutic techniques, may aid them in their efforts to approximate this ideal. Other teachers are either less anxious about their own level of psychological functioning, or are fearful of examining their own reactions or motivations.

Pupil-oriented approach. Another approach to mental health consultation owes some debt to social work methods developed in working with parents of problem children, although differing from such methods in many important ways. The major focus of attention is on the problem of the child. The relationship is one of two professionals from different backgrounds, rather than a quasi patient-doctor relationship. Every effort is made to empathize with the real difficulties confronting the teacher. At the same time, the teacher is helped to gain increased understanding of the child's behavior (that is, to gain objectivity) by looking at the situation through the eyes of the outside observer. This method, which has been developed at the Harvard School of Public Health, has been used in a number of Massachusetts communities, and it has been incorporated by the State Division of Mental Hygiene into its mental health program throughout Massachusetts.

There is little doubt but that in the future schools will make increasing use of experts in human relations coming from professions only partially related to psychiatry and the clinical fields. As this development occurs, we will be witnessing the emergence of a new and more sophisticated level of concern with children's school adjustment. Already, as was mentioned earlier, The National Education Association through its Laboratory in Group Dynamics is communicating to school administrators an understanding of group processes. The focus of concern on the individual child's personality is widening to include the child-in-the-immediate-situation. Ultimately we may secure from joint efforts of social science, psychiatry, education, public health, and other professions a much more adequate understanding of the child's personality as it is affected by the great number of forces acting on it from the family, the school, and the larger community.

Intensive observations[37] have been carried out since 1948 in one community of about 20,000 by a mental health team of experts from psychiatry, psychology, sociology, anthropology, and public health, working closely with the public schools and other community groups. Results indicate that individual personality problems — emotional disturbance of the individual — in most instances reflect a disturbance in the social system around the individual. Conversely, many disruptions in individual behavior can be ameliorated by alteration of the disruptive forces in the social milieu. Even children with marked behavior disorders — for whom prolonged psychotherapy is frequently recommended — show profound *behavioral* changes when tensions in the surrounding situation are reduced. It is of course still too early to tell whether such startling shifts are temporary in nature or whether they imply more central alterations in personality adjustment patterns. Nevertheless, the experience to date indicates how unclear are the presently-available criteria for judging certain kinds and severities of emotional disorder of children. The need for philosophies which yield fruitful hypotheses, worthy of being tested, is abundantly clear.

ASSESSMENT OF EDUCATIONAL
AND PSYCHOLOGICAL DEVELOPMENT
JOHN C. PALMER

Contemporary American education has been marked by allegiance to three concepts, so pervasive they have become pedagogical cliches. These are "the whole child," "individual differences" and "continuous growth or development." A very large proportion of the shift in professional attitude and practice from previous education to that of the mid-twentieth century has resulted from the impact of these concepts. Yet their translation from verbal consensus to the commonplace routines of most schools has only come slowly. For the several adults most concerned with the nurture and education of each child, the "wholeness" of the child is not easily perceived. The teacher, the physician, the parent each lack direct experience with some aspects of the child's life and all of them have difficulty in penetrating his inner, psychological world. Even with the best of intent, each sees the child partially and misses the psychophysical reality of the "whole" boy or girl.

Equally difficult, in any but the grossest terms, is the appraisal of the multitude of ways each child differs from others and the extent of the variation of traits within himself. The staggering complexity of an interacting pattern of physiological and psychological contributions of a unique heredity and a unique environment demands a deliberate and continuous series of observation, quantification and comparison.

The forces that inhibit the employment of a true developmental point of view in schools are built into the traditional organizational structure of American education. The segmentation of each child's experience into grades, and years, and schools shortens the teacher's perspective. The child is seen as a "second grader" or as a "sophomore," as if he were at a single stage of development with only the most meagre past history and no discernible future. As the geographical mobility of American families continues and children shift from town to town, region to region and school system to school system, this fragmentation of educational experience is exaggerated.

The universal solvent for these situations is information — observational data on every boy and girl in quantity. The concepts of "wholeness," "individual differences," and "development" only become viable in the light of a rich, detailed, diverse, accurate body of observations on each and every child, its recording and storage, and its interpretation and communication. By and large, all schools are assiduous in their observation of children; few contemporary teachers are unaware of the need to study their pupils and to make differential decisions on the basis of these observations. Schools, school systems, and teachers do differ dramatically in the degree with which the accumulated wisdom of the school is preserved, is brought to bear on the increasingly complex decisions that face each boy and girl sequentially, is systematically available through an educational and counseling process to assist the realistic enlargement of the self-concept.

When schools fail in this respect, the fault is sometimes an organizational one; too frequently it is one of the school staff being denied both the time and the equipment to perform the routine, clerical operations. One of the great tragedies in many school systems is the loss of priceless professional insights and understanding through lack of inexpensive dictating equipment and the availability of typists. Those schools that are generally acknowledged as superior have accepted the general responsibility to study all children continuously and systematically and to record and preserve these observations in order that a total developmental, differential idiosyncratic picture of each child will emerge with increasing clarity.

The role of pupil personnel services. Although the implementation of these concepts of wholeness, individuality and growth, through the gathering of the richest possible body of observations on every child, has been a general goal of good schools and their teachers, principals, and ancillary staff members, in practice the creation of the current elaborate programs of data-gathering has been and continues to be a primary responsibility of the pupil personnel or guidance services.

The history of the guidance movement is an instructive example of American empiricism at work in education. Founded as an humanitarian, protoscientific attempt to smooth the transition of the burgeoning public school populations into jobs satisfactory to the individual and the economy, guidance as a professional process, by accretion and incorporation, added appropriate dimensions from the several behavioral sciences, and especially from the applied disciplines of psychometrics and psychotherapy.[38] In its enhanced role of meeting "in a systematic and organized way, the special needs of individual pupils which cannot be met through the normal instructional practices or administrative procedures of the given school system" [39] guidance services, or in the more accurate contemporary term, pupil personnel services, have become the principal vehicle and its specialized personnel principal exponents of the concepts of "wholeness," "individual differences," and "development."

The articulation of education through guidance. Guidance services attempt to bridge systematically the several environments, school, home, and neighborhood against which the child plays out his roles. The counselor knows the parent, the teacher, the physician, the scout leader, the probation officer and mediates their several perspectives. Persistently above the often overriding group demands and allegiances of classroom or school, the guidance worker exploits individual variability and defends a personalistic approach within mass education. Above all the guidance program's most significant function is to maintain the long continuous view of the maturing boy and girl. By seeing each pupil against the backdrop of earlier experiences and accomplishments and projecting them into the anticipated challenges of the future, the guidance-pupil personnel services provide the unifying vision that tries to see a continuous meaning in the series of events. The vertical articulation of elementary, secondary, and higher stages of education for each individual girl and boy rests almost entirely on the ability of the pupil personnel program, however it may be organized or staffed, to gather, systematize, and communicate to each successive level the pertinent observations.

Thus, a primary task of the school is to study all children, steadily and continuously, from as many professional perspectives and vantage points as are physically and professionally feasible. In each school, there will be a common body of observations on *all* children. In addition, of course, children who exhibit special problems or special needs, will be studied intensively and particularly in ways suggested by their immediate symptomology. With so much of the child's daily behavior occurring in the presence of relatively sensitive and trained observers who have substantial legal prerogatives to inquire and scrutinize, the issue is selection.

Theoretical problems. The major problem is the choice of a theoretical framework which will determine what kind of information will be systematically gathered on all pupils. The interdisciplinary exchange in the behavioral sciences "toward a general theory of action" [40, 41] has not progressed far enough to give common meaning to the most ordinary events of daily life, let alone to the more technical observations of learning and social interaction. In the absence of such a unified theory of human behavior, the particular theoretical predisposition of the designers will determine what information is central, what is peripheral; what will be preserved, what discarded. Data about toilet training, position in the family, language spoken in the home, performance on a multifactor mental ability test become sharply meaningful under some hypotheses, irrelevant under others.

The most serious danger is that this lack of a controlling consensus will produce a loose eclecticism, which will declare any and all information about the child of equal significance. As the unfortunate by-product of such theoretical neutrality, only data that is accessible, easy to record, and readily quantified will be preserved.

As in any longitudinal study of human behavior, another persistent problem of selecting the significant observations to preserve involves the prediction of what information will be pertinent to decisions to be made, at least several, sometimes many, years later. The pace of development in psychology and education is sufficiently great that the thirteen years of a boy or girl's elementary and secondary school career is long enough for hindsight to show that additional or different developmental data might have been profitably recorded at an earlier age. There is no satisfactory resolution of these dynamics of time and professional advance.

Organismic age as the organizing principle. Without a basic theoretical consensus, the most promising organizing principle for the continuous study of boys and girls in schools is that of the developmental or organismic age. As explicitly developed by Olson and Hughes,[42, 43] this effort to relate the somatic, the psychosocial, and the educational progress on boys and girls represents a promising attempt to knit the observations of physicians, teachers and psychologists into a single framework, which will be inevitably "holistic." In the partial application of the organismic age concept by Millard and Rothney[44] and by Stott,[45] the linkage between physical growth and educational seems apparent, but the structure is far from complete. The search for "master curves" which will correlate the several aspects of human development into contemporary cross-sections and in longitudinal sequences is still at a primitive stage. Yet, these parallels in developmental events suggests what may be significant at each age level without a rigorous commitment to a single hypothesis of child development.

The observation of the child in school. In practice, the usable observations of children can be divided into testing procedures and nontest procedures. The psychometric approaches will include all the standardized observations which yield primarily quantitative information — individual and group explorations of mental ability, of school achievement, of personality structure. The nontest procedures embrace the myriad of observational techniques that produce qualitative information; in usual school practice, these qualitative techniques will include interviews, questionnaires, anecdotal records, sociometric surveys, samples of the child's productions, and several varieties of self-report documents. This dichotomy between quantitative and qualitative procedures is crude. Some of the testing devices, such as individual mental ability tests may produce considerable qualitative data on the child; some of the qualitative information, by the application of appropriate scaling, can be structured to produce numerical outcomes. In the current literature in education and in teacher training programs, the techniques of psychometric observation, as opposed to the nontest procedure, receive substantially greater attention than the validity of their impact on the consistent treatment of children would justify.

Nontest observations. The accumulation of information on the child generally begins before the child arrives at the school. All schools gather some kind of preschool data. Sometimes, this is restricted to a meagre summary of biographical fact, supplemented by such a record of immunizations and illnesses as state regulation may impose. In common practice a preschool registration questionnaire will be filled out by the parent and the family physician. In those school systems that have invested the most in the individualization of instruction, this questionnaire has become a rather comprehensive inquiry into the reactions of the child to the critical incidents of the preschool period feeding, toilet-training, walking, talking, accidents, illnesses, emotional traumas, sibling and peer group interactions.[46] Ordinarily, such a questionnaire will be supplemented by an interview with the mother and the simultaneous informal observation of the child by the teacher and the elementary counselor or psychologist. In a few schools this preschool visit may include a brief psychometric appraisal of the child. However, with fewer school systems attempting to manipulate the school entrance age, the consensus of good testing practice is to delay any formal measurement of the child until he is actually a pupil, so that the time and circumstances likely to produce a valid measurement can be better determined. With these data, the data on the child begins.

During the nursery, kindergarten and elementary school years, much of the daily activities of each child can be distilled into anecdotal records. The employment of this device depends on the training of the teaching staff and on the amount of time and clerical assistance they are allowed. Good anecdotal records are succinct objective recapitulations of incidents significant either because of their ability to capture the child's characteristic response to the assorted challenges of the school or because, in their wide departure from the norm of the child or the group, they reveal some previously inaccessible aspect of the child's personality. Although the spontaneous running record of behavior will be most productive through nursery school and kindergarten, during the elementary school years more structured approaches such as time samples, behavioral diaries, and various behavioral rating scales may supplement the more casual anecdotal record.

As more and more school systems include in their general procedures for reporting to the home, regular, at least semiannual, conferences between parent and teacher, the steady flow of observational information from the home, begun in the preschool questionnaire will continue. Unobjective as the parent's descriptions of the child may be, they provide a valuable series of reference points for comparative in-school behavior and disclose the emotional climate in which the child lives. In the initial stages of the development of the parent conference as the principal vehicle for communicating with the home, the interview may be largely a report by the teacher; but, as experience with this process increases for both parent and teacher, a genuine two-way interchange is created.

This accumulating file will also contain those samples of the child's school work that best summarize his mode of dealing with the intellectual and expressive opportunities, including free drawings, creative written expression, and autobiographies. Formal analyses of group interaction from sociometric devices will form a continuing part of the growing body of qualitative observations. As the school years advance, the emphasis in the qualitative record shifts. As the child gets older and more verbal, less dependence is placed on observation of external behavior and on reactions to the human and material environment. More and more will teachers and counselors record interviews, formal and casual, which show the particular meaning the child attaches to these behaviors. As time goes on the interviews with the child and the conferences with the parent will become more future-directed. Aspirations, goals, purposes, their particularization and realization will be increasingly their content. By the time the boy or girl reaches adolescence and the secondary school, much of recorded interaction between the pupil and the school will have developed the quality of that dynamic complex of relations and self-discovery, called counseling.

Included in the qualitative observations are those summary assessments of school achievement, teacher's marks. Rothney[47] summarizes their place in appraisal as follows:

There is general agreement that, although teachers' marks are often unreliable and invalid indexes of growth, they are indispensable tools. Marks are the coin of the school realm. They continue to be measures of school success — the keys that open doors of educational institutions for entrance and exit. The marks given by some classroom teachers have great value. Others may mean nothing more than that the student has official permission to forget what he has learned. In either case they seem likely to continue to be the principal basis for honor awards, promotion, and placement in schools. For a long time to come parents will accept them as the basic evaluative device.

Psychometric approaches. The growth in the use of standardized tests in American life is one of the phenomena of the twentieth century. The combination of the American passion for quantification and the successive pressures of wars, the Depression, exploding school and college populations, and rapid industrial specialization for the allocation of manpower has brought testing in fifty years from a minor tool of psychological research and a primitive distinguisher of "feeble-minded" from "normal" children to such a central role in the distribution of opportunity in an open-minded society that many commentators express alarm. Sorokin[48] expresses his concern:

We are living in an age of "testocracy." By their tests of our intelligence, emotional stability, character, aptitude, unconscious drives, and other characteristics of our personality, the testocrats largely decide our vocation and occupation. They play an important role in our promotions or demotions, successes or failures in our social position, reputation, and influence. They determine our normality or abnormality, our superior intelligence or hopeless stupidity, our loyalty or subversity. By all this they are largely responsible for our happiness or despair, and finally, for our long life or premature death.

The numbers on testing in 1959 gives substance to the "viewers-with-alarm." Approximately 125 million separate tests are now (1959) administered in American schools; many millions more under Civil Service, industrial selection and promotion, military allocation, and college admissions. The acceleration in the massive employment of standardized tests continues. The impetus of federal endorsement and federal funds under the National Education Defense Act promises an even greater expansion of large scale testing. This continuing expansion of psychometrics has occurred in spite of the failure of many standardized tests to live up to the frequently exaggerated claims of the test publishers and to the overexpectations of unsophisticated test users.

The use of tests in schools. Although in American life tests have come to have a particular mystique, in school practice they should be viewed only as another form of direct observation of the child. Certain special properties of these standardized samples of behavior — reliability or accuracy, validity or predictive power, economy of time and effort, and the normative aspect or the ability to support statements of comparison between the behavior of individuals or groups — illuminate important aspects of human behavior for the trained interpreter and contribute critical information for some of the most significant decisions of human life.

In reviewing the selection of tests for a school testing program long lists of types of standardized tests are sometimes given — intelligence tests, scholastic aptitude tests, achievement tests, diagnostic tests, prognostic tests, reading tests, readiness tests, aptitude tests, and tests of interests, preferences, temperament, values, attitudes, personality. Although dozens of tests under each one of these categories are published, these labels are frequently misleading and suggest a far greater range of outcomes from test administration than can be effected. For school practice, useful distinctions can be made between mental ability tests, achievement tests, and personality tests, although the difference between the first two is far from precise. The remainder are combinations and mutations.

Mental ability tests. Although the careful examination of the more cognitive aspects of behavior from Binet's pioneer efforts has a fifty year history, the source and nature of intelligence and the most useful ways to assess it are still the center of lively professional argument. Unfortunately, the details of the continuing controversy are largely confined to educational psychologists and test specialists. Most parents, physicians, social workers, and far too many teachers are still captured by the myth of the single, invariant I.Q., which the measurement movement oversold in its primitive, unsophisticated, and overoptimistic early days. The persistence of the fallacy of the "constant I.Q." has done enormous harm to the sound employment of tests.

The summaries[49] of the research of the last two decades into the nature of cognitive behavior and its systematic measurement suggest that psychology has a long road to travel before the conflicting evidence and hypotheses of "single factor" theory, "multifactor" theory, contemporary neurology, cybernetics, perception theory, and psychoanalytic statements about the preconscious are resolved. Out of the research and argumentation these understandings seem to have emerged. Whether intelligence has largely a unitary quality which finds its expression in a variety of forms or whether it is better viewed as a pragmatic summation of a number of largely independent traits or factors, its manifestations in the human personality are extraordinarily complex, elusive, subject to many inhibitions, and certainly cannot be captured on a single half-hour paper and pencil exercise nor even on one individual test like the Stanford-Binet or one of the Wechsler scales, however carefully administered.

We now acknowledge that variation occurs in all test performance. Some of this is accountable to chance, the "standard error of measurement" which is the property of every test; and some to individual variability, subsuming all the motivational affective, and physiological differences in the "set" each child brings to the test situation. We further recognize that many of the vehicles judged most appropriate for the assessment of mental ability — verbal facility, symbolic logic, social judgment — are culture-bound and artificially penalize those for whom the educational process has few rewards — poor readers, lower class children, withdrawn children. Substantial evidence continues to emerge that deprivation in all its forms, in nutrition, in affection, and in cultural environment severely restricts intelligence test performance.

Conversely, it is accepted, although with many more reservations and qualifications, that the reversal or removal of the inhibiting forces, if early enough, can effect some elevation of mental ability test scores. A corollary is that intelligence as we appraise it does not have the fixed upper limit in early adolescence that was originally posited but rather continues to expand under continuous educational stimulation into adulthood. Vernon[50] has recently pointed out that the older notion about the earlier ceiling on intelligence grew out of a simple sampling error.

It must be transparently clear to every test user and reader of test results that each test of mental ability is a different cross-section of measurable human behaviors which the individual test hypothesizes are the proper components of intelligence. Thus comparing performance on two discrete tests of mental ability requires not only intimate and detailed knowledge of the conditions surrounding the administration, the differences in affective "set" of the subject, but also an understanding of the distinctions in basic theory as well as correlation ratios developed on an appropriate population.

Achievement tests. Within any school system, the achievement testing program has the dual purpose of the sequential and systematic appraisal of intellectual growth within the several special instructional areas — reading, language, mathematics, social studies, science — and of the evaluation of the success of the whole school system in reaching some of the narrower educational objectives it has set for itself. In the selection of achievement measures, these purposes sometimes conflict. An achievement test battery which is the closest to the instructional objectives the school has chosen for itself may not have the item by item diagnostic power of another less broadly valid. If a single battery is used some purposes must be compromised.

As the persistently high statistical correlation between these two measures, remarked by T. L. Kelley more than three decades ago and confirmed periodically,[51] demonstrates, much of the difference between a mental ability test of high "verbal loading": i.e., emphasizing word recognition, reading facility, symbolic logic and an achievement battery purporting to appraise growth in specific subject areas — reading, arithmetic, spelling is spurious. Tiedeman and MacArthur[52] demonstrate that the all-too-common practice of comparing performance on such an intelligence test with an achievement measure to determine "underachievement" and "overachievement" probably constitutes malpractice in test use.

Achievement tests suffer from other disabilities. While useful as general reference points for the evaluation of a whole school system, the norms are frequently irrelevant for individual decisions; with the scores at the upper and lower end of the scale mere extrapolations, no true picture of educational growth emerges; the popular translation of scores into grade equivalents is the source of many misunderstandings of the actual level of accomplishment.

Personality tests. Although paper and pencil "personality" tests, self-rating questionnaires, and especially interest or preference inventories are among the most extensively used "standardized" instruments, both in schools and in business, their place in sound psychometric practice is dubious. Of the more than hundred such devices now in the standard catalogues, only a handful (i.e., the Minnesota Multiphasic Inventory, the Strong Vocational Interest Blank, and several projective procedures, like the Thematic Apperception Test and its variants) have been supported by a sufficient body of experimental evidence to suggest that they possess a minimal validity. Although each of this select group is used clinically with an occasional individual in school, no one of them has overcome its cumbersomeness of administration and scoring and its generally adult focus to be regularly employed in schools. The remainder of these "personality" tests have been largely discounted as overpretentious in their attempts at diagnostic precision, easily faked, and presented with inadequate statistics and irrelevant norms.

Test deficiencies and test strategy. In view of the many difficulties surrounding both the proper administration and, even more, the accurate interpretation of standardized tests, some in the field of measurement and guidance feel that schools should resist the trend toward wider and wider application of tests and should declare a moratorium on test construction and test use until the psychometric profession resolves its technical and ethical controversies and contradictions.[53] Even if a professional boycott or slowdown could be effected in the face of the massive commitment of colleges, businesses, and government to the greater use of all kinds of standardized measures, the writer feels that such recommendations are unrealistic and reflect an unsound strategy toward improved psychometric practice in schools.

Tests are useful; they do solve problems and contribute essential information whi h is otherwise obtained only with the greatest of difficulty. A "verbally loaded" group test of mental ability may not yield a rounded picture of a child's intelligence, but it can contribute noticeably to a prediction of scholastic success at a subsequent grade level; a nonverbal intelligence may distinguish, usefully if not precisely, which of a group of poor readers might profit from intensive remediation; a differential "multifactor" mental ability battery can discriminate sufficiently between those whose intellectual strength is in the humanities and languages and those with a mathematical-technical potential. Similarly achievement tests will not give a precise increment of instructional progress directly attributable to successful teaching, but they can support a differential diagnosis for some future instructional emphasis. Questionnaires and inventories cannot produce either a precise diagnostic categorization nor a stable description of personality; such instruments can produce static "snapshots" of the current "public" attitudes and "public" self-image. If nothing else tests administered throughout the school years are superior predictions of subsequent test performance on College Board examinations, national scholarship tests, armed forces qualification tests, industrial and business personnel selection batteries. As allocative testing plays a more determinant part in the assigning of roles in society, this is a controlled foresight of not inconsiderable importance.

A comprehensive testing program. The misuse of standardized tests in schools has its roots in overdependence on a single isolated measured test administered at one point in the child's development and over-interpreted to a significance well beyond its statistical power to reach. It is the writer's conviction, growing out of experience with the direction of a comprehensive public school program, that the soundest professional practice involves a substantial increase in the number of and frequency of tests systematically administered. In those school systems where a competent professional staff in guidance and testing has used a rigorous, cautious empiricism in the development of a "saturation" program of testing and have led the teaching staff into an understanding, fully participating relation with the whole psychometric effort, tests have made major contributions to the emergent developmental picture of each child.

A comprehensive program will involve the administration of eight or nine different measures of mental ability during the years from kinder-garten to the end of secondary school. To develop the richest possible picture of each boy and girl, the various hypotheses of intelligence — single factor dual axis, and multifactor, verbal and nonverbal, even "culture-fair" if appropriate — should be systematically exploited to produce a series of cross-sectional examples of cognitive behavior. As soon after the child's entry into kindergarten as is judged psychologically feasible, every child should be given an individually administered, rela-tively undifferentiated measure of the Binet type to serve as a reference point for later tests and to provide some impressions of the child's re-actions to standardized challenges uncontaminated by particular school successes or failures. During the elementary school grades, subsequent mental ability testing will point toward increasing differentiation. In junior high school, a differential ability battery will serve the develop-ment of appropriate educational and vocational goals. During high school, the more careful prediction of scholastic aptitude for the variety of college programs and for other post-high school education gains priority.

During elementary school, a complete testing program will employ annually two discrete achievement series covering the major learning areas, the fall achievement testing program "diagnostic" in purpose, and the end of the year "evaluative."

If their imprecisions and fallacies are accounted for and they are not taken over seriously, the casual but general administration of interest inventories have a place as a provoker of both introspection and planning. Although the mass administration of either personality questionnaires or projective devices cannot be justified, recent development in the appraisal of one noncognitive area, that of level of aspiration and of motivation, promise the emergence of new devices from the laboratory into general use. McClelland's[54] work in the achievement motive suggests a new measurable dimension of fundamental significance to the assessment of children's behavior in school.

The use of cumulative, developmental information. Though painstakingly gathered and carefully preserved, this mass of only partially edited and frequently contradictory observations will only hide the living reality of the child, his wholeness, individuality and his growth behind a wall of paper until the accumulating record is brought into the matrix of communication surrounding the child in school. When the teacher, the principal, the counselor, the parent, and most importantly the child himself, begin to draw understanding and act more rationally, more purposefully and above all more sensitively, the developmental record has begun its work.

However, the first and fundamental rule is to avoid acting too quickly on too little data. The child's school experience should be so arranged that few significant differential decisions are made until a substantial body of sequential observations have been made. Of course, the teacher will plan and modify the daily experiences of the child in the light of her best judgment from whatever information exists, however fragmentary, partial, or conflicting; minor adjustments based on partial diagnosis will be tentatively tried; occasionally a crisis in the child's school life will demand a far-reaching decision. For most elementary school children comprehensive or inflexible rearrangements of the curriculum or of his associational patterns on the basis of any single or group of observations, qualitative or quantitative, overextends their predictive power and should be avoided. Any largely irreversible decisions, like "homogeneous grouping" cannot be supported by the essential evidence until the secondary school years. Rigorous adherence to the developmental age concept as a unifying concept should act as a brake on premature judgments. During the early school years, teachers and parents must wait for the child's pattern of growth and of characteristic response to emerge slowly from the developmental record.

The nomathetic-idiographic controversy. The actual effort to bring meaning out of the body of unseemingly unrelated observations places the teacher and the counselor into the center of the nomathetic-idiographic controversy. The decisions that face each individual or are faced for him by teachers and parents can best be conceptualized as problems in prediction. Describing, labelling, classifying, categorizing are only meaningful activities when this organizing effort improves our ability to anticipate behavior in some future situation.

To the variety of predictions made for and by the individual boy and girl, the nomatheticist has a preference for "hard" objective data, external reference points, and mathematical treatment; he seeks his solutions in extensive data about the comparable behavior of other individuals in parallel situations; his principal tool is probability theory. This actuarial approach to prediction rests most comfortably and securely on the psychometric, quantitative data in the individual record.

On the other hand, the idiographic approach to the organization of the observational material seeks to make predictions on the basis of an intensive study of each individual life without comparative mathematical references; the attitudes are clinical, phenomenological, molar, non-statistical; its methodology emphasizes a search among the data for unique patterns of relationship, for internal lawfulness, for consistency and its sometimes more revealing converse, sharp discontinuities. The idiographic approach is typified by the case study or case conference.

In the handling of the complex body of quantitative and qualitative observations, the teacher or counselor who gathers, mediates, or interprets cannot take one position or the other. Both approaches must be employed simultaneously and sequentially; all the pertinent data whatever its nature should be mobilized for the variety of choices individual boys and girl must make and for the decisions that are made around them.

In pointing out that some aspects of a large number of the decisions surrounding the educational progress are purely actuarial in nature, Meehl [55] suggests that a trained clerk can make the required predictions by combining the relevant observations in the record mechanically and mathematically. This employment of statistical clerks and computing machines for norm-centered predictions would free teachers and counselors for the better handling, artistically and clinically, of the larger individual decisions through case studies and counseling.

It should be noted that recently a promising statistical procedure, Stephenson's [56] Q-technique has appeared for the mathematical treatment of idiographic materials within a single case. Cronbach [57] proposes that the newer mathematics of decision-making in games theory better serves individual decision-making than regression equations and prediction formulas.

The dispersion of organized and interpreted observations. To make the accumulating developmental record serve the needs of boys and girls, the critical information must be communicable and communicated. In whole or in selected parts, it must be transferred in a meaningful way to subsequent teachers, to other schools, to psychiatric clinics and other social agencies and, most importantly, to the individual pupil. Around each of these regular interchanges are special problems of form, language, confidentiality.

Professional communication is channeled through a dual system of records. A compact central office form, the permanent legal record, contains summarized biographical data, teacher's marks and significant test scores. A code indicates where the more detailed and confidential information is maintained. The pupil personnel folder, a partially structured file, will contain all the qualitative and quantitative assessments in their original form and is maintained by the child's teacher in elementary school and by the counselor in the secondary schools.

In spite of developmental curves, profiles, check-list reporting systems, and conferences, we still lack ways of telling parents, untrained in appraisal methodology and deeply involved in the progress of the child, what we have learned sensitively, precisely, without value loading, and within the safe limits of sound probability statements. Nor have we found secure techniques of providing children with information about their own many-sided development so that they grow toward greater congruence in their self-concept. This remains one of the great challenges of modern education.

X

THE PROTECTION
AND PROMOTION OF HEALTHY
DEVELOPMENT THROUGH
COMMUNITY HEALTH SERVICES

WILLIAM M. SCHMIDT

". . . In short, the opening of the twentieth century finds us all, to the dismay of the old-fashioned individualist, thinking in terms of communities."
Sidney Webb, *The Nineteenth Century* (1901) vol. 1.

The increasing emphasis and effort devoted to the study of child health and development in this twentieth century has been, in part, a reflection of the growing recognition of the community's influence on the well-being of children and of the community's responsibility for children. About the turn of the century a number of hitherto unrelated and relatively isolated activities on behalf of children began to find common cause, and to express themselves through organizations national in scope, and oriented to community action. The transactions of the conferences of these organizations, the documents of the first White House Conference on Children, and those relating to the act establishing the United States Children's Bureau served to awaken public interest, to lay the groundwork and promote the organization of communities on local, state, and federal levels for child health and welfare. Since those days the Children's Bureau has been guided by its mandate to "investigate and report on all aspects of child life," and through grants-in-aid since 1935, to "extend and improve" maternal and child health programs, services for handicapped children, and child welfare services. Professional societies and voluntary organizations have made important contributions. These developments are evidence of the extent to which the sense of community responsibility for children has become embedded in the fabric of opinion concerning public policy.

During this period advances in the saving of lives of mothers and children, in preventing disease, and in promoting child welfare have been spectacular. The risk of death for mothers in pregnancy and childbirth has fallen from 73 per 10,000 live births in the period 1915–1919 to less than 5 — a decrease of 95 per cent. Infant mortality has been brought down from nearly 100 infant deaths per thousand live births in 1915 by approximately 75 per cent. Deaths of children after infancy have also declined sharply. Much less information is available concerning fetal deaths, but in this respect too there appears to have been a significant decrease. The serious communicable diseases, which caused so much illness and death among children, notably diphtheria, smallpox, and typhoid and paratyphoid fever, now occur very infrequently.

Over this period of time, safeguards have been thrown up to protect children and youth from premature, hazardous, or inappropriate employment. Schooling has been extended, and whereas in 1900 one-third of the States had no school attendance laws, all now require attendance at least to age 16. Fewer children are now cared for in public institutions (because of dependency or neglect) and child welfare services, with full-time workers, have been extended to cover more than half the counties.

As advances occur in the protection and promotion of healthy development, goals too are advanced, or, at any rate, redefined and altered. We are, inevitably, always on the road toward completing the tasks set for us in former years, and always confronted with a gap between current practice and current knowledge. It is the continuous effort to narrow this gap which motivates child health workers and their colleagues in related disciplines. Before considering the present status of community organization for child health, it will be useful to restate some of the principles which have emerged in previous chapters. We may use these as bench-marks against which to measure the practices in common use today.

The continuity of growth and development. Transitions from the characteristics of one age period to another are very gradual, with the exception of a few very rapid transformations (fetus to neonate, prepubescent stage to puberty). Even in these and other episodes of rapid change the slowly evolving, orderly patterns of physical and psychological development form the determining substrate with which environmental forces interact. It is reasonable to suppose that continuity of medical, social, and related services to children by the same personnel over long periods of time would give the fullest appreciation of each child's characteristic pattern of development, and therefore the soundest basis for adapting services to each child's particular needs and potentialities.

Individual differences in rates of growth and degrees of change in development. The general patterns of progress, and the orderly sequence of changes in each period are subject to marked differences among children with respect to rate of change. These individual differences occur in infants and children who are adequate in every way. The wide range of such differences in the various developmental characteristics has been emphasized by longitudinal growth studies. Whether the individual child is manifesting a changed rate of development as a variation within expected limits or as a consequence of adverse events is a problem calling for judgment based on assessment of the individual.

Interrelations between illness experience and growth and development. In appraising a child's health it is necessary to take into account his susceptibility to illness and the rapidity of his recovery. During episodes of illness, the management of the child can be the more suitably individualized the better his individual characteristics are known. When children are under care for chronic illness or handicapping conditions, it is essential that they continue to receive complete health supervision, with special attention to the effect of the illness on the growth and development of the child, and its relation to nutritional requirements and other needs. These considerations lead to the conviction that the child should have the advantage of care by the same physician, and other personnel, for health supervision and for care during illness.

The child's physical well-being and psychological development are closely related to the health and well-being of his family. Of all the environmental factors with which he interacts, the family exerts the most profound and lasting influence upon the health and development of the child. Provision of the child's basic needs depends primarily upon the family. Illness in family members, whether infectious or not, may affect the child directly or indirectly. Progress in physical, emotional, and intellectual development are highly dependent upon the opportunities and experiences, the stimulation and encouragement which the family offers. To assess correctly the child's development and to provide fully for his health supervision, knowledge of the family is essential, and the care of the child should be an inseparable part of the plan for provision of care for the family. Pediatricians in their care of the child recognize this.

Social implications of pregnancy, and of infant and child care. Social factors are interwoven with attitudes and reactions to pregnancy and child care. Whether one considers problems such as housing or financial need, or cultural or interpersonal influences which tend to strengthen or weaken marital and family ties, their importance deserves recognition and their complexity requires skill and experience in those who are working with families. Moreover, timeliness in providing help to families with social problems is crucial, and harmony in the planning and conduct of medical and social services is indispensable. The way in which health and social services are made available to families in relation to child bearing and child rearing is therefore as important as is the availability of such services.

Reaching families to provide appropriate services for mothers and children is best achieved by a working group which includes, in addition to the physician and other professional workers, public health nurses. As with social services, so also with public health nursing: by itself its usefulness is limited; fully associated with the medical component in planning and execution, public health nursing is of great value in protecting the health of mothers and children.

We are primarily considering specific community health and social services. It must be emphasized, however, that such services operate in the framework of abundance or scarcity of community resources which meet basic needs. Stable employment with adequate income for the wage earner, adequate housing at reasonable rents, safe recreational facilities under imaginative direction, and schools sufficient in number with teaching staffs properly budgeted: these are environmental conditions of primordial importance for children. Those who are serving children professionally, even more than others in the community, may well contribute to the development of community opinion on these subjects, and to the formation of public policy.

The child population. The census of 1950 showed that about 26 per cent of the U. S. population is under 14 years of age — approximately 40 million children. The youth, from 14 to 18 years of age, form over 8 per cent of the total population — 13 million. For the U. S. as a whole there are 1.4 adults in the "productive" ages (20–64 years) for every child and youth dependent. The proportion of children had been declining since 1900, but since 1940 has again been rising. We now have nearly as great a proportion of children under 5 years as we did at the turn of the century. At the same time, the proportion of those in the age group 65 years and over has doubled. To the extent that these trends continue, we shall have relatively fewer earning and tax-paying adults, who must provide always more adequately, we hope, for the dependent age groups.

Some two-thirds of our total population is classified as of "urban" residence. In urban areas the child and youth population constitutes 31 per cent of the total, in rural nonfarm areas, 38 per cent, and in rural farm areas, 42 per cent. Thus the nonurban communities have fewer adults relative to their child and youth population, and the lower level of rural incomes adds to the difficulty of providing adequate local services. The need of such communities for State and Federal assistance was recognized in the Social Security Act, which, in its sections relating to children, expresses the purpose to extend and improve services "especially in rural areas." Urban areas have their own problems, however, since the suburbanization movement has left a larger proportion of lower income families in the central cities.

Of the 53 million children, over 4 million were living with a single parent, according to the data of the last census. The homes of 2.5 million had been broken by widowhood (1.7 million) and divorce (0.9 million). The remainder were living with a single parent because of separation, absence of a parent in military or civilian employment elsewhere, or prolonged illness of a parent. Expressed in terms of families with children, $7\frac{1}{2}$ per cent have a single parent. Of these almost half have lost a parent through death, and almost equally many because of divorce or separation. Prolonged physical or mental illness is an important factor in the remainder. This group of broken families may be considered to be at special risk, insofar as the healthy development of their children is concerned, both because of the loss of the wage-earning or care-taking parent, and because of the frequently unhappy events which have led up to the loss.

Families with three or more children constitute only 18 per cent of the population, but include 54 per cent of the child population. Family median income is lower for families with more than three children than for those with a smaller number. In order to supplement the family income both parents often seek employment. In 1950 some 15 per cent of children were in families with both parents working. This is not limited to families with older children, for about 2.5 million mothers with children of preschool age were working, in addition to 2.9 million mothers, all of whose children were of school age.

The assessment of adequacy and planning for improvement and additions to existing services must be based upon accurate knowledge of the population concerned. Census data, birth and death certificate information, housing authority surveys, school censuses and other local sources of information provide a basis for assembling the significant demographic characteristics needed. The question which those who provide services for children must ask themselves is not "How much have we done?" but rather "How much have we done in proportion to the total community need?" To the extent that the total need is not met, the limiting factors are sought by examining the structure and function of community agencies in relation to the population characteristics. Health and welfare councils, and community fund organizations logically fulfill this community-wide evaluative function. Special studies, however, may be needed, especially in the absence of such organizations of community agencies.

The general pattern of services for children. The services with which we are concerned are provided by private and public resources. Maternal care, and care of children (both preventive and curative) are, for the most part, provided by physicians in private practice. In large cities, two-thirds of maternity patients receive care from private physicians, and in smaller towns and rural areas, the proportion is even higher. For child health supervision, 9 of 10 visits are to private practitioners. Care of sick children is provided to a certain extent by pediatric clinics, but such clinics are most commonly found in the larger urban centers.

One of the most extensive studies of child health services was that of the American Academy of Pediatrics. It was published a decade ago, and although a new study would be desirable, there is reason to believe that in its broad outlines the Academy's findings still hold. It showed that, of the total volume of medical care (and health supervision) for children, over three-fourths was provided by home and office visits of physicians, a large part of the remainder by hospitals, and only a small fraction by clinics in out-patient departments or those of community health services. As one would expect, most of the private physician care of children is provided by general practitioners on a country-wide basis. Even in the larger urban centers where pediatricians and other specialists are more numerous they are providing for only a minority of the children.

Voluntary health insurance covers the cost of a part of the care mothers and children receive from private physicians and hospitals. It is reported that over 120 million individuals are covered to some extent by such insurance programs. However, some are covered only for hospital costs, fewer have coverage also for surgical and nonsurgical medical care costs, and provision for preventive services is very limited. Generally these plans affect only the means of payment for care, and not the method of organizing and providing the services. There are programs, however, which have introduced methods of group practice, established standards of care, and undertaken evaluations of the quality of services.

Public medical care programs are those provided by government and, to a great extent, are on the basis of family financial need. Such programs, with few exceptions, are administered by welfare departments, for welfare is concerned with the basic needs of families, of which medical care is one. However, the need for close relations with health departments is obvious, particularly with respect to utilization of the preventive services. For example prenatal clinics, child-health conferences, public health nursing, and other services are required by clients in the child welfare programs, aid to dependent children, and general assistance programs, and welfare workers help make such services available to the families they are serving by means of appropriate referrals. However, medical care and preventive services need be so closly interlinked that, in the minds of some, unification of such programs as a part of health department community responsibility is a logical next step.

One of the most significant of the public medical care programs in the United States is the provision of care by states, with the aid of federal funds, for handicapped children. These programs are administered in most states by the state department of public health, and in some by the state welfare department, or other agency of government. The Social Security Act, which authorizes grants-in-aid to states for these programs, and lays down the conditions for these grants does not require that a "means test" should be used to establish eligibility of families for care of their crippled children. For obvious reasons, diagnostic services are provided without a preliminary financial screening, but families are requested to participate in the actual cost of care according to their possibilities.

These programs, which served 280 thousand children in 1955, provide care for children with a wide variety of handicapping conditions and chronic illnesses. The programs provide clinic and other services of physicians, hospital care, convalescent home care, and a wide variety of auxiliary services. It must be emphasized that these programs are not mere provisions to pay for the cost of care, in full or in part, but to assure the provision of the full range of necessary services in an integrated fashion.

Mention has been made of preventive health services, often provided by state or local health agencies, by voluntary agencies, and, with respect to services for school children, often by education departments. It has been noted that prenatal clinics, and child health clinics for infants and preschool children serve a comparatively small proportion of pregnant women and of children below school age. The groups that are reached, however, include many who are at a disadvantage from the social, economic, or educational point of view. How many go without such care is not known. Special studies have shown that in large cities as many as 20 per cent of pregnant women receive no care in pregnancy, or begin care so late that it is of limited value. Moreover, it is known that many child health clinics are so understaffed and overburdened, that each child may receive only a few minutes of the physician's time. Prenatal clinics and child health clinics, with few exceptions, provide only preventive services. When medical care is needed for an intercurrent condition, or for some associated handicap or chronic illness, referral must be made elsewhere.

School systems accept a certain degree of responsibility for the health of school children either directly or through cooperative arrangements with health departments. There is no question as to the need for health education and provision for environmental health and safety. However, there are considerable differences in different school systems in the program for periodic health examinations, arrangement for examinations of pupils referred by teachers or others, and procedures for specialist consultation. In some school systems, physicians appointed by, or assigned to the school perform periodic health examinations and examine children who are referred. In others every effort is made to have such personal health services performed by physicians in private practice. The economic level of the families whose children form a given school population is one of the factors involved in determining these policies of a school health service. Differences also exist in the form of nursing service: in some systems "school nurses" are employed, in others public health nurses carry the school service as a part of their total program.

In any case the object should be an effort to assure the consistent observation of children in terms of health, growth and development, with attention to school progress and problems, and to arrange for care during illness or specialist consultation for handicapping conditions in a unified — or at the least — a well coordinated plan.

This general and necessarily incomplete account of medical care and health services for mothers and children indicates that there is unevenness and disparity of services according to social and economic groups and, it may be added, geographically, throughout the country. It is known that children in isolated counties receive less care, and less care from specialists, than do children who live in or near urban areas. Disparities exist in the proportion of handicapped children under care, and the differences are not to be accounted for entirely by differences in need. The basis exists, however, for diminishing these differences in the levels of care for children, and for improving child health programs generally. There is a nation-wide framework for evaluating services, for establishing and maintaining standards, and for planning and administering programs: the state departments of health.

The administration of child health services in the United States. In each state health department there exists a Division of Maternal and Child Health. These divisions carry the basic responsibility for planning and administration to "extend and improve" maternal and child health services, to assure the extension of such services under local administration, and to cooperate with medical, nursing, and welfare groups to these ends. Each state prepares a plan and budget periodically as a basis for the grants-in-aid it receives from federal appropriations to the Children's Bureau. These plans and budgets are the working documents which guide the state health department in its operation.

Programs will naturally vary from state to state, depending upon many factors. It is not so much the specific program activities with which we are here concerned, as with the general methods available to maternal and child health directors to work toward the program goals they have established. First is the responsibility to *investigate and report.* Reference has been made to the primary need for demographic information, and detailed knowledge of agencies serving children. Equally necessary is a continuing flow of current information on births and deaths, with detail on birth weights, complications of pregnancy, labor, and delivery, ages at death, causes of death, and other data. Local, as well as state-wide, analyses of vital records and of other reports, must be made, as well as special studies on utilization of health services, and special health and social problems. The results of such investigations must be appropriately reported, both to the professions concerned, and to the public. Such studies are intended to lead to action to *extend and improve* child health services. There are a number of forms which such action may take.

(1) Aid to localities. To be fully successful, maternal and child health services should be brought as close to the families to be served as possible. This is most readily achieved when they are administered by local health units. Not all of our counties and local administrative jurisdictions are covered as yet by full-time professional local health departments. It is self-evident that extension of local health agencies provides the basis for extension of local maternal and child health services. Existing local health agencies often need, and many receive, financial and technical aid from the state health department to strengthen their local maternal and child health services.

(2) Cooperation with professional and voluntary agency groups. Medical societies have long been interested and active in the effort to strengthen services for children, and have expressed this interest through the work of standing committees. Specialist organizations, such as the Academy of Pediatrics have made notable contributions. The cooperation of state divisions of maternal and child health with these and other professional groups has led to such valuable contributions as maternal mortality studies, and more recently, perinatal mortality studies, to accident control programs, and to education of the public concerning immunization, nutrition, and other aspects of child health protection.

(3) Establishment and maintenance of standards. Standards for maternity care, child health supervision, school health services, for care of children away from their own homes, in fact for all aspects of maternal and child health, may be established by law, regulation, or as advisory standards. In any case, the factual results of studies are secured, the expert opinion of specialists obtained, and the professional groups concerned are consulted prior to the issuance of such standards. Whatever the form of such standards, the intent is in large measure educational. The goal is to secure voluntary compliance. To this end, the issuance of standards is generally complemented by the provision of qualified consultant services to aid clinics, hospitals, or agencies to comply.

(4) Joint activities with welfare and education departments. The need for such joint activity has been presented. The implementation takes place at all levels, with the guidance and example of the state agencies. Joint planning for policy and procedure can be achieved through inter-

departmental committees, the more easily, of course, when the directors and staffs have been closely associated in case conferences, special studies, and training programs.

(5) Direct services. To the extent that areas of the state are lacking in needed services, and lacking in local resources and personnel, the state may provide direct services. It may still be necessary to rely upon itinerant clinics, travelling to outlying areas from time to time, but far to be preferred is the provision of means, including detailing of personnel, to permit on-going services to be built up locally.

Do existing services accord with the principles which have been outlined? Because of the unevenness of health services it is clear that there will be variations in the degree to which they correspond to the principles which have been developed. One may visualize the family in comfortable circumstances, whose children and other family members receive health supervision and medical care during illness from the same family physician, and who have ready access to specialist and auxiliary services as they may be needed; and, on the other extreme, the family of a migratory worker, lacking for most of the year a fixed place of abode, and with health supervision and medical care changing as the place of work shifts with the crops. Most of the population, very likely, is somewhere between these extremes.

Mobility of families is one factor which militates against continuity of care. In 1950 18 per cent of families moved within the year and 5.5 per cent to a different county. The proportion is much higher for the families with a younger head. For families in which the head of the household was under 35 years of age, 33 per cent moved within the year, and 10 per cent to a different county. We are a mobile people, and since this impediment to continuity of care cannot be eliminated, its effect must be minimized by giving thought to referral of families about to move, and transfer of pertinent information, with their consent, to the physicians or clinics from whom they will be expected to receive care in the future.

Another factor tending to run counter to the principles we have outlined is that the organization of services often tends to split health supervision from medical care during illness and to divide services according to the age groups of children. These difficulties do not exist for families who have, indeed, a family practitioner, but for many others they are real and important. For example, a family of low income or one receiving welfare assistance may have the mother under prenatal care at a city hospital, the preschool children receiving health supervision from a city child health clinic, the children of school age receiving health supervision from a school health service, and one or more members of the family receiving care during illness either from a hospital out-patient service, a private physician, or both. Moreover, even within each of these services there may be a rotation of physicians, so that, within a given year, a dozen or more different physicians may be caring for the same family. It is to be doubted that all, or perhaps any, have a reasonably complete picture of the family's health problems and of the surrounding circumstances, and the family must often find frustrating confusion in the multiple and changing relationships with physicians.

However, even when financial limitations are not involved there often is a lack of a "family doctor." No doubt sociological changes and the increasing need for specialization are at play, and one can be sure that, in many instances, exchange of information among the physicians involved helps to overcome inconsistency and confusion. But this is hardly enough, for as we have seen, it is not only an appreciation of the health problems of all the family members which is needed, but also of the social factors. Cabot expressed this when he wrote that for a complete and exact diagnosis he needed information about the patient's "home, his work, his family, his worries, his nutrition." Thus medical social work, nutrition and other disciplines have come into the picture. To supplement the medical and teaching function of the physician, the public health nurse is needed. These important, indeed in many instances, essential related professional services are not as frequently available as they should be, and may be largely lacking for patients who are seen in private practice.

As one reviews the case records of children who have developed impairment of physical or psychological development, it is clear that the concentration of skilled effort devoted to their problems and to the surrounding family circumstances often begins only when the problems are far advanced. Years may have passed during which many physicians, nurses, teachers, social workers and other individuals and agencies dealt with one or another episode in the long story of disordered development. "For all too long a period" George Baehr has said, "community effort . . . has been concentrated upon rehabilitating families approaching the end stages of social disaster. . . . Today we should be more concerned with the other end of the spectrum, the study of normal families as they exist in the community. Our orientation should be directed increasingly upon prevention and early detection of socio-medical problems within the family unit." There appears to be a potentiality for promoting healthy development of children in such an approach to comprehensive family care. A limited number of programs exist in this country which provide, to varying degrees, comprehensive care for families by groups of physicians who are aided by appropriate medical specialists, nurses, and social workers. No doubt there will be further developments in the same direction under voluntary auspices such as trade unions and other nonprofit groups, and perhaps under governmental auspices or with governmental assistance.

However, much can be done to provide for greater consistency and continuity in health supervision and medical care of children under existing patterns of care. For example, hospital maternity care might to a greater extent be so planned that the physician who sees the mother during pregnancy attends her during labor and delivery and in the postpartum period. Promptness in transferring a well-prepared abstract of the maternity case record to those who are to provide infant health supervision would help to fill the gap which often occurs at this point. Provision to unite health supervision and medical care during illness, at least for those children who must receive both from public sources can certainly be envisaged. Health services for school age children could be regularly incorporated into a general child health program, so that even if the same physicians, nurses, and others cannot continue the care of their child patients from the preschool period through the school years (which would be most desirable), the records would provide a continuous picture of development and of health status. Other approaches to coordination of care involving the community social agencies can be conceived.

In all planning for community services for children, it is the individuality of each child as expressed in his progress in growth and development which must be held firmly in mind. The programs of agencies which have the aim of meeting the health and social needs of children may be appraised in terms of the extent to which the individual developmental characteristics of children are fully taken into consideration. Are agency policies designed to avoid splitting of services according to the age of children or the type of problem? And finally, to what extent is the best type of care the community can provide available to all children of the community?

The opportunity to promote the healthy development of children is an opportunity to help them to be apt for their future family responsibilities. Thus better adaptation to environment, as environment itself changes, may be promoted.

List of Contributors

Notes and General References

Index

CONTRIBUTORS

HAROLD C. STUART, M.D. Pediatrics and Preventive Medicine: Professor of Maternal and Child Health, Emeritus, Harvard University, School of Public Health.

DANE G. PRUGH, M.D. Pediatrics and Psychiatry: Associate Professor of Pediatrics and Psychiatry, University of Rochester, School of Medicine and Dentistry.

ROBERT H. ANDERSON, Ph.D. Education: Associate Professor of Education and Director of Elementary School Internship, Harvard University, Graduate School of Education.

BERTHA S. BURKE, A.M. Nutrition: Associate Professor of Maternal and Child Nutrition, Harvard University, School of Public Health.

RUTH M. BUTLER, S.M. Social Work: Associate Professor of Social Work Research, Boston College School of Social Work.

GERALD CAPLAN, M.D. Psychiatry: Associate Professor of Mental Health, Harvard University, School of Public Health.

STANLEY COBB, M.D. Neurology: Bullard Professor of Neuropathology, Emeritus, Harvard University, Medical School.

MORRIS L. COGAN, Ed.D. Education: Lecturer on Education and Director of Secondary School Apprentice Teaching, Harvard University, Graduate School of Education.

GEORGE E. GARDNER, M.D. Psychiatry: Clinical Professor of Psychiatry, Harvard University, Medical School; Director, Judge Baker Guidance Center, Boston, Mass.

THEODORE H. INGALLS, M.D. Preventive Medicine: Professor of Preventive Medicine and Public Health, University of Pennsylvania School of Medicine.

JOHANNES IPSEN, Jr., M.D. Microbiology: Associate Professor of Public Health, Harvard University, School of Public Health; Superintendent of State Laboratory Institute, Massachusetts Department of Public Health.

SAMUEL B. KIRKWOOD, M.D. Obstetrics: Lecturer on Maternal Health, Harvard University, School of Public Health.

DONALD C. KLEIN, Ph.D. Psychology and Mental Health: Instructor in Mental Health, Harvard University, School of Public Health, and Research Associate in Psychology in the Department of Psychiatry, Medical School.

ERICH LINDEMANN, M.D. Psychiatry: Professor of Psychiatry, Harvard University, Medical School.

ELIZABETH S. MAKKAY, M.D. Psychiatry: Staff Psychiatrist, Judge Baker Guidance Center, Boston, Mass.

LOVICK C. MILLER, Ph.D. Psychology: Chief Psychologist, Louisville Child Guidance Clinic, and Associate Professor of Medical Psychology, University of Louisville Medical School, Louisville, Ky.

JOHN C. PALMER, M.A. Education and Psychology: Associate Professor of Education, Tufts University, Medford, Mass.

ELIZABETH P. RICE, M.S. Social Work: Associate Professor of Public Health Social Work, Harvard University, School of Public Health.

WILLIAM M. SCHMIDT, M.D. Pediatrics and Preventive Medicine: Associate Professor of Maternal and Child Health, Harvard University, School of Public Health.

KATHERINE SPENCER, Ph.D. Social Work: Associate Professor, Boston University School of Social Work.

PAULINE G. STITT, M.D. Pediatrics and Preventive Medicine: Assistant Professor of Maternal and Child Health, Harvard University, School of Public Health.

ISABELLE VALADIAN, M.D. Child Health and Development: Associate in Child Health, Harvard University, School of Public Health.

NOTES

NOTES TO CHAPTER I: THE PRINCIPLES OF GROWTH AND DEVELOPMENT

1. S. G. Driscoll and D. Y. Hsia, "The development of enzyme systems during early infancy," *Pediatrics 22* (1958), 785–845.

2. U. S. Public Health Service, "Monthly vital statistics report," in *Annual summary for 1958* (Government Printing Office, Washington, 1959), vol. 7.

3. *Accidents in childhood: facts as a basis for prevention* (Technical Report Series, 118; World Health Organization, Geneva, 1957).

4. R. Haggerty, "Home accidents in childhood," *New England J. Med. 260* (1959), 1322–1331.

5. *Accidental poisoning in childhood* (published for the Committee on Accident Prevention, American Academy of Pediatrics, Thomas, Springfield, Illinois, 1956).

NOTES TO CHAPTER II: DIFFERENCES IN THE CHARACTERISTICS OF CHILDHOOD
ILLNESSES AND IMMUNITY

1. H. C. Stuart, R. B. Reed, and associates, "Longitudinal studies of child health and development, Harvard School of Public Health, series II, no. 1: Description of project," *Pediatrics 24* (1959), 875–885.

2. S. D. Collins, K. S. Trantham, and J. L. Lehmann, "Sickness experience in selected areas of U. S." *Public Health Reports* (Government Printing Office, Washington, 1955), vol. 70, no. 1, monograph no. 25.

3. E. Sydenstricker, "Age curve of illness," *Public Health Report No. 42* (Government Printing Office, Washington, 1927), 1565–1576.

4. I. Valadian, H. C. Stuart, and R. B. Reed, "Patterns of illness experiences," *Pediatrics 24* (1959), 941–974.

5. I. Valadian, H. C. Stuart, and R. B. Reed, "Patterns of illness experiences by category of illness" (to be published).

6. E B.. Wilson, C. Bennett, M. Allen, and J. Worcester, "Measles and scarlet fever in Providence, R. I., 1929–1934, with respect to age and size of family," *Proc. Am. Phil. Soc. 80* (1939), 357–476.

7. W. Hammon, G. E. Sather, and N. Hollinger, "Preliminary report of epidemiological studies on poliomyelitis and streptococcal infections," *Am. J. Pub. Health 40* (1950), 293–306.

8. *Report of the committee on the control of infectious diseases* (American Academy of Pediatrics, Evanston, Illinois, 1957).

9. *Active immunization against common communicable diseases of childhood* (Technical Report Series, 6, World Health Organization, Geneva, 1950).

10. P. G. Stitt, "Usefulness of tuberculin testing in child health supervision," *J. Lancet* 79 (1959), 150–152.

NOTES TO CHAPTER III: THE PREGNANT WOMAN, THE FETUS, AND PREPARATION FOR MATERAL CARE OF THE INFANT

1. C. A. Smith, "Effects of birth processes and obstetric procedures upon the newborn infant," *Advances in Pediatrics* (Year Book Publishers, Chicago, 1948), III, 1–54.

2. Food and Nutrition Board, *Recommended dietary allowances* (Pub. 589; National Academy of Sciences–National Research Council, Washington, rev. ed., 1958).

3. B. S. Burke and H. C. Stuart, "Nutritional requirements during pregnancy and lactation," *J. A. M. A.* 137 (1948), 119–128; also chap. 15, *Handbook of nutrition* (Blakiston, Philadelphia, 2 ed., 1951).

4. K. U. Toverud, G. Stearns, and I. G. Macy, *Maternal nutrition and child health, an interpretative review* (Bull. 123; National Academy of Sciences–National Research Council, Washington, 1950).

5. H. A. Hunscher, "The life cycle and its diet," *J. Home Ec.* 49 (1957), 101–115.

6. B. S. Burke, "The dietary history as a tool in research," *J. Am. Dietet. A.* 23 (1947), 1041–1046.

7. R. B. Reed and B. S. Burke, "Collection and analysis of dietary intake data," *Am. J. Pub. Health* 44 (1954), 1015–1026.

8. B. S. Burke, S. S. Stevenson, J. Worcester, and H. C. Stuart, "Nutrition studies during pregnancy: V. Relation of maternal nutrition to condition of infant at birth: study of siblings," *J. Nutrition* 38 (1949), 453–467.

9. B. S. Burke, V. A. Beal, S. B. Kirkwood, and H. C. Stuart, "Nutrition studies during pregnancy: I. Problem, methods of study and group studied; II. Relation of prenatal nutrition to condition of infant at birth and during first two weeks of life; III. The relation of prenatal nutrition to pregnancy, labor, delivery and the postpartum period," *Am. J. Obst. & Gynec.* 46 (1943), 38–52.

10. C. A. Smith, J. Worcester, and B. S. Burke, "Maternal-fetal nutritional relationships. Effect of maternal diet on size and content of the fetal liver," *Obst. & Gynec.* 1 (1953), 46–58.

11. P. C. Jeans, M. B. Smith, and G. Stearns, "Incidence of prematurity in relation to maternal nutrition," *J. Am. Dietet. A.* 31 (1955), 576–581.

12. J. M. Woodhill, A. S. van den Berg, B. S. Burke, and F. J. Stare, "Nutrition studies of pregnant Australian women. I. Maternal nutrition in relation to toxemia of pregnancy and physical condition of infant at birth. II. Maternal diet and the duration of lactation," *Am. J. Obst. & Gynec.* 70 (1955), 987–1003.

13. M. M. Eliot, "Deaths around birth — the national score," *J. A. M. A.* 167 (1958), 945–949.

14. B. S. Burke, V. V. Harding, and H. C. Stuart, "Nutrition studies during pregnancy. IV. Relation of protein content of mother's diet during pregnancy to birth length, birth weight and condition of infant at birth," *J. Pediat.* 23 (1943), 506–515.

15. W. T. Tompkins and D. G. Wiehl, "Nutritional deficiencies as a causal

factor in toxemia and premature labor," *Am. J. Obst. & Gynec. 62* (1951), 898–919.

16. R. H. J. Hamlin, "The prevention of eclampsia and pre-eclampsia," *Lancet 262* (1952), 64–68.

17. B. S. Burke, and S. B. Kirkwood, "Problems and methods in nutrition services for pregnant women," *Am. J. Pub. Health 40* (1950), 960–965.

18. B. S. Burke, "Diet during pregnancy," *Am. J. Clin. Nutr. 2* (1954), 425–428.

19. R. Bernstein and F. E. Cyr, "A study of interviews with husbands in a prenatal and child health program," *Social Casework 38* (1957), 473–480.

20. T. Benedek, "The psychosomatic implications of the primary unit: mother-child," *Am. J. Orthopsychiat. 19* (1949), 642–654.

21. T. Benedek, *Psychosexual functions in women* (Ronald, New York, 1952).

22. F. D. Kartchner, "Study of emotional reactions during labor," *Am. J. Obst. & Gynec. 60* (1950), 19–29.

23. *Standards and recommendations for hospital care of newborn infants — full-term and premature* (American Academy of Pediatrics, Evanston, Illinois, 1954).

24. G. Dick-Read, *Childbirth without fear* (Harper, New York, rev. ed., 1953).

GENERAL REFERENCES

N. J. Eastman, *Williams obstetrics* (Appleton-Century-Crofts, New York, 11 ed., 1956).

J. Warkany, "Etiology of congenital malformations," in *Advances in Pediatrics 2* (Interscience, New York, 1947), 1–63.

T. H. Ingalls, "Preventive prenatal pediatrics," in *Advances in Pediatrics 6* (Year Book Publishers, Chicago, 1953), 33–62.

R. McIntosh, et al., "The incidence of congenital malformations in a study of 5964 pregnancies," *Pediatrics 14* (1954), 505–522.

J. Bowlby, *Maternal care and mental health* (Monograph Series, 2, World Health Organization, Geneva, 1952).

I. M. Josselyn, "The family as a psychological unit," *Social Casework 34* (1953), 336–343.

M. B. Kantor, et al., "Socio-economic level and maternal attitudes toward parent-child relationships," *Hum. Org. 16* (1958), 44–48.

K. Young, "What strong family life means to our society," *Social Casework 34* (1953), 323–329.

B. A. Wooten, "A psychosomatic approach to maternity care," *Pub. Health Nursing 44* (1952), 493–499.

NOTES TO CHAPTER IV: PHYSICAL GROWTH AND DEVELOPMENT

1. C. M. Drillien, "Studies in prematurity, part 4: Development and progress of the prematurely born child in the preschool period," *Arch. Dis. Childhood 23* (1948), 69–83.

2. A. M. Gesell, *Infant development — the embryology of early infant behavior* (Harper, New York, 1952).

3. A. M. Gesell, et al., *Vision: its development in infant and child* (Harper, New York, 1949).

4. A. H. Keeney, *Chronology of ophthalmic development* (Thomas, Springfield, Illinois, 1951).

5. W. H. Sheldon, S. S. Stevens, W. B. Tucker, *The varieties of human physique* (Harper, New York, 1940).

6. A. Gesell, et al., *The first five years of life* (Harper, New York, 1940).

7. "Report of the Committee on School Health of the American Academy of Pediatrics," *Pediatrics 18* (1956), 672–676.

8. H. C. Stuart, "Obesity in childhood," *Quart. Rev. Pediat. 10* (1955), 131–145.

9. F. K, Shuttleworth, "Sexual maturation and the physical growth of girls age six to nineteen," *Monographs of the Soc. for Research in Child Develop. 2* (1937), Serial No. 12, number 5. "The adolescent period — a graphic and pictorial atlas," *Monographs of the Soc. for Research in Child Develop. 3* (1938), Serial No. 16, number 3. (Based on data collected by Dearborn, et al. in Harvard Growth Study).

10. N. Bayley and R. Tuddenham, "Adolescent changes in body build," in *Adolescence,* Part I of 43rd Yearbook, National Society for Study of Education (University of Chicago Press, Chicago 1944), 33–54.

11. K. Simmons and W. W. Greulich, "Menarcheal age and the height, weight and skeletal age of girls age 7–17 years," *J. Pediat. 22* (1943), 518–548.

12. W. W. Greulich, et al., "Somatic and endocrine studies of puberal and adolescent boys," *Monographs of the Soc. for Research in Child Develop. 7* (1942), Serial No. 33, number 3.

GENERAL REFERENCES

A. H. Parmelee, *The management of the newborn* (Yearbook Publishers, Chicago, 1952).

E. C. Dunham, *Premature infants, a manual for physicians* (Hoeber, New York, 2 ed., 1955).

H. Koenig, "What happens to prematures?" *Am. J. Pub. Health 40* (1950), 803–807.

M. Green, J. B. Richmond, *Pediatric diagnosis* (Saunders, Philadelphia, 1955).

J. M. Tanner, *Growth at adolescence* (Thomas, Springfield, Ill., 1955).

NOTES TO CHAPTER V: NUTRITION

1. Food and Nutrition Board, *Recommended dietary allowances* (Pub. 589, National Academy of Sciences–National Research Council, Washington, rev. ed., 1958).

2. P. György, "A hitherto unrecognized biochemical difference between human milk and cow's milk," *Pediatrics 11* (1953), 98–108.

J. A. Johnston, "Protein requirements of adolescents," *Ann. New York Sc. 69* (1958), 881–901.

J. A. Johnston, "Nutritional problems of adolescence," *J. A. M. A. 137*), 1587–1589.

H. A. Waisman, J. B. Richmond, and S. J. Williams, "Vitamin require- ts in adolescence," *J. Pediat. 37* (1950), 922–925.

8. *Health of teen-agers* (Statistical Bull. 34, Metropolitan Life Insurance npany, New York, 1953).

GENERAL REFERENCES

U. S. Department of Health, Education, and Welfare, *Your child from 1 to 6* (Children's Bureau Pub. 30, Washington, rev. ed., 1956).

——— *Nutrition and healthy growth* (Children's Bureau Pub. 352, Washington, 1955).

——— *Your child from 6 to 12* (Children's Bureau Pub. 324, Washington, 1949).

E. A. Martin, *Roberts' nutrition work with children* (University of Chicago Press, Chicago, 1954).

C. A. Aldrich and M. M. Aldrich, *Feeding our old-fashioned children* (Macmillan, New York, 1941).

NOTES TO CHAPTER VI: BACKGROUND FACTORS RELATED TO

PSYCHO-SOCIAL DEVELOPMENT

1. F. Kallman, *Heredity in health and mental disorder* (Norton, New York, 1953).

2. G. Draper, C. W. Dupertius, and J. L. Caughey, *Human constitution in clinical medicine* (Hoeber, New York, 1945).

3. E. Kretschmer, *Physique and character* (Harcourt, Brace, New York, 1925).

4. W. H. Sheldon, *The varieties of temperament* (Harper, New York, 1942).

5. A. Davis, *Social class influences upon learning* (Harvard University Press, Cambridge, 1948).

6. J. H. Masserman, *Behavior and neuroses* (University of Chicago Press, Chicago, 1943).

7. K. Lewin, *Field theory in social science* (Harper, New York, 1951).

8. S. Isaacs, *Social development of young children, a study of beginnings* (Harcourt, Brace, New York, 1933).

9. J. Piaget, 1929, *The child's conception of the world* (Humanities Press, New York, 1951).

10. P. S. Sears, "Doll play aggression in normal young children: influence of sex, age, sibling status, father's absence," *Psychol. Monogr. 65* (1951), 2654.

11. A. Freud and D. T. Burlingham, *Infants without families* (International Universities Press, New York, 1944).

12. R. A. Spitz, "Hospitalism: an inquiry into the genesis of psychiatric conditions in early childhood (I)," in *The psychoanalytic study of the child* (International Universities Press, New York, 1945), I, 53–74.

3. C. A. Smith, *The physiology of the ne*
field, Illinois, 2 ed., 1951), 253–262.

4. K. Bain, "The incidence of breast feedin
States," *Pediatrics 2* (1948), 313–320.

5. I. G. Macy, et al., "Human milk studies, 2
feeding and their investigation," *Am. J. Dis. Child.*

6. F. H. Richardson, "Breast feeding comes of age,
863–867.

7. B. S. Burke and H. C. Stuart, "Nutritional req
nancy and lactation," *J. A. M. A. 137* (1948), 119–128,
book of nutrition (Blakiston, Philadelphia, 2 ed., 1951).

8. P. C. Jeans, "Feeding of healthy infants and chil
nutrition (Blakiston, Philadelphia, 2 ed., 1951), 275–298.

9. I. G. Macy, H. J. Kelly, and R. E. Sloan, *The con*
(Pub. 254, National Academy of Sciences–National Research
ington, 1953).

10. D. C. Darrow, R. E. Cooke, and W. E. Segar, "Water
metabolism in infants fed cow's milk mixtures during heat stress,'
(1954), 602–617.

11. C. A. Smith, et al., "Persistence and utilization of maternal ire
formation during infancy," *J. Clin. Investigation 34* (1955), 1391–1

12. L. E. Holt, Jr., "Breast milk, cow's milk and infant nutrition
Rev. Pediat. 10 (1955), 79–89.

13. B. S. Burke, R. B. Reed, A. S. van den Berg, and H. C. Stuart,
tudinal studies of child health and development, Harvard School of
Health, series II, no. 4: Caloric and protein intakes of children one to eig
years of age," *Pediatrics 24* (1959), 922–940.

14. U. S. Department of Health, Education, and Welfare, *Infant c*
(Children's Bureau Pub. 8; Washington, 1955).

15. C. A. Aldrich and E. S. Hewitt, "A self-regulating feeding program fo
infants," *J. A. M. A. 135* (1947), 340–342.

16. E. C. Dunham, *Premature infants: a manual for physicians* (Hoeber,
New York, 2 ed., 1955) chap. 7, 130–157.

17. G. Stearns, et al., "The protein requirements of children from one to ten
years of age," *Ann. New York Acad. Sc. 69* (1958), 857–868.

18. N. B. Talbot, E. H. Sobel, B. S. Burke, E. Lindemann and S. B. Kaufman,
"Dwarfism in healthy children: its possible relation to emotional, nutritional
and endocrine disturbances," *New England J. Med. 236* (1947), 783–793.

19. I. G. Macy and H. A. Hunscher, "Calories — a limiting factor in the
growth of children," *J. Nutrition 45* (1951), 189–199.

20. C. D. Williams, "Kwashiorkor," *J. A. M. A. 153* (1953), 1280–1285.

21. J. C. Waterlow, ed., *Protein malnutrition* (Cambridge University Press:
Cambridge, England, 1955).

22. A. M. Thomson and D. L. Duncan, "The diagnosis of malnutrition in
man," *Nutrition Abst. & Rev. 24* (1954), 1–18.

23. T. D. Spies, "Influence of pregnancy, lactation, growth, and aging on
nutritional processes," *J. A. M. A. 153* (1953), 185–193.

24. S. Dreizen, et al., "Maturation of bone centers in hand and wrist of
children with chronic nutritive failure. Effect of dietary supplements of recon-
stituted milk solids," *Am. J. Dis. Child. 87* (1954), 429–439.

13. R. A. Spitz, "Anaclitic depression: an inquiry into the genesis of psychiatric conditions in early childhood (II)," in *Ibid.*, II (1946), 313–342.

14. J. W. M. Whiting and I. L. Child, *Child training and personality* (Yale University Press, New Haven, 1953).

15. N. E. Miller and J. Dollard, *Social learning and imitation* (Yale University Press, New Haven, 1941).

16. J. Bowlby, "The nature of the child's tie to his mother," *International J. Psychoanal. 39* (1958), 1.

17. K. Z. Lorenz, "The comparative method in studying innate behavior," in *Physiological mechanisms in animal behavior* (Symposia of Society for Experimental Biology, Cambridge University Press, Cambridge, England, 1950), vol. IV.

18. F. Kallman, *Heredity in health and mental disorder* (Norton, New York, 1953).

19. M. E. Fries, "Psychosomatic relationships between mother and infant," *Psychosom. Med. 6* (1944), 159–162.

20. W. H. Jost and L. W. Sontag, "The genetic factor in autonomic nervous system function," *Psychosom. Med. 6* (1944), 308–310.

21. J. B. Watson, *Psychology from the standpoint of a behaviorist* (Lippincott, Philadelphia, 1919).

22. G. L. Engel, "Homeostasis, behavior adjustment, and the concept of health and disease," in *Mid-century psychiatry* (Thomas, Springfield, Illinois 1953).

23. S. Freud, *A general introduction to psychoanalysis* (Garden City Publishing Company, New York, 1943).

24. W. B. Cannon, *The wisdom of the body* (Norton, New York, 1932).

25. J. Warkany, "Etiology of congenital malformations," in *Advances in Pediatrics 2* (Interscience, New York, 1947), 1–63.

26. T. H. Ingalls, "Pathogenesis of mongolism," *Am. J. Dis. Child 73* (1947), 279.

27. L. W. Sontag, "Differences in modifiability of fetal behavior and physiology," *Psychosom. Med. 6* (1944), 151–154.

28. O. Rank, *The trauma of birth* (Harcourt, Brace, New York, 1929).

29. W. A. Greene, Jr., "Early object relationships, somatic, affective, and personal. An inquiry into the physiology of the mother-child unit," *J. Nerv. & Ment. Dis. 126* (1958), 225.

30. P. Greenacre, "The predisposition to anxiety," *Psychoanalyt. Quart. 10* (1941), 610.

31. J. Bowlby, *Maternal care and mental health* (Monograph Series 2, World Health Organization, Geneva, 1954).

32. F. A. Allen, "Mother-child separation — process or event," *Emotional problems of early childhood* (Basic Books, New York, 1955), 325–327.

33. M. P. Middlemore, *The nursing couple* (Hamish Hamilton, London, 1941).

34. R. Spitz, personal communication.

GENERAL REFERENCES

S. Cobb, *Emotions and clinical medicine* (Norton, New York, 1950).

S. Cobb, *Foundations of neuropsychiatry* (Williams & Wilkins, Baltimore, 6 ed., 1957).

NOTES TO CHAPTER VII: PERSONALITY DEVELOPMENT THROUGHOUT
CHILDHOOD

1. A. R. Holway, "Early self-regulation of infants and later behavior in play interviews," *Am. J. Orthopsychiat.* 19 (1949), 612–623.

2. P. A. McLendon and J. Parks, "Nurseries designed for modern maternity," *Mod. Hosp.* 65 (1945), 46–49.

3. *Health supervision of young children* (American Public Health Association, New York, 1955).

4. M. P. Middlemore, *The nursing couple* (Hamish Hamilton, London, 1941).

5. C. A. Aldrich and E. S. Hewitt, "Self-regulatory feeding program for infants," *J. A. M. A. 135* (1947), 340–342.

6. G. Dick-Read, *Childbirth without fear* (Harper, New York, rev. ed., 1953).

7. H. Thoms, *Training for childbirth* (McGraw-Hill, New York, 1950).

8. M. J. E. Senn, "Anticipatory guidance of the pregnant woman and her husband for their roles as parents," in *Problems of early infancy* (Josiah Macy, Jr. Foundation, New York, 1947).

9. N. R. Newton and M. N. Newton, "Recent trends in breast feeding," *Am. J. M. Sc. 221* (1951), 691–698.

10. H. Waller, *Clinical stress in lactation* (Heinemann, London, 1938).

11. H. Orlansky, "Infant care and personality," *Psychol. Bull. 46* (1949), 1–48.

12. S. Escalona, "Unusual sensitivities in very young infants," in *Psychoanalytic study of the child* (International Universities Press, New York, 1949), vol. III.

13. T. Benedek, "The psychosomatic implications of the primary unit: mother, child," *Am. J. Orthopsychiat.* 19 (1949), 642–654.

14. J. Bowlby, "The nature of the child's tie to his mother," *Internat. J. Psycho-analysis* 39 (1958), 350–373.

15. S. Escalona, "Feeding disturbances in very young children," *Am. J. Orthopsychiat. 15* (1945), 76–80.

16. T. Benedek, "Toward the biology of the depressive constellation," *J. Am. Psychoanalyt. A. 4* (1956), 389–427.

17. M. Ribble, *The rights of infants* (Columbia University Press, New York, 1943).

18. D. Levy, "Primary affect hunger," *Am. J. Psychiat. 94* (1937), 643–652.

19. D. Hooker, *The prenatal origin of behavior* (University of Kansas Press, Lawrence, 1952).

20. R. R. Sears, and G. W. Wise, "Relation of cup-feeding in infancy to thumbsucking and the oral drive," *Am. J. Orthopsychiat. 20* (1950), 123–138.

21. D. Levy, "Fingersucking and accessory movements in early infancy," *Am. J. Psychiat. 7* (1928), 881–918.

22. M. Massler, and A. W. S. Wood, "Thumb-sucking," *J. Dent. Child. 16* (1949), 1–9.

23. B. Spock, *The pocket book of baby and child care* (Pocket Books, New York, 1946).

24. D. G. Prugh, "Emotional problems of the premature infant's parents," *Nursing Outlook 1* (1953), 461–464.

25. M. A. Wessel, J. C. Cobb, E. B. Jackson, G. A. Harris, and A. C. Deutsch, "Paroxysmal fussing in infancy," *Pediatrics 14* (1954), 421–434.

26. L. W. Sontag, "Differences in modifiability of fetal behavior and physiology," *Psychosom. Med. 6* (1944), 151–154.

27. M. I. Levine and A. Bell, "The treatment of 'colic' of infancy by use of the pacifier," *J. Pediat. 37* (1950), 750–755.

28. H. Bakwin, "Emotional deprivation in infants," *J. Pediat. 35* (1949), 512–521.

29. R. S. Lourie, "Experience with therapy of psychosomatic problems in infants," in *Psychopathology of childhood,* P. H. Hoch and J. Zubin, eds. (Grune and Stratton, New York, 1955).

30. D. G. Prugh, "Childhood experience and colonic disorder," *Ann. New York Acad. Sc. 58* (1954), 355–376.

31. F. P. Simsarian, "Self-demand feeding of infants and young children in family settings," *Mental Hygiene 32* (1948), 217–225.

32. R. Spitz and K. M. Wolf, "The smiling response: a contribution to the autogenesis of social reactions," *Genet. Psychol. Monogr. 34* (1946), 57–125.

33. R. Spitz, "Anaclitic depression," in *Psychoanalytic study of the child* (International Universities Press, New York, 1946), II, 313–342.

34. S. Freud, *A general introduction to psychoanalysis* (Garden City Publishing Co., New York, 1943).

35. G. L. Engel, "Homeostasis, behavioral adjustment, and the concept of health and disease," in *Mid-century psychiatry,* R. R. Grinker, ed. (Thomas, Springfield, 1953).

36. R. S. Lourie, "The role of rhythmic patterns in childhood," *Am. J. Psychiat. 105* (1949), 653–660.

37. A. W. Sullivan, "The use and abuse of the pacifier (blank nipple) in infant rearing." Unpublished material.

38. E. H. Erikson, "Growth and crises of the healthy personality," in *Problems of infancy and early childhood* (Josiah Macy, Jr. Foundation, New York, 1950), supp. II.

39. W. B. Cannon, *The wisdom of the body* (Norton, New York, 1932).

40. G. L. Engel, F. Reichsman, and H. Segal, "A study of an infant with a gastric fistula. I. Behavior and the rate of total hydrochloric acid secretion," *Psychosom. Med. 18* (1956), 374–398.

41. C. M. Davis, "Self-selection of diet by newly weaned infants," *Am. J. Dis. Child. 36* (1928), 651–679.

42. M. M. Cooper, "Evaluation of the mother's advisory service," *Monographs of the Soc. for Research in Child Develop. 12* (1947) Serial No. 44, number 1.

43. B. Rank, M. Putnam, and G. Rochlin, "The significance of 'emotional climate' in early feeding difficulties," *Psychosomat. Med. 10* (1948), 279–283.

44. R. A. Spitz, "Hospitalism: an inquiry into the genesis of psychiatric conditions in early childhood," in *Psychoanalytic study of the child* (International Universities Press, New York, 1945), I. 53–74.

45. H. D. Chapin, "A plan for dealing with atrophic infants and children," *Arch. Pediat. 25* (1908), 491–496.

46. R. W. Coleman and S. Provence, "Environmental retardation (hospitalism) in infants living in families," *Pediatrics 19* (1957), 285–292.

47. J. Bowlby, *Maternal care and mental health* (Monograph Series, 2, World Health Organization, Geneva, 1952).

48. W. Goldfarb, "Infant rearing and problem behavior," *Am. J. Orthopsychiat. 13* (1943), 249–265.

49. L. Kanner and L. I. Lesser, "Early infantile autism," *Pediat. Clin. North America 5* (1958), 711–730.

50. B. Rank, "Adaptation of the psychoanalytic technique for the treatment of young children with atypical development," *Am. J. Orthopsychiat. 19* (1949), 130–139.

51. K. Glaser and L. Eisenberg, "Maternal deprivation," *Pediatrics 18* (1956), 626–642.

52. D. G. Prugh and H. Shwachman, "Observations on chronic unexplained diarrhea in infants and young children." Paper given at Joint Meeting of British Paediatric Society, Canadian Pediatric Society, and Society for Pediatric Research, Quebec, Canada, June 1955.

53. J. B. Richmond, E. Eddy, and M. Greer, "Rumination, a psychosomatic syndrome of infancy," *Pediatrics 22* (1958), 49–55.

54. D. P. Ausubel, *Theory and problems of child development* (Grune and Stratton, New York, 1957).

55. A. Gessell, and F. L. Ilg, *The infant and child in the culture of today* (Harper, New York, 1943).

56. J. E. Anderson, "The limitations of infant and pre-school tests in the measurement of intelligence," *J. Psychol. 8* (1939), 351–379.

57. M. Huschka, "The child's response to coercive bowel training," *Psychosomat. Med. 4* (1942), 301–308.

58. J. B. Watson, *Psychology from the standpoint of a behaviorist* (Lippincott, Philadelphia, 1919).

59. C. A. Aldrich and M. M. Aldrich, *Babies are human beings: an interpretation of growth* (Macmillan, New York, 1938).

60. M. E. Fries, "Psychosomatic relationships between mother and infant," *Psychosomat. Med. 6* (1944), 159–162.

61. K. E. Roberts and J. A. Schoelkopf, "Eating, sleeping and elimination practices of a group of two-and-one-half year old children. I. Introduction. *Am. J. Dis. Child. 82* (1951), 121–126.

62. M. E. Fries, et al., "The formation of character as observed in the well-baby clinic," *Am. J. Dis. Child. 49* (1935), 28–42.

63. H. Bakwin and R. M. Bakwin, *Clinical management of behavior disorders in children* (Saunders, Philadelphia, 1953).

64. J. Bostwick and M. G. Shackleton, "Enuresis and toilet training," *Australian M. J. 2* (1951), 110–113.

65. M. J. E. Senn, "On permissiveness in the early years," *Child Study 26* (1949), 67–68.

66. R. R. Sears, E. E. Maccoby and H. Levin, *Patterns of child-rearing* (Row, Peterson, Evanston, 1957).

67. B. Spock, "Chronic resistance to sleep in infancy," *Pediatrics 4* (1949), 89–93.

68. M. S. Mahler, "On child psychosis and schizophrenia: autistic and symbiotic infantile psychoses, in *Psychoanalytic study of the child* (International Universities Press, New York, 1952), vol. VII.

69. J. Piaget, *Language and thought of the child* (Routledge and Kegan Paul, London, 1926).

70. R. Strain, *New patterns in sex teaching* (Appleton-Century-Crofts, New York, rev. ed., 1957).

71. M. I. Levine and J. H. Seligman, *The wonder of life* (Simon and Schuster, New York, 1952).

72. B. Malinowski, *Sex and repression in savage society* (Harcourt, Brace, New York, 1927).

73. T. Parsons, *The social system* (Free Press, Glencoe, Ill., 1951).

74. E. Lindemann, "Modifications in the course of ulcerative colitis in relationship to changes in life situations and reaction patterns," in *Life stress and bodily disease* (Williams and Wilkins, Baltimore, 1950).

75. G. Caplan, "A public health approach to child psychiatry," *Ment. Hyg.* 35 (1951), 235–249.

76. G. Caplan, personal communication.

77. A. T. Jersild, *Child psychology* (Prentice-Hall, New York, 1947).

78. D. Levy, "Psychic trauma of operations in children, and a note on combat neurosis," *Am. J. Dis. Child.* 69 (1945), 7–25.

79. L. Jessner and S. Kaplan, "Observations on the emotional reactions of children to tonsillectomy and adenoidectomy," in *Problems of infancy and childhood* (Josiah Macy, Jr. Foundation, New York, 1948).

80. D. G. Prugh, E. M. Staub, H. Sands, R. Kirschbaum, and E. A. Lenihan, "A study of the emotional reactions of children and families to illness and hospitalization," *Am. J. Orthopsychiat.* 23 (1953), 70–106.

81. J. Robertson, *Young children in hospitals* (Basic Books, New York, 1958).

82. D. G. Prugh, "Investigations dealing with reactions of children and families to hospitalization and illness: problems and potentialities," in *Emotional disorders of early childhood*, G. Caplan, ed. (Basic Books, New York, 1955).

83. R. G. Barker, B. A. Wright, and M. R. Gonick, *Adjustment to physical handicap and illness* (Bulletin 55, Social Science Research Council, New York, 1946).

84. O. A. Faust, "Reducing emotional trauma in hospitalized children: a study in psychosomatic pediatrics," in *Reducing emotional trauma in hospitalized children* (Albany Medical College, Albany, New York, 1952).

85. J. Bowlby, J. Robertson, and D. Rosenbluth, "A two year old goes to the hospital," in *Psychoanalytic study of the child* (International Universities Press, New York, 1932), vol. VII.

86. M. Gerard, "Enuresis: a study in etiology," *Am. J. Orthopsychiat.* 9 (1939), 48–58.

87. S. D. Garrard and J. B. Richmond, "Psychogenic megacolon manifested by fecal soiling," *Pediatrics* 10 (1952), 474–483.

88. B. Bornstein, "On latency," in *Psychoanalytic study of the child* (International Universities Press, New York, 1951). VI, 279.

89. A. Adler, *Understanding human nature* (Greenberg, New York, 1927).

90. C. G. Jung, *The psychology of the unconscious* (Dodd, Mead, New York, 1927).

91. O. Rank, *Art and artist* (Knopf, New York, 1932).

92. L. Trilling, *The liberal imagination: essays on literature and society* (Doubleday, New York, 1953).

93. M. Frank and L. Frank, *How to help your child in school* (Viking, New York, 1952).

94. F. Redl, "Pre-adolescents — what makes them tick?" *Child study 44* (1943–44), 44–48 and 58–59.

95. I. Josselyn, *Psychosocial development of children* (Family Service Association of America, New York, 1948).

96. T. E. Coffin, "Television's impact on society," *Am. Psychologist 10* (1935), 630–641.

97. D. W. Winnicott, *Clinical notes on the disorders of childhood* (Heinemann, London, 1931).

98. N. Staver, "The child's learning difficulty as related to the emotion problem of the mother," *Am. J. Orthopsychiat. 23* (1953), 131–141.

99. H. S. Lippmann, *Treatment of the child in emotional conflict* (McGraw-Hill, New York, 1956).

100. G. H. J. Pearson, *Emotional disorders of children* (Norton, New York, 1949).

101. L. Eisenberg, "School probia: diagnosis, genesis, and clinical management," *Pediat. Clin. North America 5* (1958), 645–666.

102. S. Glueck and E. T. Glueck, *Unraveling juvenile delinquency* (Harvard University Press, Cambridge, 1950).

103. A. M. Johnson, "Sanctions for superego lacunae of adolescents" in *Searchlights on delinquency*, K. R. Eissler, ed. (International Universities Press, New York, 1949).

104. D. G. Prugh, "The influence of emotional factors in the clinical course of ulcerative colitis in children," *Gastroenterology 18* (1951), 339–354.

105. L. H. Taboroff and W. H. Brown, "Study of personality patterns of children and adolescents with peptic ulcer," *Am. J. Orthopsychiat. 24* (1954), 602–610.

106. M. Gerard, "Bronchial asthma in children," *Nerv. Child 5* (1946), 327–331.

107. H. Bruch, "Obesity," *Pediat. Clin. North America 5* (1958), 613–627.

108. F. Kallman, *Heredity in health and mental disorder* (Norton, New York, 1953).

109. L. Bender, "Childhood schizophrenia," *Am. J. Orthopsychiat. 17* (1947), 40–56.

110. H. C. Peck, "A new pattern for mental health services in a children's court: round table," *Am. J. Orthopsychiat. 25* (1955), 1–51.

111. A. K. Cohen, *Delinquent boys: the culture of the gang* (Free Press, Glencoe, 1955), 202.

112. A. Kinsey, W. Pomeroy and C. Martin, *Sexual behavior in the human male* (Saunders, Philadelphia, 1948).

113. H. Deutsch, *Psychology of women* (Grune & Stratton, New York, 1944), I, 91–92.

GENERAL REFERENCES

E. H. Erikson, *Childhood and society* (Norton, New York, 1950).

—————— "The problem of ego identity," *J. Am. Psychoanalyt. Ass. 4* (1956), 56–121.

I. Josselyn, "The ego in adolescence," *Am. J. Orthopsychiat. 24* (1954), 223–238.

L. A. Spiegel, "A review of contributions to a psychoanalytic theory of adolescence; individual aspects," in *The psychoanalytic study of the child* (International Universities Press, New York, 1951), VI, 375–393.

NOTES TO CHAPTER VIII: THE MODERN FAMILY AND THE SOCIAL DEVELOPMENT
OF THE CHILD

1. E. H. Erikson, *Childhood and society* (Norton, New York, 1950).
2. T. Parsons, "Psychoanalysis and the social structure," *Psychoanalyt. Quart. 19* (1950), 371–384.
3. The analysis of the American family presented here incorporates theory and principles that are current in contemporary anthropology and sociology, but primary emphasis has been placed on the work and viewpoints of Erikson, Benedict, Mead, and Parsons.
4. R. N. Anshen, ed., *The family: its function and destiny* (Harper, New York, 1949).
5. R. Benedict, "The family: genus americanus," in Anshen, *ibid.*, pp. 159–169.
6. T. Parsons, "The social structure of the family," in Anshen, *ibid.*, pp. 173–201.
7. M. Mead, *Male and female: a study of the sexes in a changing world* (Morrow, New York, 1949).
8. T. Parsons, "Certain primary sources and patterns of aggression in the social structure of the western world," *Essays in sociological theory* (Free Press, Glencoe, rev. ed., 1954).
9. M. Mead, *And keep your powder dry* (Morrow, New York, 1943).
10. M. Mead, *Coming of age in Samoa* (Modern Library, New York, 1953).
11. M. Young and P. Willmott, *Family and kinship in East London* (Free Press, Glencoe, Ill., 1957).
12. U. S. Department of Health, Education, and Welfare, *Children in a changing world,* (White House Conference on Children and Youth, Washington, 1960), Chart No. 12.
13. —— *Child welfare services: how they help children and their parents* (Children's Bureau Pub. 359, Washington, 1957).
14. —— *Protecting children in adoption* (Children's Bureau Pub. 354, Washington, 1958).
15. W. H. Stewart et al., *Homemaker services in the U. S. A., 1958* (Public Health Service Publication 644, 1958).
16. J. Regensburg, "Reaching children before the crisis comes," *Journal of Social Case Work 35* (1954), No. 3, 104–111.
17. K. Young, "What strong family life means to our society," *Journal of Social Case Work 34* (1953), 323–329.
18. R. M. Butler, "Mothers' attitudes toward the social development of their adolescents," *Social Case Work* (Family Service Association of America, New York, 1956), Part I, pp. 219–226; Part II, pp. 280–288.

GENERAL REFERENCES

E. H. Bernert, *America's children* (Wiley, New York, 1958).
P. C. Glick, *American families* (Wiley, New York, 1957).
R. M. Titmuss, "Industrialization and the family," *The Social Service Review 31* (March 1957), No. 1.

United Nations Department of Social Affairs, *Children deprived of a normal home life* (New York, 1952).

A. Gesell, *The child from five to ten* (Harper, New York, 1946).

U. S. Department of Health, Education, and Welfare, *Your child from six to twelve* (Children's Bureau Pub. 324, Washington, 1949).

———, *The adolescent in your family* (Children's Bureau Pub. 347, Washington, 1954).

B. Spock, "The middle-aged child," *Pennsylvania M. J.* 50 (1947), 1045–1052.

R. P. Knight, "Behavior problems and habit disturbances in preadolescent children: their meaning and management," *Bull. Menninger Clin.* 8 (1944), 188–199.

M. Green and J. B. Richmond, *Pediatric diagnosis* (Saunders, Philadelphia, 1955).

I. Josselyn, "Social pressure in adolescence," *Social Casework* 33 (1952), No. 5, 187–193.

I. Josselyn, *The adolescent and his world* (Family Service Association of America, New York, 1952).

J. Gallagher, *Understanding your son's adolescence* (Little, Brown, Boston, 1951).

G. Hildreth, "The social interests of young adolescents," *Child Development* 16 (1945), No. 2, 119–121.

M. Roll, "Dependency and the adolescent," *Social Casework* 27 (1947), No. 4, 123.

J. Charnley, *The art of child placement* (Univ. of Minnesota Press, Minneapolis, 1955), 163 pp. includes bibliography.

L. Young. *Out of wedlock* (McGraw-Hill & Co., New York, 1954), 261 pp.

A. L. Davis, *Children living in their own homes* (U. S. Children's Bureau, Washington, 1953), 52 pp.

NOTES TO CHAPTER IX: THE EDUCATION AND INTELLECTUAL DEVELOPMENT

OF THE CHILD

1. B. Goodykoontz, M. D. Davis, and H. F. Gabbard, "Recent history and present status of education for young children," in *Early childhood education* 46th Yearbook of the National Society for the Study of Education (University of Chicago Press, Chicago, 1947), pt. II, chap. iv, p. 44-69.

2. V. E. Herrick and M. L. Carroll, "The nursery school," *Rev. Ed. research* 23 (1953), chap. i, p. 116.

3. R. Gans, C. B. Stendler, and M. Almy, *Teaching young children in nursery school, kindergarten, and the primary grades* (World Book Company, Yonkers-on-Hudson, 1952), p. 74.

4. J. E. Nichols, et. al., "Sites, buildings, and equipment," in *Early childhood education* (University of Chicago Press, Chicago, 1947), chap. ix, p. 247–280.

5. M. Mead, "The impact of culture on personality development in the United States today," *Understanding The Child* 20 (1951), 17–18.

6. G. C. Lee, *An introduction to education in modern America* (Holt, New York, 1953), 451–465.

7. N. Headley, "The kindergarten comes of age," *J. Nat. Ed. A. 43* (1954), 153.

8. D. Snygg and A. W. Combs, *Individual behavior* (Harper, New York, 1949), p. 223–225.

9. R. H. Anderson, "The ungraded primary school as a contribution to improved school practices," *Frontiers of elementary education* II (Syracuse University Press, Syracuse, 1955), chap. iv, p. 28–39.

10. J. I. Goodlad and R. H. Anderson, *The nongraded elementary school* (Harcourt, Brace, New York, 1959).

11. F. M. Wilson, "Mental health practices in the intermediate grades," *Mental health in modern education* (University of Chicago Press, Chicago, 1955), Part II of 54th Yearbook of the National Society for the Study of Education, chap. ix, p. 195–215.

12. M. F. Farnham, *The adolescent* (Harper, New York, 1951), p. 33.

13. D. A. Prescott, *Emotion and the educative process* (American Council on Education, Washington, 1938).

14. R. J. Havighurst, M. Z. Robinson, and M. Dorr, "The development of the ideal self," in *The adolescent,* J. M. Seidman, ed. (Dryden, New York, 1953), p. 301.

15. R. J. Havighurst, *Human development and education* (Longmans, Green, New York, 1953), p. 111.

16. *Ibid.,* p. 112.

17. J. E. Horrocks, "The adolescent," in *Manual of child psychology* (Wiley, New York, 2 ed., 1954), p. 720.

18. C. M. Tryon, "The adolescent peer culture," in *Adolescence,* Part I of the 43rd Yearbook of the National Society for the Study of Education (University of Chicago Press, Chicago, 1944), p. 227.

19. H. Taba, "The moral beliefs of sixteen-year-olds," in *The adolescent* (Dryden, New York, 1953), p. 315.

20. H. E. Jones and H. S. Conrad, "Mental development in adolescence," in *Adolescence,* Part I of the 43rd Yearbook of the National Society for the Study of Education (University of Chicago Press, Chicago, 1944), p. 154.

21. N. L. Munn, "Learning in children," in *Manual of child psychology* (Wiley, New York, 2 ed., 1954), p. 432.

22. J. L. Mursell, *Development teaching* (McGraw-Hill, New York, 1949), p. 128.

23. D. McCarthy, "Child development, VII: Language," in *Encyclopedia of educational research* (Macmillan, New York, 1952), p. 167.

24. J. E. Horrocks, pp. 726–727.

25. R. C. Pooley, "English — literature," in *Encyclopedia of educational research* (Macmillan, New York, 1952), p. 400.

26. Adapted from Orr et al., *Teacher's guide to discovering new fields in reading and literature* (Scribner's, New York, 1953), bk. I, p. 3.

27. M. L. Cogan, "The relation of the behavior of teachers to the productive behavior of their pupils," unpublished Ed. D. diss., Harvard Graduate School of Education, 1954.

28. L. V. Koos, *Junior high school trends* (Harper, New York, 1955), p. 24.

29. N. Edwards, "The adolescent in technological society," in *Adolescence,* Part I of the 43rd Yearbook of the National Society for the Study of Education (University of Chicago Press, Chicago, 1944), p. 897.

30. H. D. Carter, "The development of interest in vocations," in *Adolescence*, Part I of the 43rd Yearbook of the National Society for the Study of Education (University of Chicago Press, Chicago, 1944), p. 255.

31. A. T. Jersild, "Emotional development," in *Manual of child psychology* (Wiley, New York, 2 ed., 1954), p. 897.

32. M. Krugman, ed., *Orthopsychiatry and the school* (American Orthopsychiatric Association Inc., New York, 1958).

33. D. McLelland et al., *Talent and society* (Van Nostrand, Princeton, 1958).

34. S. Gruber, "The concept of task-orientation in the analysis of play behavior of children entering kindergarten." *Am. J. Orthopsychiat. 24*, (1954), 326–335.

35. H. S. Sullivan, *The interpersonal theory of psychiatry* (Norton, New York, 1953).

36. L. M. Terman, "Psychological sex differences," in *Manual of child psychology* (Wiley, New York, 1946).

37. "Tenth anniversary report of the Human Relations Service," Wellesley, Mass., 1959 (mimeographed).

38. R. Barry and B. Wolf, *Modern issues in guidance-personnel work* (Teachers College, Columbia University, New York, 1957).

39. E. Landy and J. Palmer, *Guidance in the public schools* (Massachusetts Council for Public Schools, Boston, 1955).

40. T. Parsons and E. Shils. eds., *Toward a general theory of action* (Harvard University Press, Cambridge, 1952).

41. R. R. Grinker, ed., *Toward a unified theory of human behavior* (Basic Books, New York, 1956).

42. W. C. Olson and B. O. Hughes, *Manual for the description of growth in age units* (The Edward Letter Shop, Ann Arbor, 1950), p. 2.

43. W. C. Olson, *Child development* (Heath, Boston, 1949), chap. xii.

44. C. V. Millard and J. W. M. Rothney, *The elementary school child* (Dryden, New York, 1957).

45. L. H. Stott, *The longitudinal study of individual development* (The Merrill-Palmer School, Detroit, 1955).

46. R. Martinson and H. Smallenburg, *Guidance in elementary schools* (Prentice-Hall, New Jersey, 1958), p. 75.

47. J. W. M. Rothney, *Evaluating and reporting pupil progress* (National Education Association, Washington, 1955), p. 7.

48. P. A. Sorokin, "Testomania," *Harvard Ed. Rev. 25* (1955), 199–213.

49. "Educational and psychological testing," *Rev. Ed. Research 24* (1959).

50. P. E. Vernon, "Education and the psychology of individual differences," *Harvard Ed. Rev. 28* (1958), 91–104.

51. R. D. North, "Relationship of Kuhlman-Anderson IQ's and Stanford achievement test scores of independent school pupils," *Ed. Records Bull. 66* (1955).

52. D. V. Tiedeman and C. C. MacArthur, "Over and under achievement: if any," *13th Yearbook* (*National Council on Measurements Used in Education*, New York, 1956), pp. 135–145.

53. J. W. M. Rothney, P. J. Danielson, and R. A. Heimann, *Measurement for guidance* (Harper, New York, 1959), p. 323.

54. D. C. McClelland, J. W. Atkinson, R. A. Clark, and E. L. Lowell, *The achievement motive* (Appleton-Century-Crofts, New York, 1953).

55. P. E. Meehl, *Clinical versus statistical prediction* (University of Minnesota Press, Minneapolis, 1954), p. 16.

56. W. Stephenson, *The study of behavior: Q-technique and its methodology* (University of Chicago Press, Chicago, 1953).

57. L. J. Cronbach and G. C. Glaser, *Psychological tests and personal decisions* (University of Illinois Press, Urbana, 1957).

GENERAL REFERENCES

Encyclopedia of educational research, ed. by C. W. Harris and M. Liba (Macmillan, 3 ed., 1960) has sections on the development, organization and administration, programs, and student population of elementary education, plus many related topics.

G. Lee, *An introduction to education in modern America* (Holt, New York, 2 ed., 1958) is a thoughtful summary of the whole range of public education.

R. Gans, et al., *Teaching young children in nursery school, kindergarten, and the primary grades* (World Book Company, Yonkers-on-Hudson, 1952). Informative on programs for very young children.

V. E. Herrick et al., *The elementary school* (Prentice-Hall, New York, 1956). Deals with historical backgrounds, learning and development of children, curriculum, and administrative and organizational matters. Chap. 14, "the learning-teaching day," is a special contribution.

J. I. Goodlad and R. H. Anderson, *"The nongraded elementary school* (Harcourt, Brace, New York, 1959). An argument for abandonment of graded school structure and for more suitable ways of organizing the child's school experiences. Note chap. 7 on realistic standards and sound mental health.

Foster and Headley's *Education in the kindergarten,* rev. by N. E. Headley (American Book Company, New York, 3 ed., 1959). A standard reference on education of the 5 year old.

R. M. Thomas, *Ways of teaching in elementary schools* (Longmans, Green, New York, 1955). The opening chapters are an expert presentation of the different types of teaching and curriculum patterns found in American schools today.

Early childhood education, Part II of the 46th Yearbook (1947); *Learning and instruction,* Part I of the 49th Yearbook (1950); *Mental health in modern education,* Part II of the 54th Yearbook (1955); and *The integration of educational experiences,* Part III of the 57th Yearbook (1958) of the National Society for the Study of Education (University of Chicago Press, Chicago) can all be recommended.

The elementary school journal (University of Chicago Press) is a very useful periodical publication in the field. See pp. 1–17 of the October 1958 issue for J. Goodlad's review of recent efforts to improve elementary education.

Review of educational research (official publication of the American Educational Research Association), 29 (April, 1959), pp. 133–219, reviews the literature on "Educational Programs: Early and Middle Childhood" from 1953 to 1959.

C. M. Olson, "The adolescent: his society," *Rev. of Ed. Res.* 24 (1954), 5–10.

K. Benne and B. Muntyan, *Human relations in curriculum change* (Dryden, New York, 1951). A collection of readings in group development stemming largely from the work of Kurt Lewin and his students. This book should be of value to educators and others interested in the improvement of educational arrangements through utilization of recent findings in the group dynamics area.

L. A. Cook and E. F. Cook, *A sociological approach to education* (McGraw-Hill, New York, 2 ed., 1950). Following an introduction to sociological concepts, parts III and IV provide a valuable discussion of community-school relationships and their impact upon the school child.

E. H. Erikson, *Childhood and society* (Norton, New York, 1950). A major contribution to theory of personality development for the serious student, this work is a synthesis of psychoanalytic theory, ego psychology, and cultural anthropology. See also Erikson's thoughtful discussion of "Growth and crises of the healthy personality" in C. Kluckhohn and H. A. Murray, *Personality in nature, society, and culture* (Knopf, New York, 2 eds., 1953), p. 185–225.

J. L. Hymes, Jr., *Teacher, listen, the children speak* (New York Committee on Mental Hygiene, New York, 1949). Addressed to teachers by a well-known educator, this brief pamphlet suggests ways in which the classroom teacher can seek out the meaning of children's behavior without resorting to such stereotypes as "the lazy child," "the stubborn child," "the show off," or "the mean child."

S. L. Pressey and F. P. Robinson, *Psychology and the new education* (Harper, New York, rev. ed., 1944). A textbook of educational psychology combining basic learning theory, a dynamic view of child development, and a socioenvironmental emphasis. Of particular interest in the present context are chap. 6, which discusses teacher-pupil relationships; chap. 7, in which the advantages and limitations of sociometric devices are reviewed; and chap. 10, which contains valuable case histories of children with school adjustment problems.

A. H. Stanton and M. S. Schwartz, *The mental hospital* (Basic Books, New York, 1954). An outstanding example of the trend towards the collaboration of the student of personality and the social scientist, the book explores the distribution of power and channels of communication in a mental hospital and documents a relationship between patients' emotional upsets and staff tensions within the institution. The concepts, point of view, and methods of analysis of this pioneer study should be applicable to other institutions, such as schools.

NOTES TO CHAPTER X: THE PROTECTION AND PROMOTION OF HEALTHY
DEVELOPMENT THROUGH COMMUNITY HEALTH SERVICES

E. H. Bernert, *America's children* (Wiley, New York, 1958).

The American Academy of Pediatrics, *Child health services and pediatric education* (Harvard University Press, Cambridge, 1949).

U. S. Department of Health, Education, and Welfare, *Four decades of action for children: a short history of the children's bureau* (Children's Bureau Pub. 358, Washington, 1956).

P. C. Glick, *American families* (Wiley, New York, 1957).

Health supervision of young children (American Public Health Association, New York, 1955).

A. Moncrieff, *Child health and the state* (Oxford University Press, London, 1953).

E. R. Schlesinger, *Health services for the child* (McGraw-Hill, New York, 1953).

Administration of maternal and child health services (Technical Report Series 115, World Health Organization, Geneva, 1957).

Expert committee on maternity care (Technical Report Series 51, World Health Organization, Geneva, 1952).

Expert committee on school health services (Technical Report Series 30, World Health Organization, Geneva, 1951).

Proceedings of White House conference on the care of dependent children — 1909 (Government Printing Office, Washington, 1909).

White House conference on child welfare standards — 1919 (Children's Bureau Publication, Washington, 1919).

White House conference on child health and protection — 1930 (Century Company, New York, 1931).

White House conference on children in a democracy — 1940: Final report (Children's Bureau Pub. 272, Washington, 1941).

Proceedings of the midcentury White House conference on children and youth — 1950 (Health Publications Institute, Inc., Raleigh, 1951).

INDEX

Abnormality: 9; dwarfism, 12, 171; height-weight, 18–19; Mongolism, 59, 253; endocrine, 139; cortical, 188; behavioral, 191–192; obscure, 249. *See also* Congenital defects

Accidents: mortality, 15–17; age-incidence rates, 29–30; prevention, 108, 111; sports and, 119, 402

Acne, facial, 140–141

Adaptation: defined, 7; variability, 17–18; under one year, 104–105, 234–244 *passim;* long-circuiting, 205–206; extrauterine, 209; second year, 255–257; preschool-age, 280–283; in somatic disturbance, 288–289; school-age, 293–298. *See also* Adolescence

Adjustment of full term and premature baby, 98–101

Adolescence: 4–7; tuberculosis in, 31–32, 40; mumps in, 34; physical growth, 88–90, 125–141, 182–183, 321; three periods, 126; problems of very early or very late onset, 138–139; "nutritive failure" in, 180; diseases of malnutrition, 184–185; sex instinct in, 331–335; parental devaluation, 336–339, 374–375, 382; in "youth culture," 346–347, 373; and secondary education, 410–427; vocational choice, 425

Adolescent, The: dependence to independence, 314–318, 344–346, 367–371, 374–375; dread of isolation, 319–321; identification, 328–329; and fathers, 346–347; in family, 366–373; and mothers, 373–385; sex and social role-playing, 414–415; problem-solving, 419, 424; norms, standards, and conformity, 426–427. *See also* Boys, Girls

Adoption services, child, 354–355

Adrenal glands: cortical hormones, 11–12, 134; in menstrual cycles, 42; in pregnancy, 45; schematized, 190

Age periods: described, 4–7; *vs* developmental age, 20, 179; and illnesses, 22–40; counselling at, 85–86; growth-rate differentials, 176; need gratifications, 197, 240–250 *passim;* of conformity, 361–362, 371–372, 416

Age-specific rates for total illnesses, 27–30

Aggression: controlling, 198, 219; constructive-destructive, 240–241; and permissiveness, 260; management at three, 271–272; ambivalent adolescent, 325–329; home outlets, 344–345; nursery school, 389

Aid to dependents under Social Security, 353–354

Aldrich, C. A., 258

Allen, F. A., 212

Allergic reaction: causative factors, 13, 35; to milk protein, 154; in colic, 232

Almy, M., 390

American Academy of Pediatrics, 38, 83, 469; Committee on School Health, 120

American Orthopsychiatric Association, 428

Amino acids, 94

Amniotic fluid, 48

Analgesic in childbirth, 51, 84, 208

Androgen, 11, 134, 140

Anesthesia in childbirth, 51, 208

Anorexia, 245

Anoxia in childbirth, 51, 59, 207

Anticipatory guidance: concept, 16; situations, 72–81 *passim,* 148–149, 158–160, 164–165, 215–217, 233, 245, 292–293

Antrums and ethmoids, infant, 103

Anxiety: parental, 67, 69–72, 216–217; marital, 68–69; in pregnancy, 70, 74–76; "free-floating," 76–77, 231, 233; breast-feeding, 79, 143, 145, 159, 164, 224–225; intense infant, 237, 242–244; in six-year-old, 280–281; symptom formation, 306; school-age, 365–366; school entry, 435; family-induced, 437. *See also* Separation

Ascorbic acid, dietary intake, 52, 62, 63, 65–66, 144, 148, 156